TEXTE

CARDIAC TRANSPLANTATION

CONTEMPORARY CARDIOLOGY

CHRISTOPHER P. CANNON, MD
SERIES EDITOR

Cardiac Transplantation: The
Columbia University Medical
Center/New York-Presbyterian
Hospital Manual, edited by
Niloo M. Edwards, MD,
Jonathan M. Chen, MD,
and Pamela A. Mazzeo, 2004

Heart Disease and Erectile
Dysfunction, edited by *Robert*
A. Kloner, MD, PhD, 2004

Coronary Disease in Women:
Evidence-Based Diagnosis
and Treatment, by *Leslee J.*
Shaw, PhD, and Rita
F. Redberg, MD, FACC, 2004

Complementary and Alternative
Medicine in Cardiovascular
Disease, edited by *Richard A.*
Stein, MD, and Mehmet C. Oz,
MD, 2004

Nuclear Cardiology, The Basics:
How to Set Up and Maintain
a Laboratory, edited by *Frans*
J. Th. Wackers, MD, PhD,
Wendy Bruni, BS, CNMT, and
Barry L. Zaret, MD, 2004

Minimally Invasive Cardiac Sur-
gery, Second Edition, edited
by *Daniel J. Goldstein, MD,*
and Mehmet C. Oz, MD, 2004

Cardiovascular Health Care
Economics, edited by *William*
S. Weintraub, MD, 2003

Platelet Glycoprotein IIb/IIIa
Inhibitors in Cardiovascular
Disease, Second Edition,
edited by *A. Michael Lincoff,*
MD, 2003

Heart Failure: A Clinician's Guide
to Ambulatory Diagnosis
and Treatment, edited
by *Mariell L. Jessup, MD,*
and Evan Loh, MD, 2003

Management of Acute Coronary
Syndromes, Second Edition,
edited by *Christopher P.*
Cannon, MD, 2003

Aging, Heart Disease, and Its
Management: Facts and
Controversies, edited by
Niloo M. Edwards, MD,
Mathew S. Maurer, MD, and
Rachel B. Wellner, MPH, 2003

Peripheral Arterial Disease:
Diagnosis and Treatment,
edited by *Jay D. Coffman, MD,*
and Robert T. Eberhardt, MD,
2003

Cardiac Repolarization: Bridging
Basic and Clinical Science,
edited by *Ihor Gussak, MD,*
PhD, Charles Antzelevitch,
PhD, Stephen C. Hammill, MD,
Win K. Shen, MD, and
Preben Bjerregaard, MD, DMSc,
2003

Essentials of Bedside Cardiology:
With a Complete Course
in Heart Sounds and Murmurs
on CD, Second Edition,
by *Jules Constant, MD, 2003*

Primary Angioplasty in Acute
Myocardial Infarction,
edited by *James E. Tcheng,*
MD, 2002

CARDIAC TRANSPLANTATION

The Columbia University Medical Center/
New York-Presbyterian Hospital Manual

Edited by

NILOO M. EDWARDS, MD
University of Wisconsin,
Madison, WI

JONATHAN M. CHEN, MD

PAMELA A. MAZZEO
Columbia University College of Physicians & Surgeons,
New York, NY

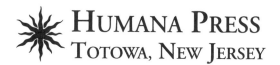

HUMANA PRESS
TOTOWA, NEW JERSEY

© 2004 Humana Press Inc.
999 Riverview Drive, Suite 208
Totowa, New Jersey 07512

humanapress.com

For additional copies, pricing for bulk purchases, and/or information about other Humana titles,
contact Humana at the above address or at any of the following numbers: Tel.: 973-256-1699;
Fax: 973-256-8341, E-mail: humana@humanapr.com; or visit our Website: www.humanapress.com

Due diligence has been taken by the publishers, editors, and authors of this book to assure the accuracy of the
information published and to describe generally accepted practices. The contributors herein have carefully
checked to ensure that the drug selections and dosages set forth in this text are accurate and in accord with the
standards accepted at the time of publication. Notwithstanding, as new research, changes in government regu-
lations, and knowledge from clinical experience relating to drug therapy and drug reactions constantly occurs,
the reader is advised to check the product information provided by the manufacturer of each drug for any change
in dosages or for additional warnings and contraindications. This is of utmost importance when the recommended drug herein is a new or infrequently used drug. It is the responsibility of the treating physician to
determine dosages and treatment strategies for individual patients. Further it is the responsibility of the health
care provider to ascertain the Food and Drug Administration status of each drug or device used in their clinical
practice. The publisher, editors, and authors are not responsible for errors or omissions or for any consequences
from the application of the information presented in this book and make no warranty, express or implied, with
respect to the contents in this publication.

Production Editor: Angela L. Burkey.
Cover design by Patricia F. Cleary.
Cover Illustration: Niloo M. Edwards.

This publication is printed on acid-free paper. ∞
ANSI Z39.48-1984 (American National Standards Institute) Permanence of Paper for Printed Library Materials.

Printed in the United States of America.   10 9 8 7 6 5 4 3 2 1
e-ISBN: 1-59259-758-0

Library of Congress Cataloging-in-Publication Data
Cardiac transplantation : the Columbia University Medical Center / New
York Presbyterian Hospital manual / edited by Niloo M. Edwards,
Jonathan M. Chen, Pamela A. Mazzeo.
    p. cm. -- (Contemporary cardiology)
Includes bibliographical references and index.
  ISBN 1-58829-181-2 (alk. paper)
  1. Heart--Transplantation--Handbooks, manuals, etc. I. Edwards, Niloo
M. II. Chen, Jonathan M. III. Mazzeo, Pamela A. IV.
Columbia-Presbyterian Medical Center. V. Series: Contemporary cardiology
(Totowa, N.J. : Unnumbered)
  RD598.35.T7C355 2004
  617.4'120592--dc22
                        2003020793

Dedication

To Dr. Keith Reemtsma, and to our patients,
their donors, and their families, for their courage and faith

Preface

Cardiac transplantation has evolved dramatically since its first human application in 1967. Since that time, as the chapters of this text collectively attest, significant progress in the areas of immunosuppression and surgical techniques have impacted substantially on posttransplant outcomes, so much so that transplantation is now considered to be the standard therapy for end-stage heart disease.

Cardiac transplantation at Columbia–Presbyterian began in 1977. Since that time, the program has grown extensively and, as of January 2004, completed its 1542nd transplant.

Faced with considerable advances in the field that have challenged our program and allowed its maturity, we decided to publish *Cardiac Transplantation: The Columbia University Medical Center/New York-Presbyterian Hospital Manual* as a compendium for the transplant clinician.

As a testament to the rapidity with which the field of transplantation progresses, many of the "cutting-edge" chapters included in this book may be partially outdated already. However, the majority of the information contained herein reflects the day-to-day practice of clinicians at Columbia–Presbyterian. It is with regret that we were not able to include chapters on topics in some ways the most critical to any transplant program: social work, psychiatry, physical therapy, and physiatry, to name a few. We hope that these and other subspecialties will be further elucidated in a future edition.

As mechanical assist devices become more refined, and progress in transplantation immunology renders immunologic tolerance a real possibility, the field of cardiac transplantation is sure to evolve even further. We hope that *Cardiac Transplantation: The Columbia University Medical Center/New York-Presbyterian Hospital Manual* will aid clinicians in caring for transplant patients preoperatively, perioperatively, and late postoperatively by adding to their knowledge the cumulative experience of the Columbia–Presbyterian heart transplant program.

Niloo M. Edwards, MD
Jonathan M. Chen, MD

CONTENTS

VALUE-ADDED eBOOK/PDA

This book is accompanied by a value-added CD-ROM that contains an eBook version of the volume you have just purchased. This eBook can be viewed on your computer, and you can synchronize it to your PDA for viewing on your handheld device. The eBook enables you to view this volume on only one computer and PDA. Once the eBook is installed on your computer, you cannot download, install, or e-mail it to another computer; it resides solely with the computer to which it is installed. The license provided is for only one computer. The eBook can only be read using Adobe® Reader® 6.0 software, which is available free from Adobe Systems Incorporated at www.Adobe.com. You may also view the eBook on your PDA using the Adobe® PDA Reader® software that is also available free from Adobe.com.

You must follow a simple procedure when you install the eBook/PDA that will require you to connect to the Humana Press website in order to receive your license. Please read and follow the instructions below:

1. Download and install Adobe® Reader® 6.0 software
    You can obtain a free copy of the Adobe® Reader® 6.0 software at www.adobe.com
    Note: If you already have the Adobe® Reader® 6.0 software installed, you do not need to reinstall it.
2. Launch Adobe® Reader® 6.0 software
3. Install eBook: Insert your eBook CD into your CD-ROM drive
    PC: Click on the "Start" button, then click on "Run"
    At the prompt, type "d:\ebookinstall.pdf" and click "OK"
    Note: If your CD-ROM drive letter is something other than d: change the above command accordingly.
    MAC: Double click on the "eBook CD" that you will see mounted on your desktop.
    Double click "ebookinstall.pdf"
4. Adobe® Reader® 6.0 software will open and you will receive the message:
    "This document is protected by Adobe DRM" Click "OK"
    Note: If you have not already activated the Adobe® Reader® 6.0 software, you will be prompted to do so. Simply follow the directions to activate and continue installation.

Your web browser will open and you will be taken to the Humana Press eBook registration page. Follow the instructions on that page to complete installation. You will need the serial number located on the sticker sealing the envelope containing the CD-ROM.

If you require assistance during the installation, or you would like more information regarding your eBook and PDA installation, please refer to the eBookManual.pdf located on your CD. If you need further assistance, contact Humana Press eBook Support by e-mail at ebooksupport@humanapr.com or by phone at 973-256-1699.

*Adobe and Reader are either registered trademarks or trademarks of Adobe Systems Incorporated in the United States and/or other countries.

CONTRIBUTORS

LINDA J. ADDONIZIO, MD, *Division of Pediatric Cardiology, Department of Pediatrics, Children's Hospital of New York, Columbia University College of Physicians & Surgeons, New York, NY*

BACHIR ALOBEID, MD, *Division of Hematopathology, Department of Pathology, Columbia University College of Physicians & Surgeons, New York, NY*

MICHAEL ARGENZIANO, MD, *Division of Cardiothoracic Surgery, Department of Surgery, Columbia University College of Physicians & Surgeons, New York, NY*

JONATHAN M. CHEN, MD, *Pediatric Cardiac Surgery, Division of Cardiothoracic Surgery, Department of Surgery, Columbia University College of Physicians & Surgeons, New York, NY*

MARIO C. DENG, MD, *Division of Circulatory Physiology, Department of Medicine, Columbia University College of Physicians & Surgeons, New York, NY*

NILOO M. EDWARDS, MD, *Department of Cardiothoracic Surgery, University of Wisconsin, Madison, WI*

HELEN HAUFF, RN, MBA, CCTC, CPTC, *Recanati/Miller Transplantation Institute, Mount Sinai School of Medicine, New York, NY*

SILVIU ITESCU, MD, *Division of Transplantation Immunology, Departments of Medicine and Surgery, Columbia University College of Physicians & Surgeons, New York, NY*

RANJIT JOHN, MD, *Division of Cardiothoracic Surgery, Department of Surgery, Columbia University College of Physicians & Surgeons, New York, NY*

TAKUSHI KOHMOTO, MD, PhD, *Department of Cardiovascular Surgery, Okayama University Medical School, Okayama City, Japan*

CHANDRA KUNAVARAPU, MD, *Division of Circulatory Physiology, Department of Medicine, Columbia University College of Physicians & Surgeons, New York, NY*

JACQUELINE M. LAMOUR, MD, *Division of Pediatric Cardiology, Department of Pediatrics, Columbia University College of Physicians & Surgeons, New York, NY*

DONNA M. MANCINI, MD, *Division of Circulatory Physiology, Department of Medicine, Columbia University College of Physicians & Surgeons, New York, NY*

CHARLES C. MARBOE, MD, *Division of Anatomic Pathology, Department of Pathology, Columbia University College of Physicians & Surgeons, New York, NY*

PAMELA A. MAZZEO, *Division of Cardiothoracic Surgery, Department of Surgery, Columbia University College of Physicians & Surgeons, New York, NY*

JEFFREY A. MORGAN, MD, *Division of Cardiothoracic Surgery, Department of Surgery, Columbia University College of Physicians & Surgeons, New York, NY*

RALPH S. MOSCA, MD, *Pediatric Cardiac Surgery, Division of Cardiothoracic Surgery, Department of Surgery, Children's Hospital of New York, Columbia University College of Physicians & Surgeons, New York, NY*

YOSHIFUMI NAKA, MD, PhD, *Division of Cardiothoracic Surgery, Department of Surgery, Columbia University College of Physicians & Surgeons, New York, NY*

SEAN P. PINNEY, MD, *Division of Circulatory Physiology, Department of Medicine, Columbia University College of Physicians & Surgeons, New York, NY*

DEON W. VIGILANCE, MD, *Division of Cardiothoracic Surgery, Department of Surgery, Columbia University College of Physicians & Surgeons, New York, NY*

1 Recipient Selection

Donna M. Mancini, MD
and Chandra Kunavarapu, MD

CONTENTS

INTRODUCTION

Cardiac transplant candidate selection involves the use of prognostic variables to identify patients with end-stage heart failure, combined with a series of empirically derived contraindications to exclude those patients with probable poor outcome from significant comorbidities or high perioperative risk. Candidate selection assumes that the treating physician has a thorough understanding of the prognosis and management of patients with end-stage heart disease. This chapter reviews the transplant evaluation process with an emphasis on cardiopulmonary exercise testing and the use of multivariable models to predict survival. Contraindications to transplant are outlined. Discussion of serial assessment of transplant candidates, criteria for removal of patients from the transplant list, retransplantation, and alternative listing are included.

From: *Contemporary Cardiology: Cardiac Transplantation:*
The Columbia University Medical Center/New York-Presbyterian Hospital Manual
Edited by: N. M. Edwards, J. M. Chen, and P. A. Mazzeo © Humana Press Inc., Totowa, NJ

ONSET OF CONGESTIVE HEART FAILURE

Epidemiology of Congestive Heart Failure

Congestive heart failure (CHF) is a major medical problem that is steadily increasing with the rising age of the general population and overall cardiovascular mortality reduction. In the United States, heart failure incidences total 500,000 patients per year, with a prevalence of 5 million Americans *(1)*. CHF now comprises the most common hospital discharge diagnosis for those over age 65 and is believed to account for 1.5% of total health care spending.

The prognosis after diagnosis worsens with the extent of myocardial dysfunction. Almost 300,000 patients die each year from heart failure or with heart failure as a contributory cause. In the medical management arm of the recent Randomized Evaluation of Mechanical Assistance for the Treatment of Congestive Heart Failure (REMATCH) trial, 1-yr survival of Class IV patients was only 25%; 2-yr survival was 8% *(2)*.

Pathophysiology of CHF

An extensive discussion of the pathophysiology and management of heart failure is beyond the scope of this chapter. Briefly, chronic heart failure consists of two components: myocardial failure and congestive failure. Myocardial failure is the initial insult and may result from chronic pressure overload (as in hypertension or obstructive valvular disease), diffuse cell loss (as in cardiomyopathy or myocarditis), or segmental cell loss (as in ischemic heart disease). The result is a reduction in cardiac output and a decrease in left ventricular ejection fraction (LVEF). Myocardial failure is best quantified by decrease in LVEF. On the other hand, CHF reflects the neurohormonal and peripheral adaptive response to reduced cardiac output. Sympathetic and renin-angiotensin activation result in heightened peripheral vascular resistance and salt and water retention, leading to congestion and edema. These peripheral changes correlate well with symptoms; CHF is best quantified by exercise performance.

The neurohormonal changes observed in heart failure, such as increased sympathetic nervous activity, help to maintain circulation early in the disease. Over time, these compensatory mechanisms become exaggerated and contribute to disease progression. Decreased renal perfusion activates the renin-angiotensin system, increasing preload by increasing salt and water retention.

Once the CHF syndrome has been diagnosed and the degree of left ventricle (LV) systolic dysfunction quantified, the evaluation focuses on the underlying disease and determining whether it has a reversible component. Management of heart failure patients is well covered in the recent 2001 American College of Cardiology/American Heart Association guidelines *(3)*.

Heart failure treatment includes both nonpharmacologic and pharmacologic strategies. Nonpharmacologic therapy is aimed primarily at sodium intake reduction. Moderate exercise should be strongly recommended, and alcohol intake should be limited. Pharmacologic therapy includes treatment with angiotensin-converting enzyme (ACE) inhibitors, diuretics, digoxin, and β-blockade. The sequence in which these agents should be added continues to evolve. ACE inhibitors are now first-line heart failure therapy, followed by treatment with diuretics, β-blockers, and digoxin. Biventricular pacing and implantable defibrillator use are becoming increasingly common in these patients. When heart failure becomes refractory, cardiac transplantation or left ventricular assist device (LVAD) placement is considered. Later in this chapter, we focus on patients with advanced structural heart disease and marked symptoms of heart failure at rest despite maximal medical therapy.

SELECTING RECIPIENTS FOR CARDIAC TRANSPLANTATION

Patient Selection Criteria

Patients listed for transplant typically are those with severe heart failure; however, patients with refractory angina and incessant life-threatening arrhythmias are also candidates. Generally, these patients have LVEFs below 20%, severely reduced functional capacity, and/or nonsurgically correctable valvular or ischemic disease with Class IIIB or IV symptoms despite maximal medical therapy. Selection hinges on identifying candidates who have a poor prognosis yet lack other comorbidities that significantly increase perioperative mortality or limit patient survival posttransplantation *(4)*.

For advanced heart failure patients who require parenteral inotropic or mechanical support, transplantation remains the best option despite recent advances in mechanical assist device therapy. Indeed, in the medically managed arm of the recent REMATCH patient cohort, the most powerful univariable mortality predictor and the only multivariable mortality predictor was dependence on parenteral inotropic support *(5)*. The definition of inotropic dependence remains somewhat nebulous. Generally, these are patients requiring sympathetic stimulation or phosphodiesterase inhibition to maintain systolic blood pressure. Without

Table 1
Exclusion Criteria for Cardiac Transplantation

- Age > 65 yr
- Fixed pulmonary vascular resistance > 6 Wood units
- Peptic ulcer disease or pulmonary infarct within 3 mo
- Brittle diabetes mellitus or diabetes with end-organ damage
- Major debilitating comorbid disease
- Symptomatic severe peripheral vascular or carotid disease
- Symptomatic hypertension requiring multidrug therapy
- Active infection
- Renal insufficiency (creatinine > 2.5 mg/dL or creatine clearance < 50 mL/min)
- Severe liver dysfunction (bilirubin > 2.5 mg/dL or transaminases > 2 × normal)
- Significant obstructive pulmonary disease (FEV_1 < 1 L/min)
- Significant intrinsic coagulation abnormalities
- Active or recent malignancy (within 2 yr)
- HIV seroconversion
- Amyloidosis
- Excessive obesity (body mass index > 35)
- Evidence of active tobacco, alcohol, or drug abuse
- History of severe mental illness or psychosocial instability

parenteral support, the patient becomes hypotensive and dyspneic and develops decreased organ perfusion (i.e., reduced urine output or decreased mental status).

In the evaluation of inotrope- or device-dependent patients, the key questions are whether there are any significant comorbidities that would limit posttransplant survival and whether the patient is too ill to survive. The chapter now discusses empirically derived exclusion factors that are examined during the evaluation process. Following this, the discussion returns to the evaluation process for patients with severe, but less advanced, heart disease.

Exclusion Criteria

A series of exclusion criteria have been formulated through experience. Generally, these exclusion criteria are comorbidities that significantly increase perioperative risk or decrease long-term survival. The traditional contraindications have been well described (2). Contraindications to transplant are listed in Table 1.

Age over 65 yr tends to be a contraindication because of concerns over increased morbidity and long-term survival in older patients. Fixed pulmonary vascular resistance (PVR) greater than 6 Wood units is problematic because of higher right heart failure risk in the perioperative period resulting from donor right ventricle dilation. Recent peptic ulcer disease is a temporary contraindication because of bleeding risk in the posttransplant period from high-dose steroid treatment and the increased risk of infection from possible colonization of the ulcer crater with cytomegalovirus (CMV) or *candida*. Recent pulmonary infarct is also a temporary contraindication because of the risk of developing a pulmonary abscess following immunosuppressive therapy institution. Symptomatic hypertension requiring multidrug therapy is generally a contraindication, as the hypertension only worsens following transplant with calcineurin inhibitor treatment.

In recent years, increasing experience has permitted a relaxation in some conventional exclusion criteria, as excellent outcomes have been demonstrated for more medically complex recipients. Transplant centers are continually trying to widen recipient criteria. There are case reports of successful cardiac transplantations in patients with a history of human immunodeficiency virus (HIV). Combined cardiac and stem cell transplants are now offered to select patients with primary amyloidosis limited to cardiac disease.

Our recent experience with diabetic patients also illustrates a relaxation of prior exclusion criteria *(6)*. From 1995 to 1999, 76 of the 374 adult cardiac transplants at our institution were performed in diabetic recipients. Of these patients, 43% were taking insulin. The only diabetic candidates rejected were those with diabetic retinopathy requiring laser surgery, intrinsic renal disease with serum creatinine greater than 2.5 mg/dL or urine protein greater than 1 g/d, autonomic dysfunction resulting in orthostasis, and/or peripheral vascular disease resulting in amputation. Of 76 patients, 42 had insulin dependence, history of diabetes greater than 10 yr, urine protein greater than 300 mg, evidence of peripheral vascular disease with an ankle to brachial ratio of less than 1, retinopathy, neuropathy, or gastroparesis. The 1- and 3-yr survival and incidence of allograft rejection, graft vasculopathy, and infection were comparable to those in the nondiabetic cohort.

Transplant Candidate Selection in Ambulatory Patients

Given the continued donor organ scarcity, cardiac transplants primarily are performed in high-priority status (Status 1A or 1B) patients dependent on inotropic or mechanical support. Only 25% of transplants performed since 1998 have been in Status 2 candidates. Wait-list mortality remains in the 20 to 25% range with the majority of deaths in high-priority groups. Elective transplant abolition, with all organs triaged to the sickest candidates within geographic zones, has been suggested, yet the current system remains. Accordingly, large numbers of ambulatory patients with heart failure are screened for transplant. It is in this patient group that knowledge of prognostic survival markers is critical. Many univariate and multivariate reduced survival predictors have been identified in patients with CHF, including a reduced LVEF, New York Heart Association (NYHA) Class, the presence of an S3, LV conduction delay on baseline electrocardiogram (EKG), reduced serum sodium, elevated serum catecholamines, increased pulmonary capillary wedge pressure, reduced cardiac index, and low peak exercise oxygen consumption (VO_2) *(7–9)*. Using Cox proportional hazards modeling in 528 patients receiving tailored therapy, serum sodium, pulmonary artery diastolic pressure, LV diastolic dimension index, peak VO_2, and the presence of a permanent pacemaker were identified as poor survival predictors *(9)*.

PEAK VO_2 AND TRANSPLANT CANDIDACY

The Prognostic Value of Peak Exercise VO_2

One variable that is particularly useful in candidate selection is peak VO_2 measurement. An algorithm for transplant candidate selection incorporates peak VO_2 as a critical branch point in the selection process (Fig. 1).

VO_2 measurement in heart failure patients was first described by Weber as a noninvasive method for characterizing cardiac reserve and functional status in these patients *(10)*. Initially, Szlachic described peak (VO_2) as a prognostic variable. Szlachic reported a 77% mortality rate at 1 yr for patients with a VO_2 less than 10 mL/kg/min and a 21% mortality rate for those with a VO_2 in the 10 to 18 mL/kg/min range in a group of 27 patients *(11)*. Other, larger studies confirmed Szlachic's findings *(7)*.

The initial application of cardiopulmonary exercise testing to the cardiac transplant selection process was done in the late 1980s. Cardiopulmonary exercise testing was prospectively performed on all ambulatory patients referred for cardiac transplantation to the University of Pennsylvania between October 1986 and December 1989 *(12)*. The 116 patients were divided into three groups based on cardiopulmonary stress test results. Patients in Group 1 had a peak VO_2 below 14 mL/kg/min and were accepted as transplant candidates (*n* = 35). Group 2 patients had a peak VO_2 greater than 14 mL/kg/min and had transplant deferred (*n* = 52), and Group 3 patients had a peak VO_2 less than 14 mL/kg/min but also possessed a significant comorbidity that precluded transplant (*n* = 27). Age, LVEF, and resting hemodynamic parameters were similar among the groups. Survival at 1 yr was 94% in the patient group with a VO_2

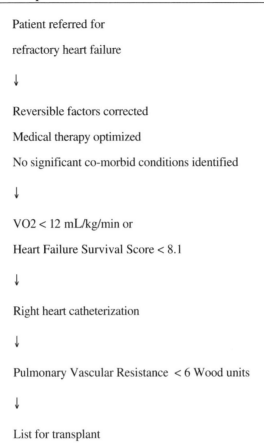

Patient referred for

refractory heart failure

↓

Reversible factors corrected

Medical therapy optimized

No significant co-morbid conditions identified

↓

VO2 < 12 mL/kg/min or

Heart Failure Survival Score < 8.1

↓

Right heart catheterization

↓

Pulmonary Vascular Resistance < 6 Wood units

↓

List for transplant

Fig. 1. Proposed algorithm for cardiac transplant recipient selection *(12)*.

greater than 14 mL/kg/min *(12)*. Accepted transplant candidates with a VO_2 less than 14 mL/kg/min had a 1-yr survival of 70%, whereas those patients with a significant comorbidity and reduced VO_2 had a 1-yr survival of 47%. Patients accepted for transplant had a falsely elevated survival, as all transplants were treated as a censored observation. If urgent transplant was counted as death, 1-yr survival fell to 48%. Using this approach, patients whose transplant could safely be deferred were identified.

Subsequent to this study, the application of cardiopulmonary stress testing for potential transplant candidate selection gained widespread acceptance in the United States *(4)*. Many studies have followed attempting to improve on this variable's predictive accuracy. Examination of this variable coupled with hemodynamic measurements or ventilatory data collected at testing time have been carefully examined.

As peak VO_2 can be affected by age, gender, muscle mass, and conditioning status *(13,14)*, whether percent of predicted VO_2 would yield better risk stratification than the absolute value has been investigated. In one study, peak exercise VO_2 normalization for predicted values added minimal prognostic information *(13)*, whereas in another study multivariable analysis selected 50% of predicted peak VO_2 as the most significant cardiac death predictor ($p = 0.007$) *(14)*. Peak VO_2 is a continuous, rather than a discrete, variable, and differences in the above two studies may be attributed to investigators attempting to assign a threshold or cut-off value to determine transplant candidacy.

Statistical analyses using stratum-specific likelihood ratios can be used to identify threshold values. Stratum-specific likelihood ratio calculation in ambulatory patients referred for cardiac transplant evaluation demonstrate a progressive increase in ratios as peak VO_2 increases without a discrete cut point *(15)*. Therefore, these stratum-specific likelihood ratios suggest that VO_2 is a strong and continuous survival predictor in this population without an absolute threshold.

In a further attempt to enhance the peak exercise VO_2's predictive power, some investigators have coupled hemodynamic monitoring with VO_2 measurements *(16,17)*. Hemodynamic parameter measurement greatly increases the testing's complexity and does not substantially strengthen the measurement's predictive value. This is not a surprising finding because the main limitations to peak exercise performance in CHF patients are peripheral factors.

Osada et al. performed multivariate analysis using all noninvasive exercise data measured during cardiopulmonary exercise testing *(18)*. Multivariate analyses of exercise and cardiopulmonary variables (i.e., peak exercise heart rate, systolic blood pressure, respiratory exchange ratio, minute ventilation, peak VO_2, percent predicted peak VO_2, and anaerobic threshold) were performed to identify the 3-yr prognostic risk. Peak systolic blood pressure above 120 mmHg ($p = 0.0005$) and percent predicted peak VO_2 at 50% or less ($p = 0.04$) were significant prognostic variables in patients with a peak VO_2 less than or equal to 14 mL/kg/min. Survival was 55% at 3 yr for patients with a VO_2 less than or equal to 14 mL/kg/min and peak exercise systolic blood pressure greater than 120 mmHg, as compared with 83% 3-yr survival in patients able to reach this exercise blood pressure ($p = 0.004$).

The ventilatory response to exercise is increased in heart failure. Chua et al. investigated this abnormal ventilatory response's use as a prognostic index of survival in 173 CHF patients *(19)*. The regression line slope relating carbon dioxide output and minute ventilation (VE–VCO_2 slope) was determined for each patient. A high ventilatory response to exercise was defined as a slope greater than 34. The patients with an increased $VE-VCO_2$ slope had a higher NYHA functional class, lower LVEF, lower peak VO_2, and lower survival rate at 18 mo (69 vs 95%; $p < 0.0001$) than those patients with a normal slope. By univariate analysis, the $VE-VCO_2$ slope was an important prognostic factor ($p < 0.0001$). Multivariate analysis including age, peak VO_2, $VE-VCO_2$ slope, and LVEF demonstrated that the $VE-VCO_2$ slope gave additional independent prognostic information ($p = 0.018$).

Exercise-Based Prognostic Scores

Although powerful as an independent variable, transplant candidate selection and stratification that is based solely on a simple dichotomization by peak VO_2 is limited. Such an approach does not efficiently use routinely obtained clinical measures of known prognostic significance such as LVEF. Pretransplant risk stratification could be improved by developing a predictive model that incorporates multiple independent mortality predictors. Univariate analysis limitations include limited accuracy, limited reproducibility, and discordant results for individual predictors. In many prior multivariable analyses, the appropriate population was not targeted, many were performed before the advent of ACE inhibition, many have not developed threshold values, and none have been prospectively validated.

Therefore, we developed a heart failure survival score (HFSS) from 467 ambulatory patients with severe CHF followed at two institutions from July 1986 to September 1994 *(20)*. The model was developed based on 268 patients at the Hospital of the University of Pennsylvania followed from July 1986 to January 1993. It was validated in 199 patients at Columbia–Presbyterian Medical Center from July 1993 to October 1995.

Eighty clinical variables on each patient derived from clinical history, physical exam, laboratory, exercise, and catheterization data were entered into the data set. Univariable survival analyses were performed using Kaplan–Meier analyses. Significant univariate factors were then analyzed with multivariate techniques. Variables were grouped and prognostic factors representing different CHF aspects were incorporated in the model. In the model's construction, the authors used clinical judgment to guide the selection process and specifically sought to include variables that incorporated multiple heart failure pathophysiology aspects.

One statistical model incorporated exclusively noninvasive parameters. The model with the fewest variables that most accurately predicted survival was derived. The best model included seven variables: presence

Table 2
Noninvasive Model Obtained From the Derivation Sample

Variable	Model coefficient	Adjusted hazard ratio (95% CI)	Wald x^2	p
Ischemic Cardiomyopathy	0.6931	2.00 (1.35, 2.97)	11.71	0.0006
Resting heart rate (bpm)	0.0216	1.02 (1.01, 1.04)	11.45	0.0007
Left ventricular ejection fraction (%)	–0.0464	0.96 (0.93, 0.98)	10.65	0.0011
Mean blood pressure (mmHg)	–0.0255	0.98 (0.96, 0.99)	8.94	0.0028
IVCD	0.6083	1.84 (1.22, 2.76)	8.55	0.0035
Peak VO$_2$ (mL/kg/min)	–0.0546	0.95 (0.91, 0.99)	6.76	0.0093
Serum sodium (mmol/L)	–0.0470	0.95 (0.92, 1.00)	4.76	0.0292

CT, confidence interval; IVCD, interventricular conduction defect.

or absence of coronary artery disease (CAD), resting heart rate, LVEF, mean arterial blood pressure, presence or absence of intraventricular conduction defect on baseline EKG, peak VO$_2$, and serum sodium. β-Coefficients were assigned from the Cox model with the hazard ratio and significance level. The noninvasive model included parameters which estimated myocardial ischemia (ischemic cardiomyopathy), the degree of systolic dysfunction (LVEF), the activation degree of the renin-angiotensin system (serum sodium), activation of the sympathetic nervous system (heart rate), the extent of myocardial fibrosis and injury (intraventricular conduction defect), and more integrative measures such as peak VO$_2$ and mean arterial blood pressure.

In addition to these variables, the invasive model included pulmonary capillary wedge pressure. It performed similarly to the noninvasive model. To calculate a prognostic score, the variable's value and the β-coefficient are multiplied and the products are added. The sum's absolute value represents the prognostic score. For noncontinuous variables (i.e., CAD or intraventricular conduction defect), their presence is assigned a value of one and their absence a value of zero. Table 2 delineates the variables used in the noninvasive model and their assigned coefficients.

VO$_2$ and HFSS in the β-Blocker Era

The efficacy of peak VO$_2$ and the HFSS to risk-stratify ambulatory patients with heart failure was evaluated prior to widespread β-blocker use for heart failure management. In the patient cohort from which the HFSS model was derived, only 13% of patients were receiving β-blockers. Whereas β-blockers improve survival in heart failure, the effect of this drug class on exercise performance has been variable *(8–10)*. Whether these parameters maintain their clinical utility in the β-blocker era is unclear.

Accordingly, we recently re-evaluated these parameters in 221 CHF patients who presented for heart transplant evaluation between 1997 and 2002. Of these patients, 65% were receiving β-blocker therapy. HFSS was calculated for each patient. Survival free from United Network for Organ Sharing Status 1 transplant or LVAD, with censoring at UNOS Status 2 transplant, was analyzed by the Kaplan–Meier method for the previously defined low-, medium-, and high-risk HFSS and VO_2 strata. Significant differences ($p < 0.01$) by HFSS strata were observed between patients for the entire cohort and for those patients treated and not treated with β-blockers. Patients treated with β-blockers had better outcomes for any given HFSS stratum than patients not receiving this therapy. By contrast, peak VO_2 did not predict survival in this small cohort of patients on β-blockers.

The fact that β-blockers considerably improve survival while having an inconsistent effect on peak VO_2 may explain why peak VO_2 did not accurately predict outcomes in patients on β-blockers in this study. However, the possibility that sample size may have been too small to detect a significant difference using VO_2 cannot be excluded. Similarly, two recent studies examined the predictive value of peak VO_2 in the β-blocker era and had discordant findings *(21,22)*. In the larger study (369 patients), peak VO_2 greater than 14 mL/kg/min trended to being an independent event-free survival predictor *(21)*, whereas a smaller study (55 patients) failed to demonstrate any discriminatory power *(22)*.

Before the β-blocker era, peak VO_2 and HFSS could be used almost interchangeably, with either a peak VO_2 greater than 14 mL/kg/min or an HFSS ≥ 8.10 sufficient to defer cardiac transplantation *(12,20)*. In the β-blocker era, the HFSS, encompassing various prognostic markers, retains the capacity to accurately risk-stratify patients and performs better than a single measure such as VO_2.

MAINTAINING PATIENTS ON TRANSPLANT LIST

Serial Assessment of Heart Transplant Candidates

If a patient is selected as a transplant candidate and activated on the regional transplant list, neither the patient nor the transplant team is obliged to proceed with transplantation. Candidate selection is a dynamic

Table 3
Guidelines for Serial Assessment of Status 2 Transplant Candidates

Repeat peak VO_2 and LVEF evaluation every 6–12 mo. Studies are done sooner if major changes have been made in medical regimen.

Panel of reactive antibodies repeated every 2 mo if level > 20% and following transfusions in all patients.

Right heart catheterization with infusion of vasodilators every 12 mo if pulmonary vascular resistance (PVR) > 3 Wood units.

Transplant is deferred if:
- Peak VO_2 is markedly improved or heart failure survival score increases to low-risk category (> 8.1)
- LVEF > 30%
- PVR becomes fixed above 6 Wood units despite parenteral inotropic therapy and optimization of vasodilators

process requiring continual reevaluation. Significant improvement as well as serious comorbidity development may preclude future transplantation (*see* Table 3).

Serial assessment of peak VO_2 has been used as a method to determine continued need for transplant. Many pharmacologic studies used exercise testing as a primary outcome measure. Stevenson et al. studied 68 patients with VO_2 less than 14 mL/kg/min with serial cardiopulmonary exercise tests after high-dose diuretic and vasodilator therapy initiation *(23)*. Patients who responded to medical therapy with an increase greater than or equal to 2 mL/kg/min in VO_2 had a good outcome and could be delisted. This study underscores the selection process' dynamic nature and the need for serial assessments of patients, particularly when medical therapy is modified. However, if medical therapy is maximized and VO_2 remains reduced, 6-mo survival remains poor *(24)*.

Exercise-based HFSS serial measurements can also guide the continued need for transplant in ambulatory patients with long waiting periods. Reevaluation of 126 patients an average of 300 d following initial assessment demonstrated that this statistical model continued to discriminate mortality *(25)*. Patients were grouped into high-, middle-, and low-risk strata using the previously defined cut-points. Survival at 1 yr was 38 ± 15%, 64 ± 7%, and 76 ± 5% (p = 0.0016) in the high-, middle- and low-risk strata, respectively. Any patient listed for transplant who was in the high-risk group initially and, with medical therapy alteration, moved to the medium- or low-risk group maintained a relatively high mortality. Thus, these patients' removal from the transplant list should occur only with major clinical status improvement. The only patients who maintained a survival better than, or comparable to, those who received transplants were those individuals who began and ended in the low-risk strata.

Status 1 Patient Management

Status 1B patients are defined as those candidates who require low-dose inotropic support or who are more than 30 d past ventricular assist device placement without a device complication. The new UNOS guidelines make it permissible for patients requiring continuous inotropic support to have a high-priority status and await transplant at home.

At our institution, inotropic therapy is started in hospitalized telemetry patients. Patients on β-blockers are generally treated with milrinone, as its action mechanism is via phosphodiesterase type III inhibition. β-Blocker intolerant patients who require inotropic support are generally treated with dobutamine. Criteria for home discharge includes treatment with low-dose parenteral inotropic infusions defined as dobutamine at a dose less than 7.5 μ/kg/min or milrinone less than 0.5 μ/kg/min. Additionally, patients must exhibit hemodynamic stability with systolic blood pressure above 90 mmHg, stable renal function (BUN below 50 mg/dL; Cr below 2.0 mg/dL), stable weight, no significant arrhythmias on telemetry, and ambulatory status *(26)*.

The impact of this change on duration and cost of hospitalization was investigated at the authors' institution from January 1999 to January 2001. During this period, 155 patients were prioritized as Status 1B. Of these candidates, 91 were discharged home. Data on cost savings, readmissions, and events at home were collected prospectively. Cost savings per patient were calculated as the hospital charge per day minus daily home care costs *(26)*. In this small patient cohort, the mean time spent at home was 87 ± 67 d. This translated into a mean cost savings per patient of more than $100,000. Fifty-nine percent of patients required at least one rehospitalization prior to transplant. The most frequent cause for readmission was worsening CHF followed by infection or line malfunction. Line infections were actually more numerous in the chronically hospitalized patients than in those who were discharged. In the patient group, home inotropic therapy was associated with a low mortality and significant cost savings, although readmission rates were high.

One major concern about the care of Status 1B patients at home is the risk for malignant ventricular arrhythmias on continuous parenteral inotropic therapy. Indeed, few transplant centers will discharge patients home because of this concern. Previous studies with outpatient dobutamine or milrinone were terminated because of excess mortality in the patients receiving inotropic therapy. In our experience, only two patients died suddenly at home. One patient received milrinone at 0.5 μ/ kg/min and the other patient dobutamine at 3 μ/kg/min *(26)*. Both patients were sent home on the wearable external defibrillator device (Lifecor vest), but both chose not to wear the device, as they found it uncomfortable. Despite the low incidence of observed arrhythmias, we strongly recommend that all discharged patients have an implanted automatic implantable cardiodefibrillator (AICD) or a wearable external defibrillator.

Patients on inotropic therapy who remain tenuous are generally upgraded to Status 1A. This involves support with a combination of high-dose inotropic agents and mechanical support (ventilation, intraaortic balloon pump). Those patients who, despite maximal inotropic support, begin to exhibit end-organ damage should undergo insertion of a LVAD as a bridge to transplant.

Despite an increase in organs allocated to high-priority recipients, outcomes posttransplant have remained stable over the past 10 yr. The excellent outcomes in this sicker population are probably attributable to advances in perioperative management, including the use of LVADs and more specific immunosuppression.

Usage indications for LVADs include both acute heart failure and CHF. A patient undergoing a high-risk coronary artery bypass graft with preoperative ventricular dysfunction may require a LVAD as a bridge to transplant if he or she cannot be weaned from bypass. A common indication for device placement is acute coronary syndrome causing profound cardiogenic shock such as extensive myocardial infarction or acute myocarditis. Patients are often referred during a critical stage of cardiogenic shock, and they frequently have multisystem failure. Determination of the end-organ damage's reversibility is not acutely possible. Assessing a patient's mental status is frequently problematic because of a combination of sedation and the aftermath of a cardiac arrest. Major neurological impairment as well as irreversible organ dysfunction should preclude patients from transplantation. Device placement in these patients is performed with the proviso that future transplant is possible only in the setting of acceptable function's return.

Patients with long-standing heart failure who deteriorate awaiting transplant are also candidates for mechanical support. Devices in these patients can be especially helpful by improving perfusion and providing a recovery period for related end-organ impairment.

Valvular pathology may complicate the decision making process for LVAD placement, but it can usually be addressed. Aortic insufficiency is a relative contraindication to LVAD placement if not repaired, as the unloaded ventricle will increase the regurgitant fraction, providing little forward flow from the device, thus negating mechanical support value. Mitral stenosis should be corrected to ensure adequate device filling from the LV. Atrial arrhythmias may be detrimental, as device filling may not be maximized. Ventricular arrhythmias can be tolerated, provided there is not severe PVR preventing a passive Fontan-type circulation. Patients with persistent ventricular arrhythmias and pulmonary hypertension may require biventricular support, and aggressive pharmacological maneuvers should be pursued to prevent these arrhythmias (27,28).

Infections are the most important long-term concern after LVAD insertion, although they rarely affect transplant outcomes. Frequently, device-related infections are superficial and involve the skin around the outflow tract. Generally, these infections are treated with local care and occasional oral antibiotics. Deeper infections involve the LVAD pocket (preperitoneal insertion site), mediastinum, or blood (device endocarditis). Pocket infections are generally manifested by low-grade fever, elevated white blood count, and mild tenderness. Blood cultures are negative, and ultrasound reveals a collection around the device. This infection type is treated with drainage and intravenous antibiotics to prevent extension. Usually, skin organisms are the culprit, and the infection is controlled but not eradicated until the device is removed.

Frequently, LVAD- referred patients are in shock following cardiac surgery, as these patients have had at least one recent sternotomy and some arrive with an open chest. They are at risk for subsequent mediastinal infections and are followed vigilantly for its development. Again, infection is generally controlled with debridement and long-term intravenous antibiotics before and after transplantation. Finally, the device itself may become infected. Clinical signs and symptoms include fevers, elevated WBC, positive blood cultures and occasional device malfunctions. Transesophageal echo can evaluate the bioprosthetic valves. Eradication comes only with device removal.

Under the current allocation scheme, patients with device-related infections can be listed as a Status 1A, because eradication is not possible without device removal, and extension threat is always present.

Finally, LVAD implantation has been associated with B-cell hyperreactivity and anti-human lymphocyte antigen (HLA) antibody development in previously negative candidates. Transplant candidates are periodically screened for preexisting antibodies that are directed against common donor HLA Class I antigens (panel-reactive antibody screen). Preformed antibodies are associated with early graft failure and poor survival. To prevent this, a donor-specific cross-match is performed at transplant in all sensitized candidates. Need for prospective donor cross-match limits the potential donor pool to local organs and significantly prolongs transplant wait time. To circumvent this problem at the authors' institution, treatment of sensitized patients begins with intravenous immunoglobin before transplant, followed by monthly cytoxan cycles to prevent antibody reaccumulation. Using this approach, waiting times for sensitized candidates were successfully reduced *(29)*.

Delisting Transplant Candidates

Patients with the greatest compromise can expect the greatest benefit from cardiac transplantation; however, preoperative condition is an important postoperative outcome determinant. Moribund patients with severe secondary end-organ dysfunction will likely have a prolonged, complicated postoperative course. Massive volume overload in patients with renal insufficiency will likely lead to postoperative problems with worsening renal function, pulmonary hypertension, prolonged intubation, coagulopathy, and hepatic dysfunction complicating recovery. For critically ill patients, close surveillance for infection and end-organ damage is needed to determine at what point they may become too ill for transplantation because of unacceptable operative risk. If a patient becomes too ill and recovery is not anticipated, transplantation should be delayed or denied.

Indeed, one of a transplant physician's most difficult decisions is a transplant candidate's removal from the active wait list when the patient develops irreversible end-organ damage as a consequence of unrelenting heart failure. Transplantation in this setting will result in a protracted intensive care hospitalization that invariably leads to death and a waste of a scarce resource. Failure to delist the patient only delays the inevitable and deprives other, more viable candidates their chance for transplant.

Alternate Transplant Candidates

Some high-volume transplant centers have developed programs that offer nonoptimal transplant candidates transplantation using organs that would otherwise not be placed. Hearts from donors with hepatitis C, or with structural abnormalities such as noncritical CAD or mild to moderate LV hypertrophy, provides a viable alternative for some candidates. Older recipients with isolated end-stage heart disease or younger patients with a comorbidity, such as significant peripheral vascular disease or coexistent HIV infection, are typical candidates for these organs. Use of these donors may also serve to gauge cardiac transplant success in patients with unusual diseases such as amyloid or primary cardiac malignancies. Initial results at UCLA and Columbia are encouraging *(30–32)*.

REFERENCES

1. Kannel WB. Epidemiologic aspects of heart failure. Cardiol Clinics 1987;7:1–9.
2. Rose E, Gelijns A, Moskowitz A, et al. Long term use of left ventricular device for end-stage heart failure. (REMATCH). N Engl J Med 2001;345:1435–1443.
3. Hunt S, Baker D, Chin M, et al. ACC/AHA Guidelines for the evaluation and management of chronic heart failure in the adult: executive summary. Circulation 2001;104:2996–3007.
4. Costanzo M, Augustine S, Bourge R, et al. Selection and treatment of candidates for heart transplanatation. Circulation 1995;92:3593–3612.
5. Mancini D, Ascheim D, Ronan N, et al. Predictors of survival in patients with end-stage heart failure. Circulation 2002;106(19):II680.
6. Lang C, Beniaminovitz A, Edwards N, et al. Morbidity and mortality in diabetic patients following cardiac transplantation. J Heart Lung Transplant 2003;22:244–249.
7. Cohn J, Johnson G, Shabetai R, et al. Ejection fraction, peak exercise oxygen consumption, cardiothoracic ratio, ventricular arrhythmias, and plasma norepinephrine as determinates of prognosis in heart failure. The V-Heft VA Cooperative Studies Group. Circulation 1993;87:VI5–VI16.
8. Lee W, Packer M. Prognostic importance of serum sodium concentration and its modification by converting-enzyme inhibition in patients with severe chronic heart failure. Circulation 1986;73:257–267.
9. Saxon L, Stevenson W, Middlekauf H, et al. Predicting death from progressive heart failure secondary to ischemic or idiopathic dilated cardiomyopathy. Am J Cardiol 1993;72:62–65.
10. Weber K, Kinasewitz G, Janicki J, et al. Oxygen utilization and ventilation during exercise in patients with chronic congestive heart failure. Circulation 1982;65:1213–1223.
11. Szlachcic J, Massie B, Kramer B, et al. Correlates and prognostic implication of exercise capacity in chronic congestive heart failure. Am J Cardiol 1985;55:1037–1042.
12. Mancini DM, Eisen H, Kussmaul W, et al. Value of peak exercise oxygen consumption for optimal timing of cardiac transplantation in ambulatory patients with heart failure. Circulation 1991;83:778–786.
13. Aaronson KD, Mancini DM. Is percentage of predicted maximal exercise oxygen consumption a better predictor of survival than peak exercise oxygen consumption for patients with severe heart failure? J Heart Lung Transplant 1995;14:981–989.
14. Stelken AM, Younis LT, Jennison SH, et al. Prognostic value of cardiopulmonary exercise testing using percent achieved of predicted peak oxygen uptake for patients with ischemic and dilated cardiomyopathy. J Am Coll Cardiol 1996;27:345–352.
15. Aaronson K, Chen T, Mancini D. Demonstration of the continuous nature of peak VO_2 for predicting survival in ambulatory patients evaluated for transplant. J Heart Lung Transplant 1996;15:S66S.
16. Chomsky DB, Lange CC, Rayos GH, et al. Hemodynamic exercise testing: a valuable tool in the selection of cardiac transplantation candidates. Circulation 1996;94:3176–3183.
17. Mancini D, Katz S, Donchez L, et al. Coupling of hemodynamic measurements with oxygen consumption during exercise does not improve risk stratification in patients with heart failure. Circulation 1996;94:2492–2496.

18. Osado N, Bernard CR, Miller LW, et al. Cardiopulmonary exercise testing identifies low risk patients with heart failure and severely impaired exercise capacity considered for heart transplantation. J Am Coll Cardiol 1998;31:577–582.

19. Chua TP, Ponikowski P, Harrington D, et al. Clinical correlates and prognostic significance of the ventilatory response to exercise in chronic heart failure. J Am Coll Cardiol 1997;29:1585–1590.

20. Aaronson K, Schwartz JS, Chen T, et al. Development and prospective validation of a clinical index to predict survival in ambulatory patients referred for cardiac transplant evaluation. Circulation 1997;95:2660–2667.

21. Peterson L, Schechtman K, Ewald G, et al. The effect of β-adrenergic blockers on the prognostic value of peak exercise oxygen uptake in patients with heart failure. J Heart Lung Transplant 2003;22:70–77.

22. Powhani A, Murali S, Mathier M, et al. Impact of β-blocker therapy on functional capacity criteria for heart transplant listing. J Heart Lung Transplant 2003;22:78–86.

23. Stevenson L, Steimle A, Fonarow G, et al. Improvement in exercise capacity of candidates awaiting heart transplantation. J Am Coll Cardiol 1995;25:163–170.

24. Aaronson K, Bowers J, Chen T, et al. Mortality remains high for outpatient transplant candidates with prolonged (>6 months) waiting list time. J Am Coll Cardiol 1999;33:1189–1195.

25. Aaronson K, Bowers J, Gonzalez J, et al. Heart failure survival model predicts survival when applied serially at subsequent reevaluation. J Heart Lung Transplant 1997;17:82A.

26. Lang C, Hankins S, Hauff H, et al. Morbidity and mortality of UNOS status 1B cardiac transplant candidates at home. J Heart Lung Transplant 2003;22:419–426.

27. Mancini D, Oz M, Williams M. Cardiac transplantation/circulatory support devices. In: Antman E, ed. Cardiovascular Therapeutics, 2nd ed. WB Saunders, Philadelphia, PA: 2002, p. 390.

28. Williams M, Joshi N, Hankinson T, et al. LVAD insertion in patients without thorough transplant evaluations: a worthwhile risk? J Thoracic and Cardiovasc Surg 2003;126(2):436–441.

29. Itescu S, Burke E, Lietz K, et al. Intravenous pulsed administration of cyclophosphamide is highly effective and safe for sensitized recipients of cardiac allograft recipents. Circulation 2002;105:1214–1219.

30. Chen J, Hammond K, Kherani A, et al. Is the alternate waiting list too high risk? The Columbia–Presbyterian Experience. J Heart Lung Transplant 2003;22:175.

31. Laks H, Marelli D. The alternate recipient list for heart transplantation: a model for expansion of the donor pool. Advances in Cardiac Surg 1999;11:233–244.

32. Laks H, Scholl FG, Drinkwater DC, et al. The alternate recipient list for heart transplantation: does it work? J Heart Lung Transplant 1997;16:735–742.

2

Donor Selection and Management of the High-Risk Donor

Jonathan M. Chen, MD and Niloo M. Edwards, MD

CONTENTS

INTRODUCTION

In light of increasing organ demand in a stable supply setting, prompt and efficacious potential cardiac donor management is of paramount importance. Since the early description of the "ideal" donor by Griepp and associates in 1971 *(1)*, the criteria by which donors are accepted—and the characteristics that determine a "high-risk" donor—have changed substantially (*see* Tables 1 and 2). Indeed, the growing acceptance of donor organs that meet so-called "extended" criteria for transplantation has further emphasized the importance of aggressive donor management by experienced individuals whose interventions can transform otherwise unusable donors into ones of low or intermediate risk.

From: *Contemporary Cardiology: Cardiac Transplantation:*
The Columbia University Medical Center/New York-Presbyterian Hospital Manual
Edited by: N. M. Edwards, J. M. Chen, and P. A. Mazzeo © Humana Press Inc., Totowa, NJ

Table 1
Griepp's Historical Criteria Describing the Ideal Cardiac Donor *(1)*

Historical donor criteria

- Age < 30 yr
- No significant medical problems
- No substance abuse
- Ischemic time < 2 h
- No evidence of infection

Table 2
Examples of Some Extended Donor Criteria

Extended donor criteria

- Age 60+ yr
- Significant echocardiographic abnormalities
- Ischemic time 7 h
- Donor/Recipient size mismatch up to 70%
- (+) Blood/Urine/Sputum cultures
- (+) Hepatitis B and/or hepatitis C
- Significant pressor/inotrope requirements
- Donor substance abuse
- Longstanding diabetes mellitus

This chapter's purpose is to review the basic practical donor management principles and to address other strategies for extending basic donor criteria to include so-called "high-risk" donors. The donor management algorithm used at Columbia–Presbyterian is reviewed as are the current recommendations of the American College of Cardiology, the United Network for Organ Sharing, and a recent consensus panel on donor use.

Ultimately, however, it must be remembered that the donor "risk" question represents a larger intellectual balance of both donor and recipient risk characteristics. Thus, the number of and extent to which donor criteria are waived ("extended") in a given circumstance often more closely represents the acuity of the recipient's condition than the actual donor utility (or risk).

IDENTIFYING THE CARDIAC DONOR

Naturally, the ideal cardiac donor is of an "appropriate" age and has suffered a catastrophic enough cerebral event to be declared brain dead, but has otherwise exhibited stable hemodynamics (and excellent cardiac function) during their hospitalization. One pursues donors whose clinical progress is notable for an absence of "major" exclusion criteria: (a) significant penetrating cardiac trauma, (b) known cardiac disease, (c) prolonged cardiac arrest (greater than 15 min) with associated chest compressions or intracardiac injections, (d) a human immunodeficiency virus (HIV)-positive history, or (e) the presence of a major extracranial malignancy. Later, this chapter discusses other "minor" criteria, as they represent areas of contention and help to define the high-risk donor.

Although generally not the purview of the cardiac surgeon or transplant team, consent for organ donation should be requested by a professional trained in its acquisition. Multiple studies have demonstrated that the consent rate for organ donation at the request of an organ procurement organization (OPO) member is favored over a physician's request *(2)*. Therefore, we strongly encourage the early involvement of such OPO-designated individuals in the transplant process.

Appropriate multiorgan donor assessment and management requires a careful balance of the solid organ transplant teams' competing clinical agendas. For example, whereas aggressive fluid infusion may favor the cardiac or renal procurement teams, it may be detrimental to those procuring lungs. Conversely, the addition of inotropes to maintain blood pressure in lieu of volume resuscitation may favor pulmonary procurement but may deplete myocardial adenosine adenosine-triphosphate (ATP) stores. Ultimately, adherence to a therapeutic algorithm that maximizes donor hemodynamic stability and end-organ perfusion generally favors all various solid organ procurement teams involved and is a goal that is easily tenable with some diplomacy.

DONOR ASSESSMENT

Formulating an accurate initial donor assessment at first referral relies on clinical practice fundamentals. Often, this task is complicated by the limited capabilities of the center where the donor resides (e.g., a small community hospital), including a lack of invasive monitoring (Swan–Ganz catheterization, serial arterial blood gas analysis) or the fact that multiple inotropes or vasopressors are not available. Under these circumstances, we have found it important to return to basic patient management principles.

What are the Vital Signs?

A blood pressure should be obtained every 2 h, as should a transduced central venous pressure (CVP) or, preferably, pulmonary artery (PA) catheter readings. Fluid "ins and outs" must be recorded hourly and accurately, and a temperature should be recorded every 4 h (temperature should be maintained above 96°F).

What Is the Blood Pressure?

All attempts should be made to maintain the systolic blood pressure above 100 mmHg. Hypotension may be treated with various colloid or crystalloid solutions (as indicated by electrolyte abnormalities) or by packed red blood cell infusion should the hematocrit fall below 30 mg/dL. Most fluids should be given through fluid warmers. Should hypotension persist despite euvolemia (CVP 10–15 mmHg), low-dose inotropic or vasopressor support may be indicated.

Are There Vasopressor Requirements?

Most centers titrate dopamine or dobutamine at 5–10 µg/kg/min to maintain the systolic blood pressure above 100 mmHg. If these requirements increase despite euvolemia, the authors have found low-dose arginine vasopressin (AVP) (0.01–0.05 U/min) to be effective in supplementing the vasopressor effect (to be discussed later) *(3)*. Neosynephrine, epinephrine, and norepinephrine may be used in low doses to counteract the vasodilation that follows brain death, but they must be titrated carefully so as not to compromise arterial inflow to the abdominal viscera. Acid/base status impacts substantially on inotrope and vasopressor efficacy, thus significant acidemia or alkalemia must be corrected.

What Is the Urine Output and How Is It Trending?

The goal is to maintain urine output greater than 2 cc/kg/h. A common pathophysiologic brain death response is diabetes insipidus, which may be reflected by (1) serum sodium greater than 150 mEq/L, (2) serum osmolarity greater than 310 osm/L, or (3) urine output greater than 7 cc/kg/h. Under these circumstances, CVP monitoring is essential, and treatment by urine output replacement cc for cc with crystalloid (D5 1/3 or D5 1/4 NS) as well as with intravenous desmopressin (DDAVP) (0.05–0.10 U/min) is indicated to maintain euvolemia and electrolyte balance.

Is the Donor Adequately Oxygenating and What Is the Acid–Base Status?

Arterial blood gas analysis is the gold standard and should be available universally. Often, however, small hospitals do not provide continuous arterial access to donors, and serial analysis may require re-emphasis of its importance with the donor intensive care unit (ICU) team. Standard ventilator management to rectify abnormalities in arterial partial pressures of oxygen (PaO_2) and carbon dioxide ($PaCO_2$) must be employed, and arterial pH must be maintained within normal limits to ensure adequate end-organ function and allow efficacious vasopressor and inotrope use.

DONOR SELECTION:
STANDARD CARDIAC PARAMETERS

All donors should have a 12-lead electrocardiogram (EKG). Nonspecific ST changes associated with brain death are common; however, major abnormalities generally require inquiry, especially if present in concert with other cardiac risk factors. Although the significance of elevated cardiac enzymes (e.g., creatinine phosphokinase-MB fractions, troponin T) in the donor referral setting has been investigated, there has been no clear consensus regarding their use. At present, we and others use serum enzyme markers as indicators that more detailed evaluation is required, should the magnitude of their elevation not correlate with other clinical findings. For example, as Grant has suggested, an otherwise acceptable donor with significantly elevated troponin T levels may warrant further echocardiographic analysis to demonstrate the absence of progressive cardiac deterioration (4). Similarly, a donor requiring significant catecholamine support but with a normal troponin T warrants further evaluation as a potentially useable source (5).

Generally, transthoracic echocardiography (TTE) is available at all designated donor hospitals, although, if necessary, portable TTE devices brought by the consulting donor team may be used for local donors for whom TTE has been absent or equivocal. Although not essential, TTE allows for the elimination of donors with intracardiac abnormalities (e.g., valvular pathology or septal defects). Clearly, a completely "normal" TTE indicates unequivocal physiologic candidacy, and, conversely, a significantly "abnormal" exam (e.g., valvular stenosis or insufficiency, substantial focal wall motion abnormalities) precludes use. However, interpreting the significance of other "intermediate" TTE abnormalities-especially mild hypokinesis-on posttransplant outcome remains difficult.

Gilbert and colleagues demonstrated TTE's use in 74 potential donor organs; of these, 21 would have been discarded had they not been cleared echocardiographically (6). Seiler et al. described complete wall motion abnormality resolution in all transplant recipients whose donors demonstrated mild to severe wall motion abnormalities. (7).

Investigators at the University of Virginia re-emphasized this finding by evaluating posttransplant "recovery" in patients whose donors demonstrated reduced left ventricular ejection fraction (LVEF) (39 ± 11%) on TTE by serial posttransplant TTE analysis. Their findings over the perioperative period revealed gradual improvement from 49 ± 8% (1 d) to 55 ± 3% (30 d) *(8)*.

Although generally not as available, often transesophageal echocardiography (TEE) clarifies contentious findings on TTE. Body habitus, trauma dressings, and operator inexperience may render TTE windows suboptimal, or at least technically difficult, where TEE may resolve such confusion. Stoddard et al. demonstrated excellent correlation (16/17) between TTE and TEE in their small cohort; however, the findings of TEE eliminated five more donors than TTE *(9)*.

Perhaps more important to donor selection than echocardiographic analysis may be the difficulty of relying on an outside echocardiogram interpretation by a referring cardiologist who is inexperienced in the common echocardiographic findings of neurologic dysfunction and brain death and who has a presumed incentive to overestimate minor echocardiographic findings (a tendency to "overcall" for fear of subsequent lawsuit or blame for posttransplant dysfunction). Lewandowski and investigators at the University of Michigan compared donor echocardiogram interpretations screened by cardiologists at referring donor hospitals to those of "experts" trained in donor heart selection. In 67 patients, they found poor correlation between two groups: minor abnormalities were 18% sensitive and 75% specific (53% agreement), major abnormalities were 33% sensitive and 94% specific (77% agreement), and the designation "unusable" was 33% sensitive and 96% specific (81% agreement); the recommendation (by the referring cardiologist) to reject a donor based on the echocardiogram was considered inappropriate (by the experts) in two patients *(10)*.

Generally, coronary angiography with left ventriculography is required for male donors greater than 45 yr and female donors greater than 55 yr based on the likelihood of coronary atherosclerosis' in these age groups. In addition, catheterization is often requested when there is a significant history of longstanding hypertension, cigarette smoking, insulin-dependent diabetes, cocaine use, or focal electrocardiographic or echocardiographic abnormalities. However, coronary angiography is frequently unavailable at small referring donor hospitals, and, in these cases, depending on the recipient's acuity and the other concomitant donor risk factors, direct coronary palpation for atheromatous plaques by an experienced donor team may represent the best alternative assay of coronary disease. In addition, mild hypokinesis evident on echocardiogram can be analyzed more closely in the operating room by needle-pressure assessment of the PA or left atrium, as indicated.

DONOR SELECTION:
OTHER STANDARD PARAMETERS

Size

Donor size is matched to recipient size on weight basis, where a discrepancy greater than 20% is generally considered significant. This crude size parameter seeks to estimate donor–recipient compatibility so that the heart is of sufficient size to support the recipient circulation, but is not so large as to preclude sternal closure or promote tamponade. Because of frequent massive recipient cardiac dilatation in the long-standing heart failure setting, it is rare for even a substantially larger donor heart not to fit in the recipient's pericardium and thus allow for chest closure (this is generally more of a pediatric recipient concern). An unusually tall recipient can infrequently require that the donor team procure more superior vena caval tissue (often up to and including the innominate vein) to allow enough length to span the intercaval vertical distance. In an effort to potentially alleviate posttransplant right ventricle (RV) failure risks, some centers purposely seek considerably larger donors for patients whose preoperative pulmonary hemodynamic profiles suggest pulmonary hypertension. However, this strategy is theoretical. The converse (using a significantly undersized heart for a recipient with high preoperative pulmonary hemodynamic indices) is not recommended, as the donor RV may not be equipped to tolerate the increased afterload posttransplant.

Despite the emphasis placed on size compatibility and functional potential, several investigators have revealed weight to be a poor heart size or function surrogate. In 1989, Hosenpud demonstrated that small hearts rely on increased heart rate and elevated filling pressures to achieve adequate cardiac output, but also showed that there is no correlation between donor weight and cardiac output or stroke volume (11). In contrast, investigators at Temple University demonstrated a gradual increase in LV mass among undersized hearts when compared with controls over a 10-wk posttransplant period (12). Also, Chan et al. evaluated the echocardiograms of 235 normal adults and demonstrated no difference in LV dimensions between 40–90 kg women or 50–99 kg men; they found major incompatibilities only at extremes of height, weight, and body surface area (13).

Weight, at present, remains one of few size parameters widely available for estimating heart size or function. Nonetheless, the transplant clinician must realize the above limitations in its consideration.

Table 3
Studies Examining the Effect
of Increasing Donor Age on Posttransplant Outcome

Study	Year	n	Age range	Findings
Schuler *(14)*	1989	74	36–54 yr	No difference in survival No difference in 1.4-yr angiogram
Mulvagh *(15)*	1989	47	35–59 yr	No difference in survival No difference in graft function
Alexander *(16)*	1991	165	45–55 yr	No difference in survival
Menkis *(17)*	1991	19	40–59 yr	No difference in survival
Luciani *(18)*	1992	18	40–55 yr	No difference in survival Higher infection rate in older group
Ott *(19)*	1994	22	40–66 yr	No difference in survival
Ibrahim *(20)*	1995	40	40–62 yr	No difference in survival
Tenderich *(21)*	1998	19	57–78 yr	No difference in survival for > 60 yr
Chen *(22)*	2000	305	27–64 yr	No difference in 30-d mortality

Age

Donor age was one of the first criteria extended in an effort to expand the donor pool. Indeed, since the Stanford Group identified the ideal donor as less than 30 yr, several investigators have reported successful heart use from donors as much as twice that age *(14–22)*. The traditional concern with older donors has been coronary atherosclerosis; however, in its absence (usually confirmed by coronary angiography), what prevents the graft from potentially functioning for another 30 yr? In other words, what is the likelihood that other competing risks posttransplant will not substantially outweigh the risk resulting from donor age alone—how can one estimate the "biological age" of the graft itself?

Table 3 collates a few major publications that have evaluated the effect of age on posttransplant survival, and, from this, it is clear that age alone does not specifically impact survival. Recently, we have accepted donors of increasing age with good result, but we generally suggest that donors greater than 50 yr be considered only if demonstrated to be free of coronary atherosclerosis by either angiography or direct palpation. Again, the impetus to accept increasingly older donor organs may often reflect the recipient's acuity or general condition (e.g., accepting a 65-yr-old donor for a 65-yr-old Status 1 recipient, not for a 25-yr-old Status II recipient), thus it represents risk balancing between donor and recipient.

Ischemic Time

Although the traditional benchmark for acceptable cold ischemic time was 120 min, this, too, has been extended so that the current benchmark is approx 240 min. Certainly, innumerable reports have documented successful ischemic times of up to 9 h, especially in the pediatric population; however, the impact of progressively long ischemic times may not be reflected easily in perioperative mortality statistics. It has been suggested that impaired (i.e., not catastrophic) preservation's "minor" effects are most often reflected by more protean manifestations (prolonged postoperative inotrope dependence, prolonged ICU stay, etc.) rather than acute graft failure. Ironically, longer ischemic times may result in more consistent, colder donor organ preservation, as shorter times necessitate wider fluctuations in temperature over a shorter time period; the significance of these differences on postoperative function is unknown.

Inotropic/Vasopressor Support

Early donor inclusion criteria often included an inotrope limitation of 10 µg/kg/min dopamine or dobutamine infusions. We currently have no exclusion criteria, and it is not uncommon for us to accept organs from donors receiving "wide open" inotrope and vasopressor infusions. Here, potentially more than anywhere else in donor management, use of experienced on-site clinicians (generally transplant coordinators) is critical. Attention to regulation of acid/base status, serum electrolyte abnormalities (especially calcium), hypothermia, oxygenation, and euvolemia often reduces or eliminates such requirements.

Natural brain death progression involves an initial surge of catecholamine release, followed by its converse, and an additional series of neurohumoral deficiencies, most of which result in hypotension. In the early 1990s, we were encouraged by the dramatic effects of intravenous triiodothyroidine (T3; 2–4 µg bolus, 2–4 µg/h infusion) as an adjunct to help reduce vasopressor and inotrope requirements; these practical efforts were based largely on by Novitsky's preliminary primate and human work demonstrating a relative thyroid hormone deficiency in the brain death setting, the rectification of which led to improved hemodynamics in this and later studies *(23,24)*. This enthusiasm waned somewhat in the late 1990s, owing to the medication's cost (and often limited availability at donor hospitals) as well as its inconsistent effect.

More recently, it was demonstrated that a substantial number of hemodynamically unstable donors display a relative deficiency in the naturally occurring hormone vasopressin *(3)*. The deficiency in this hormone is known to account for the diabetes insipidus phenomenon

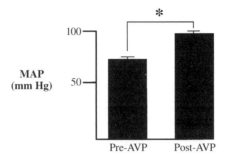

Fig. 1. The effect (MAP) of low (physiologic)-dose infusion of arginine vaso-pressin to donors on high-dose catecholamine vasopressors who demonstrated hemodynamic instability. From ref. 3 with permission.

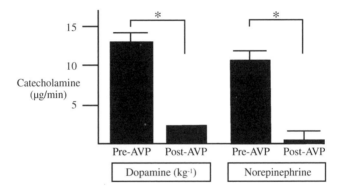

Fig. 2. The effect (catecholamine requirement) of low (physiologic)-dose infu-sion of arginine vasopressin to donors on high-dose catecholamine vasopres-sors who demonstrated hemodynamic instability. From ref. 3 with permission.

during brain death, where the treatment is a DDAVP infusion. DDAVP is a vasopressin analog with an almost exclusive effect on the vaso-pressin V_2 (renal) receptors. This central deficiency in vasopressin also accounts for a peripheral deficiency of hormone available to stimulate the vasopressin V_1 (vasoconstrictor) receptor; however, this fact was underappreciated.

Infusions of low (physiologic)-dose, commercially available AVP (which has both V_1 and V_2 effects) has helped salvage countless donors from hemodynamic instability (Figs. 1 and 2) (3). From this, we have postulated that in the setting of brain death a central vasopressin defi-ciency may lead to dramatic vasodilation unresponsive to catecholamine pressor infusion; correcting this deficiency allows for hemodynamic stability and better vasomotor tone (3).

The suggestion to add a low-dose vasopressin infusion often meets with resistance, particularly from the renal procurement teams. However, we contend that it is better physiologically to require dramatically fewer vasopressors with a small amount of AVP than to continue giving increasing doses of pressors, with their other attendant detrimental effects (e.g., lactic acidosis, end-organ hypoperfusion, etc).

ABO Compatibility/Positive Cross-Match

Although there appear to be no appreciable sequelae to transplanting across Rhesus blood groups, transplantation within ABO blood groups remains axiomatic. On occasion, we have transplanted across ABO-compatible blood groups with poor results, even with adjunctive plasmapheresis and additional immunosuppression.

Patients awaiting transplantation on our waiting list routinely undergo standard panel reactive antibody (PRA) testing at regular intervals to confirm that their reactivity is less than 20%. For those above this level, a prospective lymphocytotic cross-match is mandatory prior to transplantation, essentially limiting the potential donor pool to local donors only. Occasionally, we have transplanted across a positive cross-match (and on more occasions transplanted inadvertently across a retrospectively positive cross-match) with reasonable results. In this setting (and for those awaiting transplantation whose PRA is high), a combination therapy of cyclophosphamide, intravenous immunoglobulin, and/or plasmapheresis has been useful in lowering apparent immune reactivity (*see also* Chapter 8) *(25)*. The overall results in these settings, however, remain marginal.

Trauma

In general, most centers have avoided donors who have withstood significant chest trauma for fear of apparent or occult cardiac contusion. Additionally, some have feared the potential infectious risk of prolonged tube thoracostomy in this setting. The authors have found that, as in routine trauma patients, the cardiac contusion diagnosis can be difficult, as the findings of generalized ST abnormalities on EKG, or pericardial fluid on echocardiogram, may be evident even in atraumatic donors. Investigators have previously demonstrated neither short cardiac resuscitation episodes nor significant hemothorax/rib fractures to impact on posttransplant graft function *(26,27)*. Generally, we do not accept donors who have undergone open cardiac massage or intracardiac injection; however, we do consider donors with appreciable closed resuscitation efforts. In these situations, the experienced opinion of the harvest team (e.g., hemopericardium? overall function?) is essential.

Substance Abuse/Poisoning

It is rare to find a donor who has no history of previous substance use and/or abuse. Most commonly found is a history of cigarette use that, if chronic and substantial, may warrant coronary angiography. The second most common finding is a history of marijuana use, the significance of which is unclear. Often, marijuana use may represent additional intravenous drug use. This certainly raises the transmissible disease specter and warrants more detailed investigation.

Often, donors have a history of alcohol abuse, and it has been suggested that in these cases "preclinical" alcoholic cardiomyopathy could lead to a latent graft dysfunction postoperatively. Houyel has suggested that hearts from alcoholic donors demonstrate increased wall thickness and LV mass, with questionable LV filling impairment; this is thought to be independent of the duration of their alcoholism *(27)*. Freimark's cohort analysis (17 of 100 donors were alcoholic) demonstrated decreased survival in recipients of these organs at 1 and 2 yr (61 vs 95%) *(28)*. Unfortunately, estimating the true magnitude of a given donor's alcohol use (and thus the organ's suitability) is difficult and, unless egregious, generally is not weighted heavily.

Cocaine use is known to be correlated to vasospastic coronary disease and even myocardial infarction. As with other illicit substances, the quantity and administration method (intranasal, intravenous) is generally unclear. Freimark evaluated 112 consecutive donors at UCLA and found a 16% incidence of significant cocaine use. In this cohort, there was no evidence of prior cocaine use's impact on morbidity, mortality, or endomyocardial ischemia (by biopsy) *(29)*.

Various poisons have accounted for brain death in potential donors. Several case series have demonstrated successful heart transplantation from donors who suffered cyanide or carbon monoxide poisoning (both traditionally absolute contraindications to use) *(30,31)*. Because the history and impact of significant substance abuse or poisoning is incomplete, we have tended, in these circumstances, to rely heavily on the echocardiogram and the donor team's opinion at visualization to assess global myocardial function.

Infection

Pyrexia is a common finding of the brain-dead state, and finding positive cultures is extremely common in organ donation, owing largely to prolonged ICU support prior to the donation consent acquisition. Thankfully, in the current broad-spectrum antibiotic era, the rate of bacterial infection transferred from cardiac donor to recipient is exceedingly low. Naturally, any organisms known to have been cultured from the donor should form the basis for specific recipient preoperative and postoperative antibiotic prophylaxis. Sweeney demonstrated a lack of transmission from 17 donors with significant positive cultures *(32)*, and Jeevanandam reported 2 of 25 donors with positive cultures resulting in posttransplant infections *(33)*.

Toxoplasmosis has been transmitted in the donor graft but may not be suspected until present on posttransplant endomyocardial biopsy. For those recipients who demonstrate prior exposure, no therapy is necessary; for those who are negative and receive an organ documented to be toxoplasma-positive or who receive an organ from a donor with unknown toxoplasma status, prophylaxis with pyramethamine and folate is initiated for the first 6 wk after transplant (*see* Chapter 7). HIV positivity remains an absolute contraindication to organ donation.

The use of donors with a positive hepatitis panel remains contentious. Hepatitis B surface antibody positivity, reflecting exposure, has not been a contraindication to use. We do not consider Hepatitis B core antibody positivity, reflecting recent exposure, as a contraindication to transplantation, but, generally, this is not accepted worldwide. Traditionally, hepatitis B surface antigen positivity, indicating active infection, has represented an absolute contraindication to transplantation. We and others are currently studying this cohort to evaluate whether these hearts could be used for recipients who received the proper pretransplant immunization and who will receive appropriate posttransplant therapy.

Hepatitis C donors are equally controversial, as many studies have demonstrated poor outcome for recipients of hepatitis C-positive hearts and have shown a substantial seroconversion rate among recipients *(34,35)*. A potential solution is the use of hepatitis C-positive hearts for hepatitis C-positive recipients; however, this generally requires using an alternative list for transplantation, which is discussed later.

STRATEGIES TO BROADEN DONOR AVAILABILITY

Nonbeating Donors

Some enthusiasm has arisen from the liver and kidney procurement literature for organ use from nonbeating donors. Whereas experimental literature suggests that hearts may be harvested as long as 30 min postmortem, this process requires preservation with blood cardioplegia prior to cardiac arrest, the logistics of which in the human condition are unclear *(36,37)*. Indeed, the further legal implications of cardiac death vs brain death, the lack of good long-term results from animal studies, and the

Table 4
Consented Heart Referrals Not Recovered
in the United States in 1995 *(38)*

Reasons not recovered	Number
Infection	27
Coronary artery disease	70
Advanced age	265
Poor ventricular function	918
History of prolonged downtime	119
Total	1399

Table 5
Comparison of the Effects of Broadening the Donor Criteria vs Increasing
Consent Rates on the Number of Hearts Available Annually in 1995 *(38)*

	10%	25%	50%
Broadening donor criteria	141	351	701
Increasing consent rates	252	630	1260

need for pretreatment with heparin and/or free radical scavengers renders this an unlikely donor organ source in the immediate future.

Consent Rates

Whereas most efforts have been directed at expanding the donor pool by broadening donor acceptance criteria, it must be remembered that potentially the largest impact may be made by increasing consent rates. Rayburn investigated the national recovery of consented heart referrals for 1995 and collated the reasons donors were declined (*see* Table 4). Although difficult to estimate, clearly a proportion of these donors would surely have been used today, albeit potentially as "high risk." Rayburn then estimated the number of hearts that would be made available by either broadening donor criteria or increasing consent rates by 10, 25, and 50%, respectively (*see* Table 5). As demonstrated, the effect of increasing consent rates is nearly double that of extending donor criteria *(38)*. Furthermore, of this proportion, not all would be marginal donors, hence the increase in usable donors would likely be greater. Thus, it is imperative that transplant clinicians consistently make efforts toward community education to promote an increase in organ donation consent.

Alternate List

Since 1996, investigators from UCLA have promoted the alternate transplantation waiting list concept, in which candidates who would not be considered for transplantation under standard criteria on an age basis or other "minor" exclusion criteria (e.g., diabetes, hepatitis), might receive hearts that otherwise would have been discarded *(39,40)*. According to their scheme, a standard donor heart would first be offered to the appropriate Status I recipient. If declined, it would then be offered to the next Status II recipient. If declined again, it would be offered to the appropriate alternate list recipient. Similarly, if a "marginal" heart became available, but was declined by the first Status I recipient on the list, it would be offered to an alternate list recipient. Marginal hearts would not be offered to Status II patients. The results of this format have been promising and have demonstrated few complications attributable solely to recipient comorbidities.

We have also employed an alternate list based on similar schema. The alternate list concept is particularly appealing in that it may use normal hearts that otherwise would be discarded for lack of an appropriate recipient. However, the transplant clinician must be careful of "stacking risks" for those hearts that are more high-risk, for the marginal donor and marginal recipient combination clearly creates a marginal outcome. For the authors' alternate list, this has meant restricting the defining (alternate) criterion to one (e.g., a 67-yr-old patient, not a 67-yr-old patient with hepatitis) and resisting the tendency to list significantly high-risk recipients with multiple comorbidities.

CONCLUSION

Such donor–recipient mismatching as promoted by the alternate list represents the consideration central to every potential donor referral acceptance. Extending donor criteria to include "riskier" donors has largely stemmed from the acuity of the Status I list. Indeed, as medical heart failure management has improved over the past two decades, so, too, have the patients on the Status I list become potentially sicker. Thus, whether to consider the donor with minor TTE changes, chronic alcoholism, and a possible history of cocaine use derives largely from whether the designated recipient is a Status I patient dying in the ICU, a Status II patient otherwise well at home, or a patient from the blood group O alternate list. We continue to advocate aggressive marginal donor management, in particular because of a programmatic sense that many are actually poorly managed reasonable donors. We also continue to push comorbidity limits by which we may accept patients on their waiting list. However, as Copeland suggested *(41)*, cost effectiveness is a social imperative in these situations, and we must constantly remember that the donor use assessment always represents the critical evaluation of the donor–recipient combination, rather than individual donor characteristics alone. Ultimately, this combination accounts for posttransplant survival and, therefore, equitable scarce resource use.

REFERENCES

1. Griepp RB, Stinson EB, Clark DA, et al. The cardiac donor. Surg Gyn Obst 1971;133:792–798.
2. Niles PA, Mattice BJ. The timing factor in the consent process. J Transplant Coord 1996;6:84–87.
3. Chen JM, Cullinane S, Spanier TB, et al. Vasopressin deficiency and pressor hypersensitivity in hemodynamically unstable organ donors. Circulation 1999;100(suppl 19):II244–II246.
4. Grant JW, Canter CE, Spray TL. Elevated cardiac troponin I: a marker or acute failure in infant heart recipients. Circulation 1994;90:2618.
5. Riou B, Dreux S, Roche S, Arthaud M, et al. Circulating cardiac troponin T in potential heart transplant donors. Circulation 1995;92:409–414.
6. Gilbert EM, Krueger SK, Murray JL, et al. Echocardiographic evaluation of potential cardiac transplant donors. J Thorac Cardiovasc Surg 1988;95:1003–1007.
7. Seiler C, Laske A, Gallino A, et al. Echocardiographic evaluation of left ventricular wall motion before and after heart transplantation. J Heart Lung Transplant 1992;11:867–874.
8. Kron IL, Tribble CG, Kern JA, et al. Successful transplantation of marginally acceptable thoracic organs. Ann Surg 1993;217(5):518–524.
9. Stoddard MF, Longaker RA. The role of transesophageal echocadiography in cardiac donor screening. Am Heart J 1993;125:1676–1681.
10. Lewandowski TJ, Aaronson KD, Pietroski RE, et al. Discordance in interpretations of potential donor echos. J Heart Lung Transplant 1997;17:100.
11. Hosenpud JD, Pantely GA, Morton MJ, et al. Relation between recipient: donor body size match and hemodynamics three months after heart transplantation. J Heart Transplant 1998;8:241–243.
12. Mather PJ, Jeevanandam V, Eisen JH, et al. Functional and morphologic adaptation of undersized donor hearts after heart transplantation. J Am Coll Cardiol 1995;26:737–742.
13. Chan BBK, Fleischer KJ, Bergin JD, et al. Weight is not an accurate criterion for adult cardiac transplant size matching. Ann Thorac Surg 1991;52:1230–1236.
14. Schuler S, Warnecke H, Loebe M, et al. Extended donor age in cardiac transplantation. Circulation 1989;80(suppl III):III.133–III.139.
15. Mulvaugh SL, Thornton B, Frazier H, et al. The older cardiac transplant donor. Relation to graft function and recipient survival longer than 6 years. Circulation 1989;80(suppl III):III.126–III.132.
16. Alexander JW, Vaughn WK, Carey MA. The use of marginal donors for organ transplantation: the older and younger donors. Transplant Proc 1991;23(1):905–909.

17. Menkis AH, Novick RJ, Kostuk WJ, et al. Successful use of the "unacceptable" heart donor. J Heart Lung Transplant 1991;10:28–31.
18. Luciani GB, Livi U, Faggian G, et al. Clinical results of heart transplantation in receipinets over 55 years of age with donors over 40 years of age. J Heart Lung Transplant 1992;11:1177–1183.
19. Ott GY, Herschberger RE, Ratkovec RR, et al. Cardiac allografts from high-risk donors: excellent clinical results. Ann Thorac Surg 1994;57:76–82.
20. Ibrahim M, Masters RG, Hendry PJ, et al. Determinants of hospital survival after cardiac transplantation. Ann Thorac Surg 1995;59:604–608.
21. Tenderich G, Koerner MM, Stuettgen B, et al. Extended donor criteria. Hemodynamic follow-up of heart transplant recipients receiving a cardiac allograft from donors ≥ 60 years of age. Transplantation 1998;66(8):1109–1113.
22. Chen JM, Rajasinghe HR, Sinha P, et al. Do donor characteristics really matter? Analysis of consecutive heart donors 1995–1999. J Heart Lung Transplant 2002;21(5):608–610.
23. Novitzky D, Cooper DK, Reichart B. Hemodynamic and metabolic responses to hormonal therapy in brain-dead potential organ donors. Transplantation 1987; 43(6):852–854.
24. Mullis-Jansson SL, Argenziano M, Corwin S, et al. A randomized double-blind study of the effect of triiodothyronine on cardiac function and morbidity after coronary bypass surgery. J Thorac Cardiovasc Surg 1999;117(6):1128–1134.
25. John R, Lietz K, Burke E, et al. Intravenous immunoglobulin reduces anti-HLA alloreactivity and shortens waiting time to cardiac transplantation in highly sensitized left ventricular assist device recipients. Circulation 1999;100(suppl 19): II.229–II.235.
26. Schuler S, Parnt R, Warnecke H, et al. Extended donor criteria for heart transplantation. J Heart Transplant 1988;7:326–330.
27. Houyel L, Petit J, Nottin R, et al. Adult heart transplantation: adverse role of chronic alcoholism in donors on early graft function. J Heart Lung Transplant 1992;11: 1184–1187.
28. Freimark D, Aleksic I, Trento A, et al. Hearts from donors with chronic alcohol use: a possible risk factor for death after transplantation. J Heart Lung Transplant 1996;15(2):150–159.
29. Freimark D, Czer LSC, Admon D, et al. Donors with a history of cocaine use: effect on survival and rejection frequency after heart transplantation. J Heart Lung Transplant 1994;13:1138–1144.
30. Tenderich G, Koerner MM, Posival H, et al. Hemodynamic follow-up of cardiac allografts from poisoned donors. Transplantation 1998;66:1163–1167.
31. Koerner MM, Tenderich G, Minami K, et al. Extended donor criteria. Use of cardiac allografts after carbon monoxide poisoning. Transplantation 1998;63:1358–1360.
32. Sweeney MS, Lammermeier DE, Frazier OH, et al. Extension of donor criteria in cardiac transplantation: surgical risk versus supply-side economics. Ann Thorac Surg 1990;50:7–11.
33. Jeevanandam V, Furukawa S, Prendergast TW, et al. Standard criteria for an acceptable donor heart are restricting heart transplantation. Ann Thorac Surg 1996; 62:1268–1275.
34. Zein NN, McGreger CG, Wendt NK, et al. Prevalence and outcome of hepatitis C infection among transplant recipients. J Heart Lung Transplant 1995;14:865–869.
35. Ong JP, Barnes DS, Younossi ZM. Outcome of de novo hepatitis C infection in heart transplant recipients. Hepatology 1999;12:93.

36. Gundry SR, Fukushima N, Eke CC, et al. Successful survival of primates receiving transplantation with "dead" nonbeating donor hearts. J Thorac Cardiovasc Surg 1995;109:1097–1102.

37. Martin J, Sarai K, Yoshitake M, et al. Successful orthotopic pig heart transplantation from non-heart beating donors. J Heart Lung Transplant 1999;18:597–606.

38. Rayburn BK, Burton TM, Wannenburg T, et al. Are efforts at expanding the donor pool misdirected? J Heart Lung Transplant 1998;17:998–1003.

39. Drinkwater DC, Laks H, Blitz A, et al. Outcomes of patients undergoing transplantation with older donor hearts. J Heart Lung Transplant 1996;15:684–691.

40. Laks H, Scholl FG, Drinkwater DC, et al. The alternate recipient list for heart transplantation: does it work? J Heart Lung Transplant 1997;16:735–742.

41. Copeland JG. Only optimal donors should be accepted for heart transplantation: protagonist. J Heart Lung Transplant 1995;14(6 pt. 1):1038–1042.

3   UNOS Policy and Transplant Coordination in Practice

Helen Hauff, RN

INTRODUCTION: HISTORICAL PERSPECTIVE

Origins of the United Network for Organ Sharing

The United Network for Organ Sharing (UNOS) was established in 1977 to provide a computerized sharing network for transplant centers that were not South-Eastern Regional Organ Procurement Program (SEROPP) members. The need for a computerized system became evident with the discovery that outcomes dramatically improved for kidney recipients when human leukocyte antigen (HLA) matching was performed. SEROPP began this work when it was awarded a contract by the Kidney Disease and Control Agency of the Public Health Service in 1969 and provided services for eight transplant centers, which later expanded to 18 centers. SEROPP demonstrated that appropriately matched, procured, and preserved kidneys could improve graft survival and ultimately improve patient outcomes (1).

UNOS had access to SEROPP's computerized registry and began offering the service on a national level, as well as maintaining a registry for other organs. The UNOS that is familiar to all in the transplant world

From: Contemporary Cardiology: Cardiac Transplantation:
The Columbia University Medical Center/New York-Presbyterian Hospital Manual
Edited by: N. M. Edwards, J. M. Chen, and P. A. Mazzeo © Humana Press Inc., Totowa, NJ

today began to take shape in 1982, when SEROPP and UNOS combined forces to create the "Kidney Center." This later evolved into the "Organ Center," as it is currently known. Status codes were established along with policies and procedures, as all organs were placed through the Organ Center. UNOS began maintaining a national registry and coordinating organ placement as well as collecting outcome data. UNOS then became a private, not-for-profit, voluntary organization with a defined mission, and, in 1986, it was awarded the federal contract to operate the national registry as well as to establish the Scientific Registry, where all transplantation and donation data are stored and compiled. By 1987, UNOS was the sole organ center operator. During this time, transplant centers were required to be members of the UNOS-operated Organ Procurement and Transplant Network (OPTN) under the Omnibus Reconciliation Act of 1986 and thereby abide by the policies and procedures set forth by UNOS. Under this regulation, centers could not receive federal Medicare/Medicaid funds if they continued to transplant as nonmembers.

Organization

After these changes took effect, a board of directors was established consisting of 15 transplant surgeons and physicians and 16 nonphysician members, including patients, public members, and voluntary health organization members, as well as representatives from the tissue-typing laboratories and independent organ procurement organizations. The 15 transplant physicians were representatives from the 10 UNOS regions including 5 members of the board: president, immediate past president, vice president, treasurer, and secretary. The board later grew to 16 physician-members when a thoracic member was added *(1)*. The board structure was designed to represent both the transplant industry and the community it was to serve. The organization's administrative component was established with an executive director and an assistant executive director leading operational management. Eleven regions were established, each with a regional administrator who communicated with the standing UNOS committees and the board of directors. National committees and ad hoc committees were established to guide policymaking on transplantation and procurement issues. Fifteen permanent standing committees exist today: Communications, Ethics, Finance, Membership and Professional Standards, Thoracic Organ Transplantation, Histocompatibility, Kidney and Pancreas Transplantation, Liver and Intestinal Organ Transplantation, Transplant Administrators, Pediatric Transplantation, Patient Affairs, Organ Procurement Organization

(OPO), Organ Availability, Minority Affairs, and Data Advisory. This structure ensures that UNOS remains abreast of current practices at the operational level, with each committee receiving regional and national input.

Policymaking

UNOS policies and procedures continue to evolve, as does the transplantation field itself. Usually, changes to current policies and procedures originate from the transplant/donation community. Opportunity also exists for public comment on any changes to UNOS practices. Final policy decisions are made only after regional and national review by all parties concerned.

By 1998, the role of UNOS was again under review. The OPTN awarded two separate contracts for operating the Organ Allocation System and the Scientific Registry for 3-yr periods. In 2000, the contract for the Scientific Registry was awarded to the University Renal Research Education Associates, with UNOS charged to maintain and promote an equitable organ sharing system.

CURRENT UNOS POLICY AND PROCEDURE

As wait times for transplant increase and the mortality rate rises for those waiting, it is no surprise that the thoracic organ distribution system is constantly reviewed and revised to promote equitable policy and ensure that those in urgent clinical need are transplanted. Of all transplant lists, the cardiac wait list is probably the most dynamic. A patient's clinical status can change rapidly, and the patient's wait list status needs to be adjusted accordingly. In 1999, the change in UNOS policy for listing heart recipients came into effect to ensure that the sickest patients had the greatest transplant opportunity.

Current Thoracic Allocation Policy (2002)

Patients are listed as Status 1A when they meet the following criteria (UNOS Policy 3.7, Allocation of Thoracic Organs):

1A(a). Mechanical circulatory support for acute hemodynamic decompensation that includes at least one of the following devices. Patients meeting this criterion may be listed for 30 d at any point after being implanted as Status 1A once the treating physician determines that they are clinically suitable for transplant. Admittance to the transplant center hospital is not required.
   i. Left and/or right ventricular assist device

    ii. Total artificial heart

    iii.Intra-aortic balloon pump

    iv.Extracorporeal membrane oxygenation (ECMO)

1A(b). Mechanical circulatory support for more than 30 d with objective medical evidence of significant device-related complications, such as thromboembolism, device infection, mechanical failure, and/or life-threatening ventricular arrhythmia. (Patient desensitization is not an appropriate device-related complication for qualification as Status 1A under this criterion.)

1A(c). Mechanical ventilation

1A(d). Continuous infusion of a single high-dose intravenous inotrope (e.g., dobutamine ≥ 7.5 mcg/kg/min or milrinone ≥ 0.50 mcg/kg/min), or multiple intravenous inotropes, in addition to continuous hemodynamic monitoring of left ventricle (LV) filling pressures

1A(e). A patient who does not meet the criteria specified above may be listed as Status 1A if the patient is admitted to the listing transplant center and has a life expectancy without a transplant of less than 7 d

All patients listed as a Status 1A must have a "justification form" submitted to UNOS within 24 h. Any delay in justification form receipt will result in the patient being downgraded to the next lower category. The justification form is a certification process that renews a patient's status. For categories (a), (b), and (c), the patient needs to be recertified every 14 d.

Category 1A(a) now includes additional criteria, as the 1A time commences when the physician determines that the patient is ready for transplant, and not simply at insertion of the left ventricular assist device (LVAD). The issue of when to transplant a patient who has received an LVAD is not new. Originally, these patients were listed as a Status 1A immediately at insertion of the LVAD and remained at 1A status for 30 d postimplantation. After 30 d, the patient was automatically downgraded to Status 1B. However, in clinical practice, this does not benefit the patient. Many patients requiring a LVAD are debilitated during the immediate postoperative phase and can not tolerate transplant during this time. The LVAD allows for hemodynamic recovery *(2)*. Additionally, some patients may experience ventricular recovery, and it may not be in their best interest to proceed directly to transplantation without a full exploration of their options *(3)*.

Categories (d) and (e) are more complicated. The certification for category (d) is valid for 7 d and is only renewed for an additional 7 d for each occurrence. In practice, if the patient is not transplanted within this period, the patient remains a 1A, but the category is changed to 1A(e). The 1A(e) category is valid only for 7 d and is renewed only once for an

additional 7-d period. However, any further extension requires a conference call with the applicable UNOS Region Review Board. The board
is comprised of all of the region's transplant center members and effectively acts as a peer review committee to ensure that the criteria for
listing remain valid.

Patients not listed as Status 1A may fall into the next three categories:
Status 1B, Status 2, or UNOS Status 7. Status 1B patients may be at home
or in the hospital and must fulfill one of the following criteria:

1B(a). Left and/or right ventricular assist device implanted1B(b).
Continuous infusion of intravenous inotropes

A justification form is required from the attending physician and must
be received within 24 h; otherwise, the patient is downgraded to Status 2.
Additionally, a patient who does not meet the criteria stated above is
assigned Status 1B if the patient's clinical condition warrants listing
under this category. After a justification form is submitted, the Regional
Review Board decides if the listing is appropriate. For example, this can
occur with patients suffering from ischemic heart disease who require
continuous intravenous infusions of vasodilators such as nitroglycerin
and cannot be managed on oral medications. This is considered as an
exception and the decisions of the Regional Review Board are submitted
to the Thoracic Organ Transplantation and Membership and Professional
Standards Committees to determine consistency within the regions.

Currently under discussion is nesiritide use (Natrecor, Scios Inc.,
Sunnyvale, CA) and its clinical application in heart failure. Certainly,
this will lead to some revision of the criteria in the near future, as greater
experience is gained with this therapy. Use of intravenous nesiritide,
nitroprusside (Nipride, Roche, Basel, Switzerland), or nitroglycerin
without inotropes does not fulfill the criteria for listing a patient as a
Status 1A or 1B.

Patients who do not meet the criteria for Status 1A or Status 1B are
assigned Status 2 unless they are considered temporarily unsuitable for
transplant, in which case they should be listed as UNOS Status 7. No
justification forms are currently required for these two categories. The
coordinator must be aware that assigning a patient a UNOS Status 7
should be temporary only. Patients should not be assigned to the UNOS
Status 7 category if it is determined that the patient will never receive a
transplant, and, in fact, these patients should be completely delisted.
Leaving patients on the list as UNOS Status 7 only adversely affects the
mortality rate pretransplant.

The procedure for pediatric patient listing is similar to that for adult
listing but is outside this chapter's scope. However, the adult clinical
coordinator should be aware that, if a pediatric patient is listed prior to

his or her 18th birthday and subsequently turns 18, the patient remains listed under the pediatric criteria. Often, pediatric programs follow their congenital patients well past 18 yr. The pediatric team should realize that subsequent patient listing needs to occur under adult (and not pediatric) criteria, although the patient remains under pediatric team care.

Interpretation of UNOS Policy

All transplant coordinators must familiarize themselves with UNOS policies and procedures. Often, issues arise in the middle of the night, during a transplant, when there is limited time for clarification. Prior knowledge is needed on the actual policies and their interpretation. The coordinator needs to be aware of the following:

- Listing criteria must be fully understood. The listing criteria for adults and pediatric patients are different. A patient is considered pediatric up to age 18 yr (UNOS policy 3.7.3, Adult Patient Status).
- The transplant coordinator must be aware of the minimum cardiac donor information that is required by UNOS for the OPO to make an offer (UNOS policy 3.7.12, Minimum Information for Thoracic Organ Offers).
- The transplant center has only 1 h after receiving the information in which to accept or decline an offer. An offer can be removed by the OPO and the organ is then offered to another center (UNOS policy 3.4.1, Time Limit for Acceptance).
- Acceptance of an offer without condition is binding and cannot be relinquished unless there is mutual agreement. Occasionally, at the request of the OPO and another transplant center, a center is asked to relinquish an organ on compassionate grounds. Should this situation occur, the accepting surgeon must agree to the organ being offered elsewhere (UNOS policy 3.3.6, Center Acceptance of Organ Offers).
- Operating room (OR) times are mutually arranged; however, if a center cannot agree to a time, the offer can be removed and the organ is placed elsewhere. This requires a highly mobile team if time constraints are to be met (UNOS Policy 3.4.2, Multiple Organ Retrieval).
- Cardiac catheterizations, creatine phosphokinase (CPK) levels, troponin levels, and echocardiograms are desirable, but not required, to make an offer. Additionally, the coordinator should understand the transplant center's policy on paying for additional testing and ensure that additional testing is required before tests are requested (UNOS Policy 3.7.12.2, Desirable Information for Heart Offers).
- Refusal codes are applied to each declinature and need to be verified once submitted by the OPO. These are public data and should always be verified to ensure that the correct code is used. Coordi-

nators need to know the refusal codes and be clear on reasons for turning down an organ. (*See* Appendix at the end of this chapter.)

- Once an organ is accepted at one center, an additional offer is made to the transplant center with the next patient on the list. This ensures that the organ can be transplanted if, for any reason, the accepting center cannot transplant the organ. The same rules of acceptance apply both to the primary and the backup offer. However, if additional information is forthcoming when the organ is re-offered to the backup center, the backup center can decline the organ. In reality, backup offers for hearts rarely come to fruition unless the backup offer is made when the patient for the primary offer requires a cross-match (UNOS Policy 3.7.1.1, Exception for Sensitized Patients). Organs declined in the OR are usually declined for organ-related issues rendering the organ untransplantable, rather than for recipient-related issues (UNOS Policy 3.3.5, Transplant Recipient Backup for Organ Offers).
- A high panel reactive antibody (PRA) level necessitating a prospective cross-match is not a justification for making a patient a UNOS Status 1A (UNOS Policy 3.7.1.1, Exception for Sensitized Patients).
- An OPO can bypass a center if a cross-match is required and if, because of distance, it is not possible to cross-match the patient prospectively, or if time constraints on the donor side prevent the transplant center from performing a cross-match.
- Domino hearts must be re-allocated according to UNOS policy and cannot be used for another patient on the list in the transplanting center (UNOS Policy 3.7.16, Allocation of Domino Donor Hearts).
- Guidelines for wait-time accumulation and application in each status must be understood. When a patient enters a higher status, his or her time begins again in that status. The previous time accumulated in the lower status does not move with the patient. However, if a patient had previous time in the higher status, that is added to the new accumulated time, pushing a patient higher on the list. When a patient is downgraded, the accumulated wait-time in the higher status goes with the patient (UNOS Policy 3.7.9.1, Waiting Time Accrual for Heart Candidates).
- O blood-type hearts will be offered to O and B blood-type recipients first. If no O or B blood-type recipients are available *in that status*, the heart is offered to the A blood-type recipient in the same status group before the organ is offered to the patients in the lower status (UNOS Policy 3.7.8, ABO Typing for Heart Allocation).
- A pediatric heart (less than 18 yr) is first offered to all pediatric patients in the accepted weight range. Only if no pediatric recipients are found in that status is the heart offered to the adults in that status and then offered to a pediatric patient in the lower status (UNOS Policy 3.7.4, Pediatric Patient Status, and UNOS Policy 3.7.5, Allocation of Adolescent Donor Hearts to Pediatric Heart Candidates).

- Occasionally, a recipient's condition deteriorates rapidly and the transplant center calls the OPO for any available organ. If an organ becomes available and the recipient is not the highest candidate on the list, the transplant center needs to contact each transplant center in the sharing region to request that each center relinquish the organ to the requesting center on compassionate grounds. This should be confirmed in writing, signed by all program directors, and submitted to UNOS, preferably prior to the allocation of the organ. If this occurs in the middle of the night, a verbal agreement may be obtained and followed by written confirmation the next day.
- Transplant coordinators must list potential recipients appropriately. Exaggerating weight ranges and the distance the transplant center is willing to travel is pointless if the organ cannot be transplanted.
- When a patient transfers to another center, the new listing center requests the wait time from the previous transplant center via UNOS. UNOS notifies the previous center that the patient is delisted when the transfer of time is completed (UNOS Policy 3.2.2.1, Waiting Time Transferal).
- Clerical and program errors affecting wait time are adjusted after the coordinator's completion of a wait time modification form and submission of the form to UNOS for consideration (UNOS Policy 3.2.1.8.1, Waiting Time Modification for Urgent Status Patients).
- Patients may be listed at multiple centers, provided that the centers are not in the same OPO region (UNOS Policy 3.2.2, Multiple Listings Permitted).
- UNOS policy allows for Local and Alternative Local Unit establishment for organ allocation, provided it is established that an inequity in organ allocation exists in a given region. This also accommodates individual state laws that may require statewide organ sharing first. Attention must be paid to any variances that exist in a given region (UNOS Policy 3.1.7, Local and Alternative Local Unit).
- Foreign nationals can be transplanted. However, only 5% of total transplant recipients can be foreign nationals. The transplant center is subject to an audit if more than 5% of its recipients are foreign nationals (UNOS Policy 6.3, Audit).
- The OPO is responsible for providing a donor evaluation written record, a donor maintenance record, consent documentation, death pronouncement documentation, and donor quality documentation (UNOS Policy 2.1, Host OPO).
- The OPO is responsible for ensuring that teams have appropriate transportation to and from the local airport (UNOS Policy 2.6.8, Organ Procurement Quality).
- Transplanted or deceased patients should be delisted within 24 h (UNOS policy 3.7.14, Removal of Thoracic Organ Transplant Candidates from Thoracic Organ Waiting Lists when Transplanted or Deceased).

- The transplant surgeon has the final decision of transplanting the organ in his or her patient.

LVAD and UNOS Policy

The original listing criteria for the LVAD patient (granting the patient 30 d at Status 1A from the date the device was inserted) evolved from the rationale that LVAD patients experience a short time period before complications arise from the device *(4)*. These complications include coagulation problems, infections, and multisystem organ failure. Patients who develop these complications can have their 1A status extended (UNOS Policy 3.7.3 Adult Patient Status). The system's intention was to transplant these patients before complications arose and before the nonsensitized patient became sensitized, producing autoantibodies resulting in high PRA reactivity.

In 2002, this thinking changed. In practice, these patients often require a recovery period from LVAD insertion before they can be transplanted, in order to regain hemodynamic recovery and improve end-organ perfusion, problems that are a consequence of congestive heart failure *(2)*. Also, granting immediate 1A status did not give the patient adequate time to regain ventricular recovery from acute events such as myocardial infarction *(5)*. This window of opportunity for transplant was too short before the patient was downgraded to Status 1B.

The change to UNOS Policy 3.7.3, Status 1A(a) allows the patient to be listed as a Status 1B and upgraded to Status 1A when the medical team determines that the patient is physically and mentally prepared for transplant and that all other treatment options have been explored. It has not been determined if this change will significantly impact the wait time to transplant for this patient category, although survival is expected to improve.

UNOS Reporting Requirements

Generally, the day-to-day reporting required by the OPTN is the transplant coordinator's responsibility. Reporting is required at listing time, transplant, and at annual intervals. In addition, justification forms are required for patients in the Status 1A and Status 1B categories, as well as verification of the declinature codes used when an organ is declined (UNOS Policy 7.0, Data Submission Requirements). The data collected from these disclosures comprise the largest transplantation database in the United States. The current reporting requirements are under review and will be broadened to capture more data on the wait list as well as to obtain more accurate and reliable survival and morbidity data after transplant. The intention is to accurately follow those patients waiting for transplant and ensure that allocation policies meet the needs of those waiting for transplant. These data are also publicly available and needs to be accurate if they are to truly reflect outcomes at specific centers.

THE ROLE OF THE
CARDIAC TRANSPLANT COORDINATOR

As the transplantation field has evolved, so, too, has the coordinator role. It has evolved into a multifaceted, highly complex, nursing role. Most transplant coordinators practice in pretransplant care, post-transplant care, mechanical assist device management, research, or a combination of all four, depending on the transplant center's size. The role is highly autonomous, requiring experienced nurses with excellent clinical skills who are able to educate and manage complex patients and develop acute management skills to execute transplant coordination.

This highly specialized, distinctive role has led to the development of a professional body of transplant professionals who now have a certification process through the American Board of Transplant Coordinators, established in 1988. Practice standards have been determined by the North American Transplant Coordinators Organization, and, currently, there is lobbying for recognition of the coordinator's role within the UNOS bylaws. Transplant coordinator certification has become commonplace in transplant centers, as they strive to become centers of excellence and acquire more managed care contracts; the Certified Clinical Transplant Coordinator examination has become the minimum standard for all practicing transplant coordinators.

The primary goal of coordinating a transplant is to minimize the organ's cold ischemic time through precise transplant team coordination. During a transplant, the coordinator is the team leader. This is the only person who has all relevant information and can guide the process. To achieve excellence in this area, the coordinator must communicate effectively with all transplant team members. Also, the coordinator needs to have an in-depth working knowledge of UNOS policies, as described earlier, and understand donor management's impact on cardiac donation.

Donor Management for the Cardiac Transplant Coordinator

Few clinical transplant coordinators have had the privilege of working with donor families or have an in-depth understanding of donor management and donor evaluation. Often, applying donor management and evaluation to clinical coordination is also missing in most clinical coordinators' education or orientation programs. The impact of the cause of death, sequelae of brain death, donor management, underlying disease processes, and their subsequent impact on potential organ donor cardiac evaluation from the clinical perspective are important to understand *(6)*.

The OPO is called to the potential donor's hospital at some point during the declaration process, depending on each institution's policies, in accordance with the required referral laws in each state *(7)*. The OPO performs a full donor evaluation and assesses the donor's suitability for donation (UNOS Policy 2.1, Host OPO). The injury mechanism is an acute anoxic injury to the brain by direct impact, trauma, or intracranial hemorrhage. The medical care rendered at this time attempts to preserve all cerebral function with hyperventilation, diuresis, steroid therapy, induced barbiturate coma, the maintenance of a negative fluid balance, and the control of hypertension secondary to cerebral damage.

However, once herniation and brain death occur, profound hypotension follows because of severe vasodilatation, hypothermia, electrolyte imbalance, and volume depletion resulting from diabetes insipidus *(8)*. The clinical coordinator should take an in-depth report to assess the consequences of these findings on cardiac function (UNOS Policy 3.7.12, Minimum Information for Thoracic Organ Offers).

Donor Management in the Field

The initial donor management that occurs in the field is intended to stabilize the donor hemodynamics, to correct any electrolyte imbalance, and to maintain circulatory and ventilatory support. The procurement team achieves this by replacing any fluid deficit that occurred prior to brain death confirmation, correcting any underlying acidosis, correcting any electrolyte imbalance (especially in the presence of diabetes insipidus), and commencing appropriate inotropic support of the circulatory system.

Once consent for organ donation is obtained, UNOS is contacted and the list is run that matches the donor to the recipients in the local geographic area. If no heart recipients are found in the local area, the list will extend to the Zone A catchment area, which is a 500-mile geographic radius around the donor hospital. Again, if no recipient is found, the list is extended to Zone B and Zone C, which are in a 1000- and 1500-mile radius, respectively (UNOS Policy 3.7.10, Sequence of Heart Allocation).

The recipient center is contacted and an in-depth report is given regarding the donor. The minimum information that the clinical coordinator can expect to receive falls into two categories:

1. Essential information (UNOS Policy 3.7.12.1, Essential Information):
   * Cause of death
   * Details of any documented cardiac arrest or hypotensive episodes

- Vital signs, including blood pressure, heart rate, and temperature
- Cardiopulmonary, social, and drug activity histories
- Serologies for human immunodeficiency virus (HIV), hepatitis B and C, and cytomegalovirus (CMV).
- Accurate height, weight, age, and sex
- ABO type
- Interpreted electrocardiogram (EKG) and chest radiograph
- History of hospital treatment, including vasopressor and hydration treatments
- Arterial blood gas and ventilator settings
- Echocardiogram, if donor hospital has facilities

The thoracic organ procurement team must have the opportunity to speak directly with intensive care unit (ICU) personnel or the on-site coordinator to obtain current first-hand information about the donor physiology (UNOS Policy 3.7.12.1). This is an important point to remember, as the OPOs further develop the in-house coordinator role to place organs, and more current detailed information may be required from the on-site personnel.

2. Desirable information for heart offers (UNOS Policy 3.7.12.2, Desirable Information for Heart Offers):
   - Coronary angiography for male donors greater than age 40 yr and females greater than age 45 yr
   - Central venous pressure or Swan–Ganz instrumentation
   - Cardiology consult
   - Cardiac enzymes, including CPK isoenzymes

It is important to note that UNOS policy does not require obtaining CPK results or troponin levels. Additionally, coronary angiography is not essential to place a heart but may be requested by the accepting center when the clinical picture calls for it. Many OPOs have standing protocols in place for when a coronary angiography is performed. When requesting a coronary angiography, the transplant center should always have a specific patient identified for the heart.

Once the information is received, the clinical coordinator needs to assess this information's impact on the potential heart donation. Using set acceptance criteria for cardiac transplantation has, in recent years, become obsolete, as transplant centers try to expand the donor pool by considering high-risk donors. Many centers have policies permitting them to consider all donor offers on a case-by-case basis. The only possible rule-out criteria at this time are HIV1, HIV2, human T-cell lymphotrophic virus (HTLV)1, HTLV2, active sepsis, active extracranial malignancy, active hepatitis B, active hepatitis C, and diagnosed cardiac disease resulting in the heart being unsuitable for donation.

However, some centers challenge even these criteria as organ shortage becomes more acute. As heart transplant centers become more aggressive, it may not be uncommon to accept hearts with minimal coronary artery disease (CAD) or older donors up to age 65 yr. Less emphasis is placed on social history and more emphasis is placed on the clinical physiologic findings of the donor team at the offer time. All offers *must* be considered in the context of the recipient for whom the heart is considered. For this reason, many centers steer away from any set criteria for donor heart acceptance; acceptance is dependent on the recipient and not the donor.

The clinical coordinator needs to assess the following areas in detail when obtaining a donor report.

CAUSE OF DEATH

Often, donors with gunshot wounds to the head are the most unstable donors, necessitating quick donor team deployment. Donors who have been ejected from a vehicle may present cardiac contusion and pericardial effusion on echocardiogram; depending on donor age and contusion severity, this may be reversible. Donors with intracerebral bleeds following a cerebral vascular accident may have plaque in the cerebral arteries and, also, may have plaque in the coronary arteries. This may lead the team to consider asking for a coronary angiogram in these donors.

CARDIAC ARREST OR HYPOTENSION

Often, downtime lasts for extended periods, especially in donors whose death was unwitnessed. The downtime episode needs to be assessed in terms of its impact on current cardiac function. If the downtime occurred 2 d earlier, the myocardium may have had sufficient recovery time. This is considered along with donor age (i.e., the younger the donor, the more resilient the heart). Additionally, the coordinator will need to know if cardiopulmonary resuscitation (CPR) was performed and for how long. If CPR was performed, a pericardial effusion may be evident on the echocardiogram. Cardiac arrest and downtime alone are not contraindications to transplant.

VITAL SIGNS, BLOOD PRESSURE, HEART RATE, AND TEMPERATURE

Organ donors do not have autonomic nervous system autoregulatory control and are extremely fluid- and pressor-sensitive. A donor with a negative fluid balance is tachycardic and pressors are higher, as inotropes require euvolumia to be effective. Additionally, during the brain death process, the massive surge of catecholamines released as the body attempts to maintain circulatory support often results in tachycardias as high as 120–160 beats per minute. These arrhythmias should resolve when the donor stabilizes. Therefore, it is important to understand when brain death occurred.

The donor may be hypertensive during the acute management of the injury and then become severely hypotensive after brain death, requiring inotropic support. Donors are often labeled as hypertensive because of high blood pressure recorded at admission to the hospital. However, this hypertension may be secondary to the acute event and not a chronic condition.

Also, the donor may be hyperthermic during the acute injury phase and rapidly become hypothermic after brain death. Attention should be paid to a donor who remains febrile after brain death with an elevated white blood cell (WBC) count and bandemia, bearing in mind that steroid therapy can also elevate a WBC count. Any evidence of infection should be investigated.

CARDIOPULMONARY, SOCIAL, AND DRUG ACTIVITY HISTORIES

A documented cardiac history may exclude the donor from eligibility. However, less emphasis is placed on social history. Homosexuality was considered an exclusion criterion a few years ago but is not currently.

Drug abuse histories must be extensive and taken under consideration when assessing the donor, but alone they do not contraindicate donation. However, donors with drug abusive histories of may be more arrhythmogenic, and detailed cardiac rhythm histories should be taken. Additionally, donors with a histories of alcohol abuse should not be excluded unless alcoholic cardiomyopathy resulted from the abuse.

The social and medical history is important from the standpoint of identifying cardiac risk factors in donors. Smoking, diabetes, hypertension, and hypercholesterolemia are risk factors for heart disease, and the team may decide that the donor's clinical picture warrants a cardiac angiogram, especially in male donors greater than age 40 yr and female donors greater than age 45 yr (9). Medical contraindications based on pre-existing disease have changed tremendously, and many centers do not abide by specific rules, as the donor pool is constantly expanded. Donors with mild CAD may well be considered for selected higher-risk patients (10). Results from UCLA show that donor hearts with CAD are acceptable for transplantation in select recipient groups, even hearts that required revascularization prior to transplant with acceptable outcomes (11).

SEROLOGIES

Active hepatitis B and C remain contraindications to transplant. However, evidence of old infections should not exclude the donor. Although the use of hepatitis C donor hearts remains limited, some centers are beginning to use these donors, considering them on a case-by-case basis in conjunction with the recipient's clinical picture. HIV and HTLV remain exclusions to donation. Toxoplasmosis is often not tested, and the procurement team should return a vial of donor blood so that this test can be done at the transplant center. Also, the clinical coordinator needs to be aware that excessive fluid resuscitation in the donor can lead to dilution and give false negative serology reports. Thus, the coordinator should request *pre*transfusion serology results.

ACCURATE HEIGHT, WEIGHT, AGE, AND SEX

Recipients' body weights are listed with a 30% lower limit and a 50% upper limit for the donor match. However, special consideration should be given to donor size for recipients who have high pulmonary vascular resistance, as they may need donors to be larger rather than smaller. The recipient needs to be listed appropriately. Height is a key component for matching the recipient to the donor, and it needs to be accurate. Advanced age alone is not a contraindication, and, often, donors are considered up to age 65 yr, given that the available heart donor pool has remained static during recent years.

ABO TYPE

The OPO should confirm blood typing, and the coordinator should be aware that, in some circumstances, recipients may be listed across all blood groups. Occasionally, this occurs for pediatric recipients, incurring a high hyperacute rejection risk for these patients. These patients may require plasmapheresis pretransplant and/or subsequent exchange transfusions if the transplant is to be a success.

INTERPRETED EKG AND CHEST RADIOGRAPH

EKG interpretation is essential to identify any acute myocardial injury as well as to identify old injuries. However, it should not replace the echocardiogram and full cardiac history. Often, left ventricular hypertrophy (LVH) is diagnosed by EKG when it is not significant or evident on the echocardiogram. The EKG should correlate with the echocardiogram and the donor history and not be considered in isolation. Additionally, brain death causes S-T segment abnormalities that may be misinterpreted and are often temporary *(6)*. The donor EKG will most often be reported as abnormal and can be misdiagnosed as myocardial infarct or ischemia *(12)*. Also, cardiac arrhythmias may be present in donors with subarachnoid hemorrhage *(12)*.

The chest X-ray remains important to determine heart size and to detect any signs of infection. Blood, urine, and sputum cultures are taken at donation time, and the results should be available to the transplant center to ensure that the recipient receives appropriate antibiotic therapy. Evidence of a pulmonary infection on the chest X-ray alone is not a contraindication to heart donation. Additionally, the coordinator should be aware that organ donors may have evidence of neurogenic pulmonary edema secondary to brain death, and a report of pulmonary edema is not uncommon; this is not pulmonary edema associated with cardiac dysfunction.

HISTORY OF TREATMENT IN HOSPITAL INCLUDING VASOPRESSOR AND HYDRATION HISTORY

The donor's medical history should be consistent with the donor's clinical picture. Often, donors receive large volumes of fluid and inotropes during the resuscitation phase after brain death, especially if diabetes insipidus is present. This can lead to electrolyte imbalances. To manage diabetes insipidus, the donor may receive intravenous vasopressin (Pitressin) (Monarch Pharmaceuticals, Bristol, TN) or subcutaneous desmopressin (DDAVP) (Aventis Pharmaceuticals, Inc., Bridgewater, NJ). In donor management, dopamine is the pressor of choice. However, if the donor cannot be managed on dopamine, additional pressors may be added.

The transplant center needs to assess whether the pressor support is acceptable for heart donation *(7)*. Many centers shy away from donors receiving high-dose pressors. Dobutamine has not been a favored inotrope for the cardiac donor, as it potentially masks poor myocardial function because of its positive inotropic effect. However, this view is changing, as studies show that low-dose dobutamine improves cardiac function if the dysfunction is reversible and associated with the neuro-hormonal effects of brain death *(13)*. The importance of pressors needs to be assessed in the context of the echocardiogram and the donor's fluid status. Optimal donor management should allow for a reduction in pressor agent use. Often, thyroid hormone replacement protocols are implemented to reduce pressor agent need and maintain hemodynamics *(7)*.

ARTERIAL BLOOD GAS AND VENTILATOR SETTINGS

Always obtain a recent arterial blood gas. Adequate oxygenation, in part, indicates good perfusion of all organs. Acidosis has an adverse impact on cardiac function and the team's ability to maintain the donor's hemodynamic stability. Additionally, acidosis compromises the effectiveness of inotropic or pressor support. Donors may be on high-dose pressors in the presence of acidosis *(6)*.

ECHOCARDIOGRAM

Echocardiogram is considered the gold standard for assessing cardiac function. Increasingly, it should be used as a tool to guide donor management, but, often, it is used only to acquire sufficient information to place the heart. The echocardiogram must absolutely be considered because of the donor management issues described earlier. Acidosis can produce hypokinesis in the donor heart, and, therefore, an arterial blood gas should be obtained when the echocardiogram is performed. The fluid balance needs to be considered, as a volume-depleted donor has inadequate filling pressures and myocardial depression is exacerbated *(14)*. A fluid-overloaded donor may exhibit right ventricular dilatation if cardiac output is not maximized. Additionally, the echocardiogram needs to be considered in the context of donor pressor/inotropic support *(6)*.

Any LVH reports should be correlated with myocardium measurements to aid the team's decision to accept or refuse the heart. LVH alone may not be a contraindication to transplant; however, the preservation technique and the anticipated cold ischemic time require consideration, depending on donor location. Suboptimal echocardiograms may need to be repeated if donor management is not optimized. Some centers now recognize that obtaining repeat echocardiograms may be difficult for the on-site coordinator and perform their own echocardiogram to further assess the donor. Valvular structures should always be assessed by echocardiogram. In the absence of an echocardiogram, Swan–Ganz measurements are useful in assessing cardiac function, and in Great Britain this is the favored cardiac assessment tool *(15)*.

Additionally, when a cardiac angiogram cannot be performed, the team may rely on visual inspection of the heart. Again, an experienced surgeon needs to determine if CAD is palpable. These issues need to be considered with the potential recipient in mind. Often, a more aggressive approach is taken when considering hearts for Status 1A patients, as there are strong data to support using hearts with suboptimal echocardiograms; LV function often recovers over time and these patients have a limited window of opportunity for transplant *(16)*.

CARDIAC ENZYMES

Often, enzymes are elevated in brain death and trauma and, to be considered significant, need to be correlated with the clinical history, the echocardiogram, and the EKG. Studies document elevated cardiac enzymes in the acute setting of a subdural hemorrhage. Troponin levels are more cardiac-specific but, again, need to correlate with the clinical picture and also can be elevated *(17)*. Abnormal cardiac enzymes and troponin levels in the presence of normal echocardiographic findings should not preclude a heart from transplant consideration. Additionally, it is documented that troponin levels are elevated in myocardial dysfunction *(18)*. If these are abnormal in the presence of an abnormal echocardiogram, then the impact of the neurohormonal changes, donor management, and the use of low-dose dobutamine echocardiography needs to be assessed *(17)*. Additionally, special consideration needs to be given to donor hearts with marginal echocardiograms in the presence of elevated troponin levels. Often, these donor hearts are discarded; however, myocardial dysfunction is reversible if the dysfunction results from brain death's neurohormonal effects. Thus, the *entire* picture needs to be considered along with the recipient's clinical situation. No single issue should exclude a potential donor.

The Coordination Process

The keys to effective transplant coordination are good communication skills, acute problem solving abilities, quick thinking, an effective team effort, and, above all else, cold ischemic time minimization. The clinical coordinator is the key person in orchestrating a transplant and directing the transplantation process. Large volume centers that perform transplants every day still have issues and problems that need to be resolved with each transplant, as will the smaller centers. An effective team is one that maintains high communication levels and whose team members are highly skilled at performing their roles.

Communication with all transplant team members is a key coordination factor. Confusion and misunderstanding occurs when team members are not clearly directed or if they do not understand fully their roles in the process. It is the coordinator's responsibility to ensure that all the team members are aware of the plan for each transplant, and to communicate this plan effectively to all key members.

Transplant setup would be relatively simple if each transplant went according to plan. Generally, this is not the case. Problems that arise can be both internal and external. The terrorist attacks of September 11, 2001 presented some unique problems at our institution, when a donor team landed just 10 min before the George Washington Bridge closed in New York City. The donor team crossed the bridge before it closed, but, as the phone lines were down and cellular phones were without service, the donor team could not confirm that they landed. There was no means of communication with the team during that time.

On another occasion, the George Washington Bridge was closed because of a terrorist alert, and the donor team decided to return across the bridge with the heart. The team was then driven in by the New York Police Department (NYPD) on the other side of the bridge. In the summer of 1999, a power outage forced the hospital to consider moving the transplant team and patient to a sister hospital to perform the transplant. Emergency generators were on but were insufficient to safely perform a transplant. This transplant was aborted when, logistically, it was unsafe for the recipient to undergo the transplant.

Transportation can always produce interesting problems. Twice, a helicopter has made emergency landings because of bad weather, and the NYPD drove the team back to New York City. These issues affect the delicate art of coordination.

Other coordination issues affect the donor side of the equation. Often, donation is delayed when a trauma is present at the donor hospital. Families request that donation occur within specific times, creating time constraints. Additionally, other transplant teams need to prepare their recipients, and the actual procurement may take longer than expected. It is important for the clinical coordinator to know when additional organs are procured, as this affects transplant timing. Multiple transplants occurring simultaneously at the transplant center can cause confusion and requires that the transplanting center be able to mobilize multiple teams at any time.

The art of coordination lies in dealing with these issues as they arise and minimizing cold ischemic time. The goal is to explant the heart just as the donor heart is brought to the recipient's OR. To achieve this goal, the team needs to be in place and ready to operate at the surgeon's designated time, considering all factors involved with each donation. This time is determined by the donor OR time, the travel time to the donor hospital, the estimated visualization and cross-clamp time at the donor hospital, and the recipient's clinical condition, as well as the recipient's location. Designation of this time is achieved by considering the following:

- Establish the operating time for the donor. Arrangements are made to ensure that the team arrives at the designated time. If a delay is foreseen, the abdominal team should begin dissection pending the heart team's arrival. This may occur for donors in other states where the team needs to travel by air.
- Establish with the surgeon the time required to open the chest and explant the recipient's heart. This varies depending on the surgeon and the recipient's previous surgeries. A recipient who is not a re-op requires less time than a patient with a LVAD *in situ*. This time varies from 45 min to 2 h.

- Depending on the number of procured organs, establish a tentative visualization time with the donor team.
- Establish a potential cross-clamp time with the donor team. The donor team must never cross-clamp without final confirmation from the coordinator, whose role is now to ensure that the patient is on time for the OR at the transplant center.
- Estimate the expected return arrival time at the transplant center, including air and ground time.
- The recipient operation begins at the time the organ is expected back at the center minus the time the surgeon needs to open the chest.
- Anesthesia time varies depending on the patient's clinical condition. A patient who is already in the ICU with a Swan–Ganz and intubated needs less preparation time than a Status 2 patient coming from home.
- If the donor becomes unstable at any time during the process, the donor team must proceed directly to cross-clamp to procure as many organs as possible, even if the heart cannot be procured.
- The donor team returns a copy of the donor chart and two 10 mL red-topped tubes of donor blood, five lymph nodes, a spleen wedge, and 40 mL of blood for HLA tissue-typing and prospective cross matching. If the spleen cannot be recovered, 8 lymph nodes are provided. In the absence of spleen and peripheral blood, 12 lymph nodes are provided. If nodes and blood are not available, then 2 × 4 cm spleen wedges are made available (UNOS Policy 2.6, Organ Procurement Quality).

Figure 1 shows the calculation of the OR time for the recipient. The algorithm is adjusted for each transplant and for delays that occur during the process. The timing is also adjusted if the donor team arrives to an open donor chest. The time to visualization is shorter. If the travel time is short, it is possible that by using this method the incision time for the surgeon can occur prior to visualization. In this instance, the recipient goes to the OR at the same time as the donor, and the surgeon waits for visualization confirmation and ensures that the donor heart is good before opening the chest. Also, consideration needs to be given to timing when the donor is in the transplant center. Effectively, the operations happen almost simultaneously once the heart is inspected. If the donor is stable and young, the surgeon may decide to proceed with anesthesia prior to visualization to save time. Conversely, long travel times give the surgeon more time to begin the transplant. As in Fig. 1, the surgeon needs to make the first incision when the donor team leaves the donor hospital to have the recipient heart explanted by the time the team returns.

The algorithm is a guide for coordinating the transplant and many complications can occur. Invariably, the timing is pushed back on the recipient side, as delays occur on the donor side. Delays can also occur

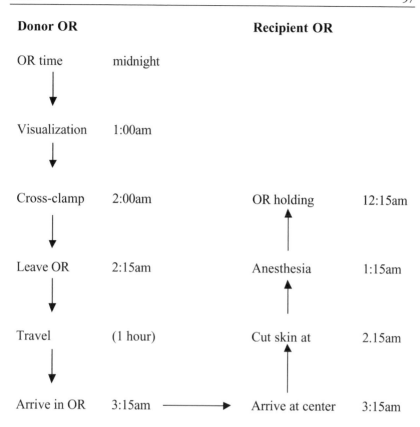

Estimated minimum cold ischemic time 2 h 15 min.

Fig. 1. Example of calculations of the recipient OR timing.

on the recipient side. Occasionally, the heart is more difficult to explant than expected, causing a delay. Travel issues for the returning donor team may require that the surgeon slow down, as the return is taking longer than expected. (This nearly always occurs when coordinating a transplant when the New York Yankees are in the World Series!) The experienced coordinator is able to anticipate the delays and act accordingly. Knowing the patient, donor team, donor process, and surgical team allows the coordinator to make quick decisions and effectively coordinate a transplant.

Coordinator Education and Development

The coordinator needs to have an orientation program that provides experience in the relevant areas. He or she should:

- Attend all UNOS regional meetings and, if possible, visit the Organ Center at UNOS.
- Participate in donor runs to see the donor process in action.
- Spend time with the local OPO and work with a procurement coordinator in the field.
- Participate in orientation programs provided by the local OPO.
- Attend educational and professional seminars.
- Take advantage of preceptorship programs offered (if none is available, then spend time at a high-volume center as a part of the orientation process).

CONTINUING ISSUES

As UNOS policies evolve and transplantation continues to expand the donor pool, many issues are under consideration. For example, HIV patients demand a right to transplantation. Some are willing to accept organs from HIV-positive donors. Will this be incorporated into practice in the near future? As donors become older, additional evaluative testing will be requested more often. Will this change UNOS policy such that desired information becomes essential information?

Variances, regional sharing agreements, and state laws affect allocation. Current practices need constant review if equitable sharing is to be achieved. Sharing policies and donor strategies need to be reconsidered in the future if all donors are to be maximized and the greatest number of organs transplanted. Discussion continues over transplantation of Status 2 patients over a neighboring region's 1A patients *(19)*. Also, it remains to be seen how nesiritide use will affect UNOS policy. The transplant coordinator needs to be aware of the constantly changing environment in which the coordinator practices and remain abreast of the changes as they occur.

REFERENCES

1. In: Phillips MG ed. Organ Procurement, Preservation, and Distribution in Transplantation. 1st Ed. United Network for Organ Sharing: Richmond, VA: 1991.
2. Camp D. The left ventricular assist device (LVAD). A bridge to heart transplantation. Crit Care Nurse 2000;12(1):61–68.
3. Mancini DM, Beniaminovitz A, Levin H, et al. Low incidence of myocardial recovery after left ventricular assist device implantation in patients with chronic heart failure. Circulation 1998;98(22):2383–2389.
4. Warner Stevenson L. The continuing evolution of donor heart allocation. In: Norman DJ, Turka LA, eds. Primer on Transplantation. American Society of Transplantation, New Jersey: 2001, pp. 341–344.
5. Chen JM, De Rose JJ, Slater JP, et al. Improved survival rates support left ventricular assist device implantation early after myocardial infarction. J Amer Coll Cardiol 1999;33(7):1903–1908.

6. Holmquist M, Chabalewski F, Blount T, et al. A critical pathway: guiding care for organ donors. Crit Care Nurse 1999;19(2):84–97.

7. Stuart FP, Abecassis MM, Kaufman DB. Organ Transplant. Landes Bioscience, Georgetown: 2000.

8. Graham JM. Adult and Pediatric Donor Management(c). 1998, unpublished.

9. Baldwin JC, Anderson JL, Boucek MM, et al. 24th Bethesda Conference: Cardiac Transplantation. Task force 2: donor guidelines. J Amer Coll Cardiol 1993;22:15–20.

10. Laks H, Marelli D. The alternate recipient list for heart transplantation: a model for expansion of the donor pool. Adv Cardiac Surg 1999;11:233–244.

11. Marelli D, Laks H, Bresson S, et al. Results of transplantation using donor hearts with pre-existing coronary artery disease. J Thorac Cardiovasc Surg 2003;126(3):821–825.

12. Sommargren CE. Electrocardiographic abnormalities in patients with subarachoid hemorrhage. Amer J Crit Care 2002:11(1):48–56.

13. Kono T, Nishina T, Morita H, et al. Usefulness of low-dose dobutamine stress echocardiography for evaluating reversibility of brain death induced myocardial dysfunction. Amer J Cardiol 1999;84(5):578–582.

14. Deng MC. Cardiac transplantation. Heart 2002;87(2):171–184.

15. Wheeldon DR, Potter CD, Oduro A, et al. Transforming the "unacceptable" donor: outcomes from the adoption of a standardized donor management technique. J Heart Lung Transplant 1995;14:734–742.

16. Zaroff J, Babcock W, Shiboski SC, et al. Temporal changes in donor left ventricular function: results of a serial echocardiography. J Heart Lung Transplant 2003;22(4):383–388.

17. Deibert E, Aiyagari V, Diringer MN. Reversible left ventricular dysfunction associated with raised troponin I after sub-dural hemorrhage does not preclude successful heart transplantation. Heart Engl 2002;84(2):205–207.

18. Riou B, Dreux S, Roche S, et al. Circulating cardiac troponin T in potential heart transplant donors. Circulation 1995;92(3):409–414.

19. Deng M, Smits JM, Packer M. Selecting patients for heart transplantation: which patients are too well for transplant? Curr Opin Cardiol 2002; 17(2):137–144.

Appendix:
UNOS Donor Refusal Codes

Code	Refusal reason	Description: Recipient-related reasons
901	Recipient ill	Recipient too sick to attempt transplant at the time of offer.
902	Recipient unavailable	Recipient cannot be contacted, is not ready for transplant, or has died at the time of offer
903	Recipient refused	Recipient refused transplant at the time of offer
904	Multiple-organ transplant required	Recipient requires multiple organ transplants, other required organ(s) not available from the specified donor at the time of offer
905	Recipient transplanted/ inactive	Recipient already transplanted or is on the inactive list at time of offer
906	Positive cross-match	Cross-match results between donor and recipient positive
907	HLA mismatch unacceptable	HLA mismatch between donor and recipient unacceptable
908	Recipient testing results unavailable, not done, or unacceptable	Recipient requires a cross-match at time of offer, high PRA, no current typing, or any other recipient testing
909	Patient's condition improved, transplant not needed	Recipient's condition has improved and transplant is currently unnecessary
911	Program too busy or surgeon unavailable	Program unable to accept an organ for transplant at the time of offer because of heavy work load or unavailability of transplant surgeon
912	Administrative	Physician judgement, transportation, logistics, distance, exceeded 1-h response time, or other administrative reason

Code	Refusal reason	Description: Recipient-related reasons
921	Donor quality	Hypertension, prolonged hypotension, high vasopressor/medication dosage, cardiac arrest, evidence of infection/positive cultures, non-heart not beating, etiology of death, donor unstable, donor diabetes, other medical history
922	Donor age	Donor too old or too young
923	Donor size/weight	Donor too large or small, weight incompatible with recipient
924	Donor ABO	Donor ABO group incompatible/unacceptable
925	Donor social history	History of high-risk sexual behavior, alcohol or intravenous drug use

926	Positive serological tests	CMV, HBV, HCV, HIV, HTLV, VDRL, etc. donor testing is positive
927	Organ preservation	Method/Quality of preservation, length of cold ischemic time, length of warm ischemic time, possible organ contamination, inadequate typing material, labeling/packaging problems
928	Organ anatomical damage or defect	Surgical damage, nonsurgical trauma, diseased organ, organ vasculature, en bloc kidney's or any other anatomical reason

Code	Refusal reason	Description: Organ-specific donor issues: heart
950	Cardiac function test results unavailable, not done, or unacceptable	Test results relating to cardiac function are not available, or tests relating to cardiac function were not performed
951	Abnormal echocardiogram	Echocardiogram shows wall motion abnormalities or valvular lesions
952	Abnormal coronary angiography	Presence of CAD
953	Abnormal EKG results	Q-waves, ST-T abnormalities or conduction disease
954	Abnormal hemodynamics	Elevated filling pressures or reduced cardiac output

Code	Refusal reason	Description: Other
991	Medical urgency	Recipient(s) bypassed because of medical urgency or OPO time constraints
992	Multiorgan placement	Previous recipients bypassed for priority multiorgan transplant
993	Directed donation	Use for recipients who receive an organ from a directed donation
994	Military donor	Use for recipients who receive an organ from a military donor
995	ALU Sharing Agreement, variance	Self-explanatory
996	Extrarenal placed with kidney	Self-explanatory
998	Other, specify	Use only if the refusal reason does not fit the above categories. Be sure to write in the other reason; UNOS staff will review the OTHER reason and may recode if necessary

Abbreviations: HLA, human leukocyte antigen; PRA, panel reactive antibody; HBV, hepatitis B virus; HBC, hepatitis C virus; HIV, human immunodeficiency virus; HTLV, human T-cell lymphotrophic virus; VDRL, veneral disease research laboratory test; CAD, coronary artery disease; EKG, electrocardiogram; OPO, Organ Procurement Organization; ALU, alternative local unit; UNOS, United Network for Organ Sharing.

4 Techniques of Cardiac Transplantation in Adults

Jeffrey A. Morgan, MD
and Niloo M. Edwards, MD

INTRODUCTION

Shumway and Lower introduced orthotopic heart transplant in 1960, and the technique they described has had few changes since its inception *(1)*. This chapter reviews the surgical techniques and their modifications and also reviews our approach to the transplant recipient at surgery time. It is worth noting that the majority of our transplant recipients have had previous cardiac surgical procedures; therefore, heart transplantation is as much about the techniques of reoperations as it is about the techniques of transplantation itself. Despite this added layer of complexity, 1-, 3-, 5-, and 10-yr survivals of 84, 79, 72, and 53%, respectively, are attainable *(2)*.

PREPARING THE RECIPIENT FOR TRANSPLANTATION

A detailed history and physical examination, with frequent updates, are necessary because transplants often occur at night with little time for

From: *Contemporary Cardiology: Cardiac Transplantation:*
The Columbia University Medical Center/New York-Presbyterian Hospital Manual
Edited by: N. M. Edwards, J. M. Chen, and P. A. Mazzeo © Humana Press Inc., Totowa, NJ

a complete system review. This should not preclude a careful update at transplant admission time to determine any new problems. Our practice is to retain copies of their transplant evaluation forms, clinical updates, and any pertinent prior operative notes in their cardiac surgical intensive care unit, where they may easily be obtained at night. Additionally, routine blood tests (including a complete blood count with a differential and platelet count, electrolytes, liver function tests, coagulation tests, and a type and cross) are sent to the laboratory. A chest X-ray is also performed at admission.

We admit transplant recipients directly to the operating room (OR), where venous and arterial lines can be placed while awaiting confirmation from the procurement team that the heart is visualized and suitable for transplantation. This has allowed us to shorten recipient preparation time and allows us to capitalize on heart offers that become available on short notice.

INTRAOPERATIVE TECHNIQUES

Perioperative medications include immunosuppressive agents (*see* Chapter 8) and a first-generation cephalosporin antibiotic. Following donor team confirmation that the heart is suitable, the recipient is intubated, a Foley catheter is inserted, and a Swan–Ganz catheter is floated into the pulmonary artery (PA). A median sternotomy is performed. We avoid using bone wax for hemostasis, because the marrow bleeding often abates with heart decompression, and the bone wax, as a foreign body, is a putative infection source. For patients who have undergone a previous sternotomy, the femoral vessels can be dissected in the event that emergency cannulation is required. We do not dissect out the femoral vessels routinely, because we have found that groin cannulation sites are frequent complication sources and that, if necessary, available cannulae allow for easier percutaneous cannulation.

The pericardium is opened with a vertical incision extending from the diaphragm to the pericardial reflection at the aorta. The pericardium is tacked using 2–0 silk sutures that are tied to the sternal retractor to expose the myocardium and great vessels *(3–5)*.

The recipient is then heparinized and cannulated for bypass. Aprotinin is routinely used for all transplants; prior to loading dose administration, a 1 cc test dose is administered following aortic cannulation.

Cannulation

Aortic cannulation should be high on the lesser curvature, especially in previous coronary artery bypass surgery patients, in whom the proximal aorta may be excised. Higher cannulation is facilitated by using wire-reinforced flexible arterial cannulae and taking down the pericardial reflection at the great vessels. The venae cavae are also cannulated as distally as possible, and umbilical tape snares are placed around the vessels and cannulae. Right-angle metal-tip cannulae are preferable for venous cannulation, as they allow for smaller cannulation pursestrings and room for sewing the bicaval anastomoses.

Explantation

Recipient excision timing is at the discretion of the surgeon, who may chose to wait until the donor heart is in the OR or until the donor team is 30 min from the hospital.

The superior vena cava (SVC) and inferior vena cava (IVC) are snared, the aortic cross-clamp is applied, and the patient is placed on bypass and cooled to 32°C. The aorta and PA are separated, and the aorta is divided just above the right coronary artery's origin. The back wall of the aorta is divided, with care to avoid the right PA.

Then, the PA is divided just distally to the pulmonary valve; care is taken to keep the division plane perpendicular with the base of the heart to avoid beveling the PA and, thereby, shortening the back wall of the vessel. Pericardial silk sutures placed through the adventitia of the aorta and PA aid in holding these divided vessels out of the way.

In preparation for a bicaval anastomosis, the atrioventricular groove is opened, and the dissection is extended under the SVC. The right atrium is divided proximally to the SVC, leaving an atrium cuff on the proximal end of the cava. When dividing the PA and SVC, care must be taken to avoid transecting the Swan–Ganz catheter. The right atrium is divided just proximally to the IVC, with care to leave a long posterior cuff that tends to retract, following transection, toward the diaphragm.

An incision is made in the left atrial dome below the aorta. The incision is extended counterclockwise across the atrial septum, including the fossa ovalis, to the coronary sinus base. The remainder of the atrial transection is easiest when performed clockwise, from the incision in the atrial dome to the coronary sinus, staying below the base of the left atrial appendage and just below the coronary sinus.

If the operation is a standard biatrial implantation, following transection of the aorta and PA, an incision is made in the left atrial dome just below the aorta. This incision is extended counterclockwise into the atrial septum; the right atriotomy is made just below the base of the appendage and connected with the septal incision, which is extended to the coronary sinus base. The remainder of the left atrial transection is

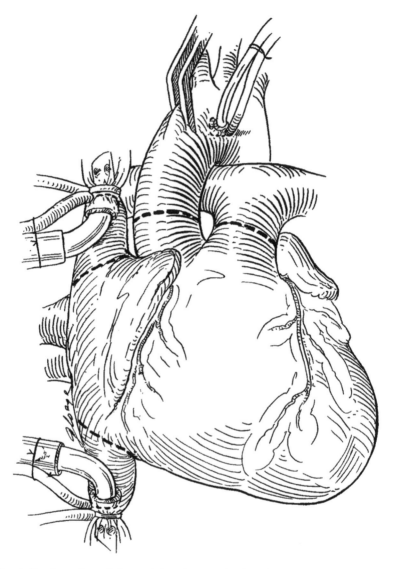

Fig. 1. Explantation of the recipient heart. The dotted lines represent the incisions in the right atrium and great vessels. From ref. *4* with permission.

easiest if performed in a counterclockwise direction from the atrial dome to the coronary sinus, below the level of the left atrial appendage and the coronary sinus (Fig. 1) *(4)*.

Hemostasis following explantation is extremely important, because many sites are no longer visible following implantation. Care is taken to electrocauterize the edges of the atria and, in reoperations, the posterior pericardium. Further, the pulmonary veins should be examined for debris and thrombus, and old coronary proximal sites on the aorta should be oversewn.

Preparing the Donor Heart for Transplantation

The donor heart is carefully inspected for abnormalities, in particular a patent foramen ovale (PFO), valvular anomalies, and debris. The SVC and PA are identified and separated from each other with sharp dissection. The pulmonary vein openings are connected, creating one large left atrial cuff, and the excess atrium is trimmed. The mitral valve is inspected for abnormalities. Excess aorta and PA are trimmed. Using a coronary probe, the fossa ovalis is examined for a PFO. If a PFO is discovered, it is closed in two layers from the right atrial side using 4–0 polypropylene monofilament suture.

In preparation for a biatrial procedure, the SVC is doubly ligated, and the right atrium is opened from the lateral IVC toward the right atrial appendage, thereby avoiding the sinus node. This is not performed if a bicaval operation is planned, although the donor SVC is trimmed below the azygous vein opening.

Recipient Anastomoses: Bicaval Technique

The left atrial anastomosis is performed first; the sequence of the other anastomoses can be changed to decrease the ischemic time. Donor left atrial cuff is sutured to the recipient left atrium using an extra long 3–0 prolene suture. This begins at the base of the donor left atrial appendage, above the orifice of the recipient's left superior pulmonary vein, and run toward the IVC (Fig. 2) (4). A second suture is placed at the left atrial corner and the IVC on the donor heart and through the corresponding region on the recipient atrium. After clamping this suture to the drape and the applying tension to the anastomosing suture, the exposure to the lateral atrial suture line is improved and inadvertent left atrial anastomosis rotation is avoided. Attention is paid to averting the atrial edges to minimize the raw suture line exposed inside the left atrium.

Once the lateral suture line is complete, the tacking stitch placed through the IVC is removed, and the left atrial anastomosis is completed by sewing counterclockwise using the anastomosing suture's opposite end. This prevents placing the knot under the PA where repair sutures, if needed, are particularly hard to place. Some advocate introducing a catheter in the left atrium via the left atrial appendage. To avoid cardiac rewarming, cold saline is run through the catheter into the left atrium. The catheter is also used for venting after the aortic cross-clamp is removed. The authors' practice is to place an ice saline-soaked laparo-

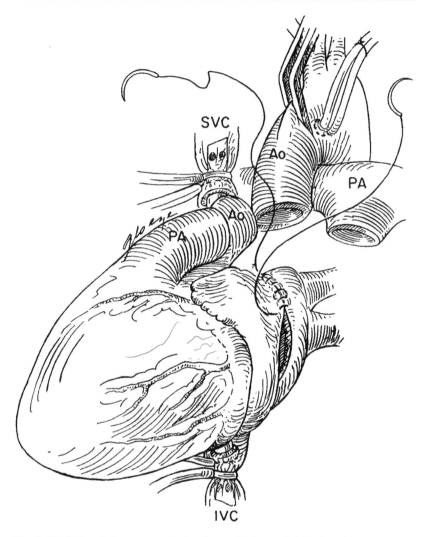

Fig. 2. The left atrial anastomosis begins at the base of the left atrial appendage and is continued inferiorly. From ref. *4* with permission.

tomy sponge around the heart to retard premature heart rewarming. It is also their practice to run continuous carbon dioxide into the pericardial well from the time of the sternotomy to displace air and aid the de-airing process.

The Swan–Ganz catheter is manually guided through the SVC, right atrium, and right ventricle (RV) using a large-angled clamp. Then, the donor IVC and SVC are anastomosed to the recipient IVC-atrial cuff and SVC-atrial cuff, respectively. This is performed in an end-to-end manner using 4–0 polypropylene suture. To avoid constricting or rotating the anastomosis, each of these anastomoses may be performed with two separate sutures. Excessive suture length or tension can cause a caval constriction (Fig. 1).

Then, the donor and recipient PAs are trimmed to avoid excess length and possible kinking. The PAs are anastomosed end-to-end using running 4–0 monofilament suture. Again, attention must be paid to avoid constricting or rotating the anastomosis.

The donor and recipient aortas are anastomosed end-to-end with running 4–0 monofilament suture (Fig. 3) *(4)*. Often, the aorta's medial border, between the aorta and PA, is denuded of adventia and likely to bleed; therefore, reinforcing this quadrant by incorporating a pledget of autologous or donor tissue at the time of the anastomosis can be beneficial. Prior to completion of the aortic anastomosis, the aorta's back wall should be examined for cardioplegia needle injury. This is more likely if the heart was transported with the cardioplegia needle in the ascending aorta.

Recipient Anastomoses: Standard, Biatrial Technique

With the standard, biatrial technique, the left atrial anastomosis is initiated as stated earlier, starting at the left atrial appendage base and using a second suture at the inferior left atrial septum border to aid in lateral suture line exposure. The medial wall of the donor left atrium is sewn to the atrial septum, and the left atrial suture line is completed, leaving the other end of the suture to finish anastomosing the left atrial domes in a counterclockwise direction. The suture can be left untied to facilitate air removal from the heart.

The right atrium is opened from the right side of the IVC orifice to the base of the right atrial appendage. The incision is extended from the right toward the right atrium's base to avoid the sinus node. Prior to right atrial anastomosis initiation, the Swan–Ganz catheter is passed through the RV into the PA. The suture line for the right atrial anastomosis starts at the superior aspect of the atrial septum, and, in essence, the donor right atrium is sewn to the septum over the previous suture line. Care should be taken not to handle the sinus node during anastomosis.

The PA and aortic anastomoses are performed as described in the previous section.

Taking Recipient Off Bypass

Once the anastomoses are complete, the patient is placed in a head-down position, and the aortic cross-clamp is removed. All air is carefully removed from the heart. The transesophageal echocardiogram is invalu-

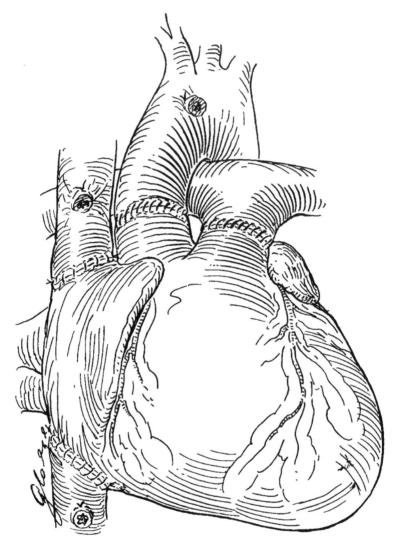

Fig. 3. The donor heart after implantation completion. From ref. *4* with permission.

able for confirming ventricular function and air removal. When sinus rhythm initiates at 100 beats per minute and the air is evacuated, the patient is slowly weaned from cardiopulmonary bypass. Even in the face of good cardiac function, the authors place all patients on inotropic support (either dobutamine or milrinone) in anticipation of a nadir in cardiac function at 6–8 h following implantation.

Temporary pacing wires (two on the right atrium and two on the RV) are placed. Hemostasis prior to implantation (when the heart is out of the chest) aids meticulous posttransplant hemostasis, which is crucial. Straight and right-angled chest tubes remain in place to drain the anterior and posterior pericardium, respectively.

HETEROTOPIC HEART TRANSPLANTATION

During heterotopic transplantation, initially performed by Losman and Barnard in 1974, the recipient heart remains in its native location *(6)*. This transplant type may be necessary in situations when there is irreversible high pulmonary vascular resistance or significant donor–recipient size mismatch *(3)*.

There are numerous differences in donor heart harvesting and handling for a heterotopic transplant. Greater lengths of SVC, aorta, and PA are harvested. The SVC should be harvested to innominate vein level. The aortic arch should be harvested along with the proximal aspect of all three head vessels. It is especially important to harvest as much PA as possible to allow a direct donor–recipient anastomosis and avoid the need for a Dacron interposition graft. The tissue separating the left pulmonary veins is divided, connecting their orifices and creating a single, large left atrial cuff.

Cannulation is slightly different than orthotopic transplantation. The aortic cannula should be placed as distally as possible in the ascending aorta. SVC cannulation is achieved through the right atrial appendage. Finally, IVC cannulation is performed at the IVC–diaphragmatic junction. Venous inflow occlusion is achieved by snaring the SVC and IVC. The native heart in the recipient is then cross-clamped.

The donor heart is placed in the right pleural cavity with the heart's apex angled to the right. The left atrial anastomosis is performed first using 3–0 monofilament polypropylene suture, attaching the donor left atrium to the incision in the recipient left atrium. The recipient's SVC is opened with a vertical incision, and the anastomosis is performed attaching the donor SVC to the recipient SVC. The aortic anastomosis is performed using 4–0 monofilament suture in an end-to-side manner. Either the right or left PA branch is oversewn, with the other participating in the anastomosis with the donor PA. This is performed using running 4–0 monofilament suture. A prosthetic graft may be required if the donor PA length is not adequate *(3)*.

After air is removed from the heart chambers using standard de-airing maneuvers, the patient is weaned off bypass. The chest is then closed with sternal wires followed by a subcuticular closure using absorbable suture.

BICAVAL VS STANDARD TECHNIQUE

The standard technique for cardiac transplantation, developed by Lower and Shumway, involves anastomoses of the donor atrial cuffs to the recipient's atrial cuffs —a biatrial anastomosis *(1,7)*. This technique avoids the putative technical difficulty of separate caval anastomoses. However, several problems may result from this approach. A biatrial anastomosis results in an abnormally enlarged atrial cavity and distorted atrial geometry, producing atrioventricular (AV) valvular insufficiency *(8–11)*. Additionally, bradyarrhythmias may arise because of the close proximity of the right atrial suture line to the sinus node, resulting in node injury *(12–14)*.

Over recent years, there has been growing interest in alternative techniques. Yacoub and Banner modified the standard technique described by Lower and Shumway *(15)*. A bicaval approach preserves the donor atria and combines the standard left atrial anastomosis with a separate bicaval anastomosis *(16–18)*.

Another approach is total orthotopic heart transplantation. This approach was described by Webb and Neely in 1959 and introduced by Dreyfus and Yacoub in 1991 *(15,17,19)*. It involves complete recipient atrial excision with complete AV transplantation, in addition to separate bicaval and pulmonary venous anastomoses *(20,21)*. This technique's major disadvantages are the additional time required to complete the six anastomoses and the technical challenge of performing the pulmonary vein island anastomoses.

There are many studies in the literature comparing the bicaval approach to the standard approach. Milano et al., reporting on 75 cases, demonstrated an increase in postoperative cardiac index, a decrease in postoperative epinephrine requirements, less tricuspid regurgitation (TR), a decrease in temporary pacing requirements, and fewer arrhythmias associated with the bicaval approach *(22)*. The bicaval group had a shorter hospital stay; however, there was no difference in survival between the two groups.

In a prospective, randomized study by Sievers et al., eight bicaval patients were compared to 10 biatrial patients. The data showed that bicaval patients had a smaller right atrial size and less TR with exercise postoperatively, as well as better preserved atrial dimension at 3 yr, when compared to the standard group *(10)*.

El-Gamel et al. compared 40 bicaval with 35 standard patients. Bicaval patients had lower atrial pressures, fewer atrial arrhythmias, decreased requirements for temporary pacing, less mitral regurgitation (MR), and shorter hospital stays *(23,24)*.

Aziz et al. published a randomized trial comparing 96 bicaval cases with 105 standard cases, with 5-yr follow-up. They found an improvement in 1-, 3-, and 5-yr actuarial survival, left ventricular ejection fraction, and TR in the bicaval group *(25)*.

A randomized trial by Deleuze et al. comparing the bicaval approach with the standard approach found that patients who underwent a bicaval approach had a significantly decreased requirement for postoperative pacemakers (12.5% for the standard group vs 0% for the bicaval group) *(12)*.

Other studies comparing the bicaval with the biatrial approach showed an improvement in hemodynamics, cardiac chamber dimensions, and exercise capacity associated with the bicaval approach *(11,12)*. The bicaval approach is also associated with a decreased incidence of postoperative atrial arrhythmias, both early and late, as compared to the standard approach *(26)*. Traversi et al., in studying 22 bicaval and 27 standard patients, found that bicaval patients had greater right and left atrial emptying and pump fractions, right atrial ejection force, and less MR and TR *(27)*. Grande et al., in comparing 46 bicaval and 71 standard patients, found that bicaval patients had decreased postoperative pressor requirements and blood loss *(28)*.

Potential disadvantages of the bicaval approach involve prolonged ischemic time and the potential to develop a stenosis at the SVC–IVC anastomosis. However, the latter is rare. In the series reported by Milano et al., no patients required a revision of the SVC–IVC anastomosis either surgically or with percutaneous techniques *(22)*. Similarly, in the 27 patients studied by Leyh et al. over 36 mo, there were no incidences of caval stenoses or thromboses *(11)*.

Aziz et al. performed a worldwide survey of 210 International Society for Heart and Lung Transplantation (ISHLT) centers regarding operative techniques; they received a response rate of 70% *(29)*. The survey demonstrated that the bicaval approach is the most widely used. Because of its simplicity and effectiveness, it has been accepted as the replacement technique for the standard Lower and Shumway approach. A bicaval approach retains the normal atrial morphology, and it preserves synchronous atrial contractility, sinus node function, and AV valvular competence. Also, the bicaval approach avoids some potential problems

Table 1
Studies Comparing Total and Standard Techniques

Authors	Journal	Year	No. of patients	Findings
Blanche et al. (*31*)	Ann Thorac Surg	1994	40 total; 64 standard	Bicaval patients had less postoperative tricuspid regurgitation, bradyarrhythmias, and pacemakers, as well as improved survival at 1, 6, 12, and 18 mo.
Bouchart et al. (*32*)	Eur J Cardiothorac Surg	1997	30 total; 65 standard	Bicaval patients had fewer left atrial thrombi and embolic events.
Blanche et al. (*33*)	J Cardiovasc Surg	1997	117 total; 64 standard	Bicaval patients had lower right atrial mean, pulmonary arterial systolic, pulmonary arterial mean, pulmonary capillary wedge pressures, tricuspid regurgitation, postoperative arrhythmia, and pacemaker requirement, as well as improved 1-, 2-, 3-, and 4-yr survival.

associated with the total technique, such as bleeding from inaccessible suture lines in the posterior pulmonary veins and twisting or narrowing of the pulmonary veins, causing a narrowed pulmonary anastomosis.

The ISHLT survey by Aziz et al. also found that the total technique is infrequently employed (29). This may be because of the technical difficulty in performing a separate pulmonary venous anastomosis. Additionally, it is difficult to preserve adequate quantities of donor left atrial tissue.

However, the total orthotopic transplantation data seem positive. A study by Trento et al. retrospectively analyzed 100 total orthotopic heart transplants (30). Early, 1-yr, and 3-yr survivals were 100, 98, and 96%, respectively. All patients were discharged in normal sinus rhythm, and no permanent pacemakers were required in the first 6 postoperative mo. One yr after transplantation, 22% of patients had greater than or equal to 2+ MR and 36% had greater than or equal to 2+ TR, which is lower than much data in the standard technique literature (8,9).

A number of studies have been conducted comparing standard with total techniques (see Table 1) (31–33). To further evaluate the issue of which technique is best, a randomized trial comparing a bicaval approach with a total approach is necessary.

Currently, a bicaval approach is the authors' preferred approach for orthotopic cardiac transplantation. As compared to the standard technique, a bicaval approach provides anatomic and functional advantages, with a consequent improvement in hemodynamics and patient survival.

REFERENCES

1. Shumway NE, Lower R, Stofer RC. Transplantation of the heart. Adv Surg 1966;2:265–284.
2. Robbins RC, Barlow CW, Oyer PE, et al. Thirty years of cardiac transplantation at Stanford University. J Thorac Cardiovasc Surg 1999;117(5):939–951.
3. Shumway SJ, Shumway NE. Thoracic Transplantation. Blackwell Science, Inc., Oxford, England. 1995, pp.163–180.
4. Kapoor AS, Laks H. Atlas of Heart–Lung Transplantation. McGraw Hill, Inc., New York, NY. 1994, pp. 51–85, 103–116.
5. Kirklin JW, Barratt-Boyes BG. Cardiac Surgery. 2nd ed., Churchill Livingstone, Philadelphia, PA. 1993, pp.1658–1667.
6. Losman JG, Barnard CN. Hemodynamic evaluation of left ventricular bypass with a homologous cardiac graft. J Thorac Cardiovasc Surg 1977;74:695–708.
7. Lower RR, Stofer RC, Shumway NE. Homovital transplantation of the heart. J Thorac Cardiovasc Surg 1961;41:196.
8. Angermann CE, Spes CH, Tammen A, et al. Anatomic characteristics and valvular function of the transplanted hearts: transthoracic versus transesophageal findings. J Heart Transplant 1990;9:331–338.

9. Stevenson LW, Dadourian BJ, Kobashigawa J, et al. Mitral regurgitation after cardiac transplantation. Am J Cardiol 1987;60:119–122.
10. Sievers HH, Leyh R, Jahnke A, et al. Bicaval versus atrial anastomoses in cardiac transplantation. J Thorac Cardiovasc Surg 1994;108:780–784.
11. Leyh RG, Jahnke AW, Kraatz EG, et al. Cardiovascular dynamics and dimensions after bicaval and standard cardiac transplantation. Ann Thorac Surg 1995;59: 1495–1500.
12. Deleuze PH, Benvenuti C, Mazzuccotelli JP, et al. Orthotopic cardiac transplantation with direct caval anastomosis: is it the optimal procedure? J Thorac Cardiovasc Surg 1995;109:731–737.
13. Trento A, Czer LSC, Blanche C. Surgical techniques for cardiac transplantation. Semin Thorac Cardiovasc Surg 1996;8(2):126–132.
14. Forni A, Faggian G, Luciani GB, et al. Reduced incidence of cardiac arrhythmias after orthotopic heart transplantation with direct bicaval anastomosis. Transplant Proc 1996;28(1):289–292.
15. Yacoub M, Mankad P, Ledingham S. Donor procurement and surgical techniques for cardiac transplantation. Semin Thorac Cardiovasc Surg 1990;2:153–161.
16. Sievers HH, Weyand M, Kraatz EG, et al. An alternative technique for orthotopic cardiac transplantation with preservation of normal anatomy of the right atrium. Thorac Cardiovasc Surg 1991;39:70–72.
17. Dreyfus G, Jebara V, Mihaileanu S, et al. Total orthotopic heart transplantation: alternative to the standard technique. Ann Thorac Surg 1991;52:1181–1184.
18. Sarsam MA, Campbell CS, Yonan NA, et al. An alternative technique in orthotopic cardiac transplantation. J Cardiovasc Surg 1993;8:344–349.
19. Webb WR, Howard HS, Neely WA. Practical method of homologous cardiac transplantation. J Thorac Surg 1959;37:361–366.
20. Blanche C, Valenza M, Aleksic I, et al. Technical considerations of a new technique for orthotopic heart transplantation: total excision of recipient's atria with bicaval and pulmonary venous anastomosis. J Cardiovasc Surg 1994;35:283–287.
21. Couetil JP, Mihaileanu S, Lavergne T, et al. Total excision of the recipient atria (TERA) in orthotopic heart transplantation (OHT) as a new clinical procedure: technical considerations and early results. J Heart Lung Transplant 1991;10(suppl 1):179.
22. Milano CA, Shah AS, Van Trigt P, et al. Evaluation of early postoperative results after bicaval versus standard cardiac transplantation and review of the literature. Am Heart J 2000;140(5):717–721.
23. El-Gamel A, Yonan NA, Grant S, et al. Orthotopic heart transplantation: a comparison between the standard and the bicaval Wythenshawe technique. J Thorac Cardiovasc Surg 1995;109:721–730.
24. El-Gamel A, Deiraniya AK, Rahman AN, et al. Orthotopic heart transplantation hemodynamics: does atrial preservation improve cardiac output after transplantation? J Heart Lung Transplant 1996;15:564–571.
25. Aziz T, Burgess M, Khafagy R, et al. Bicaval and standard techniques in orthotopic heart transplantation: Medium-term experience in cardiac performance and survival. J Thorac Cardiovasc Surg 1999;118(1):115–122.
26. Brandt M, Harringer W, Hirt SW, et al. Influence of bicaval anastomosis on late occurrence of atrial arrhythmia after heart transplantation. Ann Thorac Surg 1997;64:70–72.
27. Traversi E, Pozzoli M, Grande A, et al. The bicaval anastomosis technique for orthotopic heart transplantation yields better atrial function then the standard technique: an echocardiographic automatic boundary detection study. J Heart Lung Transplant 1998;17(11):1065–1074.

28. Grande AM, Rinaldi M, D'Armini A, et al. Orthotopic heart transplantation: standard versus bicaval technique. Am J Cardiol 2000;85(1):1329–1333.

29. Aziz TM, Burgess MI, El-Gamel A, et al. Orthotopic cardiac transplantation technique: a survey of current practice. Ann Thorac Surg 1999;68:1242–1246.

30. Trento A, Takkenberg JM, Czer LSC, et al. Clinical experience with one hundred consecutive patients undergoing orthotopic heart transplantation with bicaval and pulmonary venous anastomoses. J Thorac Cardiovasc Surg 1996;112(6):1496–1503.

31. Blanche C, Valenza M, Czer LS, et al. Orthotopic heart transplantation with bicaval and pulmonary venous anastomoses. Ann Thorac Surg 1994;58(5):1505–1509.

32. Bouchart F, Derumeaux G, Mouton-Schleifer D, et al. Conventional and total orthotopic cardiac transplantation: a comparative clinical and echocardiographical study. Eur J Cardiothorac Surg 1997;12(4):555–559.

33. Blanche C, Nessim S, Quartel A, et al. Heart transplantation with bicaval and pulmonary venous anastomoses. A hemodynamic analysis of the first 117 patients. J Cardiovasc Surg 1997;38(6):561–566.

5 Techniques of Cardiac Transplantation for Congenital Heart Disease

Jonathan M. Chen, MD,
Jeffrey A. Morgan, MD,
and Ralph S. Mosca, MD

CONTENTS

INTRODUCTION
DONOR OPERATION
RECIPIENT OPERATION
ANOMALOUS CONDITIONS
OTHER CONSIDERATIONS
CONCLUSION
REFERENCES

INTRODUCTION

Cardiac transplantation for complex congenital heart disease incorporates aspects of both reparative and replacement surgery *(1–10)*. Whereas intracardiac congenital malformations are replaced and, therefore, pose few obstacles to the transplant surgeon, extracardiac malformations (be they congenital, acquired, or iatrogenic) present a major challenge to the operative team. Traditionally, the majority of these patients range in age from infancy to young adolescence. However, more recently, survival into adulthood of those with congenital heart disease and a lack of suitable alternative therapies for end-stage

From: *Contemporary Cardiology: Cardiac Transplantation:*
The Columbia University Medical Center/New York-Presbyterian Hospital Manual
Edited by: N. M. Edwards, J. M. Chen, and P. A. Mazzeo © Humana Press Inc., Totowa, NJ

heart disease have generated a substantial population of adult congenital transplant candidates.

Not surprisingly, the transplantation technique in patients with myopathic congenital heart disease is not different from that performed in adults. However, the disease spectrum and the limitless combinations of congenital defects (and prior palliative operations) can significantly complicate the recipient operation. Pretransplant, a full comprehension of the operative plan for the management of each patient (and his or her lesion) is essential for the donor team so that they may harvest donor tissue of appropriate amounts to allow for adequate reconstruction and potential conduit formation. This understanding also extends to the perioperative recipient teams—especially in adult congenital patients—where the cardiac anesthesia team, in particular, may be less familiar with congenital lesions and their perioperative concerns.

For infants and children with congenital heart disease, donor–recipient size matching can be difficult and generally requires some liberalization of the standard criteria. We have extended the donor–recipient mismatch up to 200% to enlarge the potential donor candidate pool. Often, the recipient's cardiomegaly allows for organ replacement from a substantially larger donor. When necessary, adjunctive procedures, such as opening both pleural spaces, reducing tidal volumes, or delaying sternal closure, can accommodate significantly oversized donor hearts.

DONOR OPERATION

The donor operation proceeds as routine for heart transplantation, except for the frequent need for additional donor tissue to reconstruct the recipient. In general, there are three anatomic concerns for recipient reconstructive techniques. First, donor procurement for a recipient with a persistent left superior vena cava (LSVC) may require the mobilization and extirpation of the entire donor innominate vein. Second, reconstruction of the recipient's main pulmonary artery (PA) after Rastelli reconstruction, or with branch PA stenosis, may mandate harvesting the donor's entire intrapericardial main and branch PAs. Finally, donor procurement for recipients with aortic arch hypoplasia or other arch abnormalities can require full mobilization and removal of the aortic arch, arch vessels, and portions of the descending aorta if necessary (Fig. 1).

Our institutional preference is using Celsior solution for preservation, at a dose of 20 cc/kg of the donor, infused at 80 mmHg. For donors greater than 50 kg, we administer 1 L of solution at a systolic pressure of 150 mmHg (80 mmHg in infants and children). As with standard transplant procedure, the organ is stored in saline in multiple sterile containers at 4°C for transport.

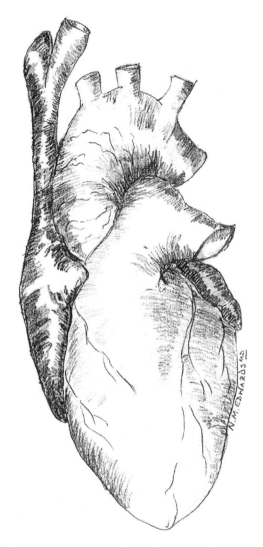

Fig. 1. Result of donor procurement for recipients with aortic arch hypoplasia or other arch abnormalities.

RECIPIENT OPERATION

In patients with multiple prior procedures, and for those in whom cardiomegaly and volume overload may significantly complicate reoperative dissection, peripheral cardiopulmonary bypass is often instituted through femoral artery and vein cannulation, when patient size permits. When safe entry in the chest is accomplished, and the great vessels and atria are dissected, it is not uncommon to recannulate the patient centrally to ensure sufficient flow at low-line pressure. Naturally, aortic cannulation, when performed centrally, must be done sufficiently distally along the aortic arch for appropriate reconstruction in cases requiring aortoplasty. In addition, those infants with ductal-dependent circulation may benefit from an additional cannula in the main PA and directed through the ductus. Iatrogenic venous considerations (e.g., Glenn shunt) may also require proximal cannulation for venous drainage.

If a relatively straightforward procedure and short ischemic time are anticipated, the recipient is cooled to 32°C. However, for complex cases requiring significant reconstruction and for recipients with increased bronchial venous return, more profound hypothermia, or even deep hypothermic circulatory arrest at 18°C, may be used.

ANOMALOUS CONDITIONS

Atrial Anomalies

Essentially, there are three types of atrial anomalies: (a) those involving size discrepancies between donor and recipient, (b) those created by iatrogenic surgical distortion, and (c) viscero-atrial situs inversus, in which the donor and recipient atria are spatially inverted.

For donor–recipient atrial discrepancies, we employ two techniques (often in concert) to better align the atria. First, the recipient atrium may be reduced by oversewing the cephalic atrium, thereby extending the recipient's superior vena cava (SVC) length (Fig. 2). Second, the donor right atrial incision may be performed in the sinus venosus region of the right atrium, just posterior to the sinoatrial node (Fig. 3). Then, this paraseptal incision may be extended to increase the donor's right atrium as needed. Interestingly, in our experience, the latter technique has not resulted in an increased incidence of atrial arrhythmias.

Often, patients who have undergone Mustard or Senning atrial inversion procedures develop significant atrial distortion. First, in such patients, the right atrium may be abnormally large and the left atrium abnormally small, and the venae cavae are often drawn to the left side. Therefore, after baffle excision, the cavae orifices tend to align in close proximity to the pulmonary vein orifices. The size discrepancies of donor

---

Fig. 2. (*top right*) Technique for reducing atrial cuff size for donor–recipient atrial discrepancy. From ref. *1* with permission.

Fig. 3. (*bottom right*) Technique to increase donor atrial cuff size for donor–recipient atrial discrepancy. From ref. *1* with permission.

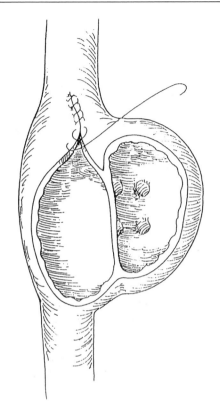

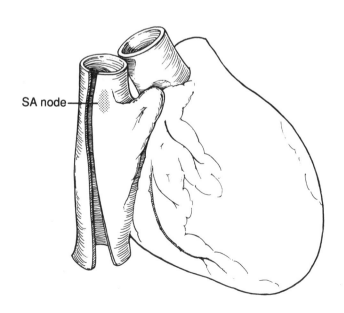

SA node

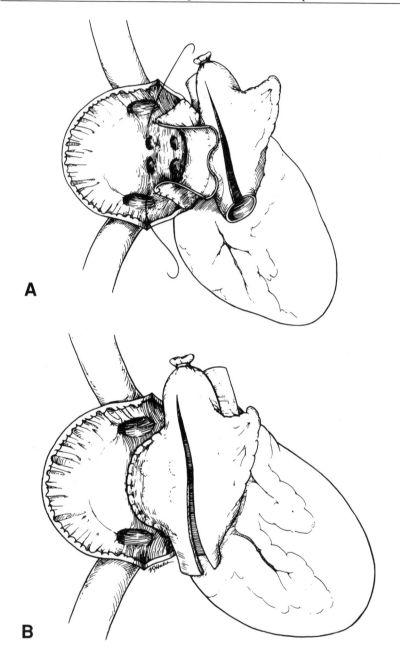

A

B

and recipient atria may be addressed with the two techniques described earlier. The donor heart's interatrial septum may be used to fashion a new atrial septum in the recipient's common atrium (Fig. 4A–C), or, as

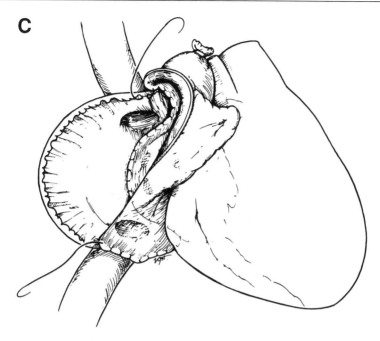

Fig. 4. Technique for adjusting for patients with prior atrial inversion procedures. **(A)** left atrial anstomosis, **(B)** elongation of the donor right atrial cuff **(C)** right atrial anastomosis. From ref. *1* with permission.

has been suggested, the inclusion of a "tongue" of left atrial wall on the right side may allow for atrial septation when anchored to the posterior atrial wall (common atrium) or to a septal remnant.

Viscero-atrial situs inversus represents an anatomic variant for which several complicated techniques have been described. One method, which may be used in the setting of bilateral SVCs with the LSVC and inferior vena cava (IVC) entering to the right of the pulmonary veins, allows for interatrial septum excision and creation of a lateral "T" incision in the left atrium (Fig. 5A). Two baffles may then be created along the common atrium's back wall to bring the vena caval return rightward and, therefore, allow for standard left and right atrial anastomoses (Fig. 5B,C).

Anomalies of Systemic and Pulmonary Venous Return

We have encountered two types of anomalies of systemic and pulmonary venous connections: (a) left SVC and (b) deficiencies of SVC tissue from prior operations. For those patients with a left SVC, in which the vena cava drains into a coronary sinus not in communication with the left atrium, we have found that the recipient cardiectomy may be performed

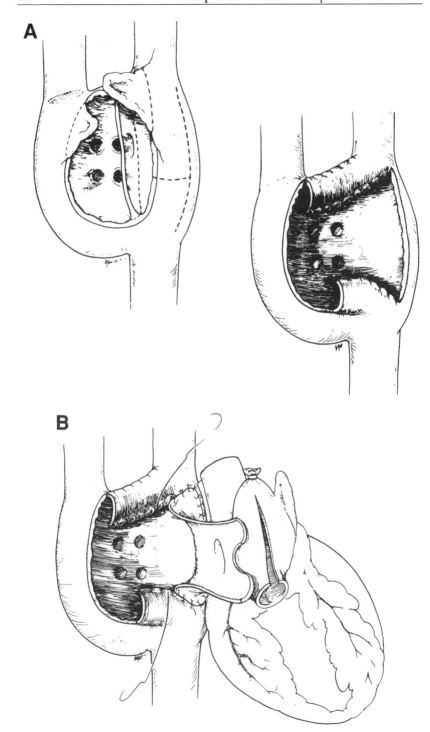

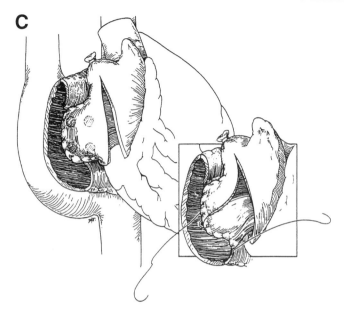

Fig. 5. Technique for reconstructing the atria in a recipient with bilateral SVCs. **(A)** interatrial septum excision and creation of a "T" incision in the left atrium that ultimately baffles flow from the left-sided SVC and left IVC to the new right side, **(B)** left atrial anastomosis, **(C)** right atrial anastomosis. From ref. *1* with permission.

leaving the coronary sinus intact. However, here, the middle cardiac vein must be transected and oversewn prior to completing the left atrial anastomosis (Fig. 6). Whereas, for those patients in whom the coronary sinus is unroofed, the left SVC may be ligated, divided, and subsequently anastomosed directly to the donor innominate vein (Fig. 7) or baffled to the right atrium using additional adjacent recipient left atrial tissue (Fig. 8).

Those single-ventricle patients who have undergone cavopulmonary shunts or have bilateral SVC may be reconstructed easily using donor SVC and innominate vein to anastomose the left and right vena cavae, respectively. Naturally, cannulation must be sufficiently high along the SVC for the necessary dissection, mobilization, and reconstruction.

Anomalies of the Great Arteries

These anatomic variants represent anomalies of position, size, and surgical distortion, in addition to anomalies produced by aortopulmonary collateral arteries. Simple malposition can be reconstructed easily with harvesting of additional donor great vessels. The most severe size dis-

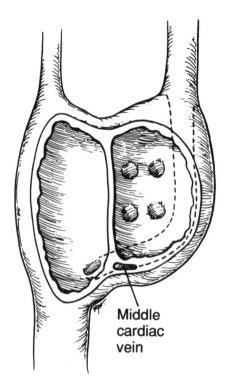

Fig. 6. Management of the patient with L-SVC to the coronary sinus (oversewing of the middle cardiac vein). From ref. *1* with permission.

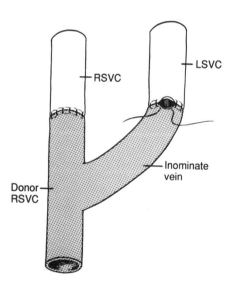

Fig. 7. Alternative management of the recipient with an L-SVC (use of donor innominate vein to baffle flow from the recipient L-SVC to the right atrium). From ref. *1* with permission.

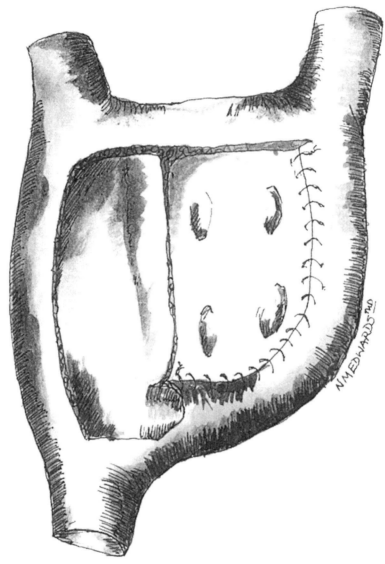

Fig. 8. Management of the patient with an unroofed coronary sinus using left atrial tissue to reconstruct the coronary sinus roof.

crepancy is seen in hypoplastic left heart syndrome, although other abnormalities of the arch and descending aorta may be encountered where repair is similar (Fig. 9A,B).

PA reconstruction may be necessary because of (a) position abnormalities, (b) pulmonary outflow obstruction abnormalities, or (c) previ-

A

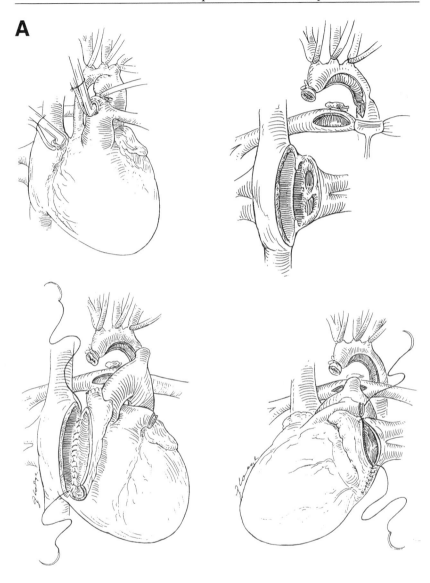

ous cavopulmonary, atrial pulmonary, or systemic pulmonary shunts. Either or both branch PAs may be congenitally atretic or stenotic, or, alternatively, they may have areas of acquired stenosis or distortion from prior shunt procedures mandating reconstruction. In addition, we have performed transplantation in individuals with only one "functional" PA (the other having been rendered nonfunctional by congenital unilateral atresia), a condition which requires "baffling" of the donor PA for

B

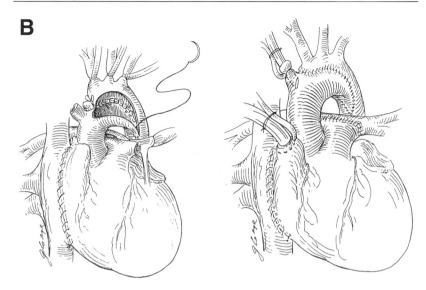

Fig. 9. (**A**) and (**B**) Use of donor aortic arch to reconstruct the hypoplastic arch of a recipient with hypoplastic left heart syndrome. From ref. *11* with permission.

unobstructed, unilateral pulmonary blood flow (Figs. 10A,B). In general, PA abnormalities may be bypassed completely or augmented via patch angioplasty or with additional donor PA tissue.

For those with L-TGA (congenitally corrected transposition of the great arteries) who received prior reconstructions with PA conduits, the conduit may be transected distally to the prosthesis (and the donor PA anastomosed directly end-to-end to the remaining conduit), or, preferably, the entire conduit tissue may be removed and the PAs may be reconstructed and enlarged, if necessary, with extended donor PA tissue.

For those patients with pulmonary outflow obstruction who have undergone Waterston shunts or PA banding procedures, or have pulmonary stenosis or atresia at baseline, PA reconstruction may be performed with band removal, and partial pulmonary arterioplasty may be performed with either bovine pericardium or extended donor PA. Alternatively, Waterston shunts may be repaired from within the aorta, and PA band tissue may simply be excised, and the PA anastomosis may be performed directly to the PA bifurcation (Fig. 11). Prior modified Blalock–Taussig shunts may be ligated or oversewn from within the PA, and the cavopulmonary shunts may be reconstructed bilaterally, the PAs may be repaired, and the venae cavae may be reconstructed end-to-end with extended donor SVC and/or innominate vein.

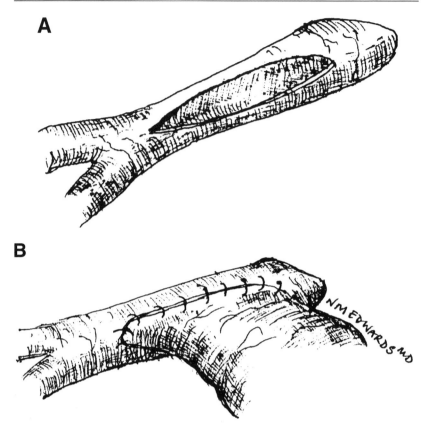

Fig. 10. Demonstration of the use of donor main pulmonary artery (PA) to reconstruct the front wall of the recipient PA in a patient with one functional PA **(A)** after donor excision and **(B)** after recipient anastomsis.

Additionally, often those who have had a right classic Glenn cavopulmonary anastomosis in conjunction with a Fontan to the left or main PA can often have a significant gap between the right PA orifice and the main or left PA. This requires reconstruction with donor PA tissue at transplant time.

OTHER CONSIDERATIONS

Heterotaxy Syndromes

Children with heterotaxy syndromes have ambiguous visceral and atrial situs with associated anomalies of both systemic and pulmonary venous return, presenting a significant challenge at transplant. Bilateral SVC is common, as is an absent IVC with azygous continuation, with

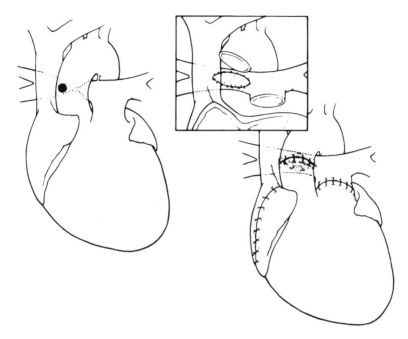

Fig. 11. Management of the patient with a prior Waterston shunt (treated by excision of the previous shunt, reconstruction of the pulmonary artery. From ref. *1* with permission.

aberrant hepatic venous drainage in a sizeable proportion. In such cases, a preoperative cardiac catheterization to elucidate the anatomy is essential.

Generally, recipient cardiectomy is modified such that some reconstruction of the recipient atrium is necessary prior to implant (Fig. 12). The majority of atrial tissue is used to reconstruct the left atrium, and both SVC and IVC are disconnected at their respective atriocaval junctions. This large left atrium may require reduction atrioplasty prior to implant to make size discrepancies less egregious and to avoid atrioventricular valve distortion or incompetence. The caval anastomoses are performed in a standard fashion. In essence, by devoting the majority of atrial tissue to left atrial reconstruction, this technique accounts for, and repairs, anomalous pulmonary venous return without sacrificing caval tissue.

Biatrial vs Bicaval Anastomosis

Many studies have been performed in adults comparing biatrial with bicaval techniques. Unlike the bicaval approach, biatrial anastomosis is associated with distorted right ventricle (RV) geometry, RV dilatation,

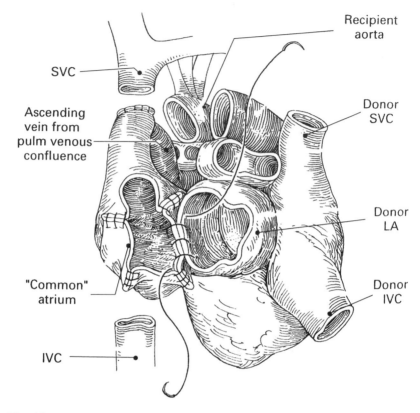

SVC

Ascending
vein from
pulm venous
confluence

"Common"
atrium

IVC

Recipient
aorta

Donor
SVC

Donor
LA

Donor
IVC

Fig. 12. Reconstruction of the donor heart in anticipation of implantation into a patient with heterotaxy sundrome. From ref. 2 with permission.

and abnormal septal motion. Hemodynamic studies in adults who have undergone a bicaval approach have demonstrated less tricuspid regurgitation, more normal right atrial dimension and function, and decreased requirement for postoperative pacemakers *(10)*. We favor the bicaval approach wherever possible, for the above reasons and because of the common need to reconstruct prior caval anastomoses. However, whereas the possibility of caval stenosis is rare in larger children and adults, its potential in neonates and small children is real and must be taken into consideration.

CONCLUSION

Cardiac transplantation for congenital heart disease offers various of challenges to traditional heart replacement techniques. Incorporating the reparative methodology of congenital heart surgery, transplantation in this setting often requires extracardiac great vessel reconstruction as well as intracardiac baffling to ameliorate anomalous systemic and pulmonary venous return. With the advent of therapeutic adjuncts to aid perioperative management of critically ill patients, many patients with congenital heart disease can anticipate survival comparable to patients with acquired heart disease. Because of the growing cohort of adult congenital patients, this population is certain to be more prominent in the near future.

REFERENCES

1. Addonizio LJ, Kichuk MR, Chen JM, et al. Benefits and pitfalls of transplantation for patients with congenital heart disease. In: Franco KL, ed. Pediatric Cardiopulmonary Transplantation. Futura Publishing, Armonk, NY. 1997, pp. 115–148.
2. Huddleston CB. Heart trasnplantation in infants and children—indications, surgical techniques, and special considerations. In: Cooper DKC, Miller LW, Patterson GA, eds. The Transplantation and Replacement of Thoracic Organs. Kluwer Academic Publishers, Dordrect, Netherlands. 1996. pp. 367–377.
3. Turrentine MW, Kesler KA, Caldwell R, et al. Cardiac transplantation in infants and children. Ann Thorac Surg 1994;57:546–554.
4. Schlechta B, Kocher AA, Ehrlich M, et al. Outcome of pediatric heart transplantation. Transplant Proc 2001;33:2834–2835.
5. Bauer J, Thul J, Kramer U, et al. Heart transplantation in children and infants: Short-term outcome and long-term follow-up. Pediatr Transplant 2001;4:457–462.
6. Kanter KR, Tam VHK, Vincent RN, et al. Current results with pediatric heart transplantation. Ann Thorac Surg 1999;68:527–531.
7. Donato RMD, Carlo DD, Squitieri C, et al. Pediatric heart transplantation: changing indications and improved results. Transplant Proc 2001;33:1595.
8. Parisi F, Squitieri C, Carotti A, et al. Ten-year follow-up after pediatric transplantation. J Heart Lung Transplant 1999;18(3):275–277.
9. Sundararaghavan PE, Strasburger JF, Mitchell BM, et al. Impaired exercise parameters in pediatric heart transplant recipients: comparison of biatrial and bicaval techniques. Pediatr Transplant 2000;4:268–272.
10. Haas GS, Bailey L, Pennington DG. Pediatric cardiac transplantation. In: Baue, ed. Glenn's Thoracic and Cardiovascular Surgery. Appleton and Lange, Stamford, CT. 1992, pp. 1297–1317.
11. In: Kirklin J, Barrett-Boyes B, eds. Cardiac Surgery, 2nd ed., vol 2. Churchill Livingstone, New York, NY. 1993.

6 Pathology and the Transplant Patient

Charles C. Marboe, MD
and Bachir Alobeid, MD

CONTENTS

THE INTERNATIONAL SOCIETY FOR HEART AND LUNG
    TRANSPLANTATION GRADING SYSTEM
HUMORAL REJECTION
TRANSPLANT CORONARY ARTERY DISEASE
TRANSPLANTED HEART REINNERVATION
POSTTRANSPLANT LYMPHOPROLIFERATIVE DISORDERS
OTHER VIRUSES AFFECTING GRAFT SURVIVAL
ALTERNATIVE REJECTION MARKERS
OTHER PATHOLOGY RESULTING FROM THERAPY
REFERENCES

THE INTERNATIONAL SOCIETY FOR HEART AND LUNG TRANSPLANTATION GRADING SYSTEM

In August 1990, under the guidance of Margaret Billingham, FRCPath, then president of the International Society for Heart and Lung Transplantation (ISHLT), a group of pathologists met to establish a universal grading system for the interpretation of transplanted heart biopsies. This grading system *(1)* was quickly and widely adopted by transplant centers and has provided some uniformity for communication, publication, and multicenter clinical trials.

From: *Contemporary Cardiology: Cardiac Transplantation:*
The Columbia University Medical Center/New York-Presbyterian Hospital Manual
Edited by: N. M. Edwards, J. M. Chen, and P. A. Mazzeo © Humana Press Inc., Totowa, NJ

Technical Considerations

If a standard adult bioptome is used, a minimum of four pieces of myocardium must be obtained. Each piece must be greater than or equal to 50% myocardium and not scar or prior biopsy site. Experienced operators can distinguish red-brown myocardium from clot or white fibrous scar tissue. A minimum of four different sites on the right side of the interventricular septum must be sampled; a single large piece of tissue must not be cut in half to count as two pieces. If a smaller bioptome must be used because of the patient's age or problems with access, a minimum of six myocardial biopsies should be retrieved.

Fixation in commercially available 10% neutral buffered formalin is adequate for routine histology. Electron microscopy is not necessary for the diagnosis of rejection. At least one myocardial biopsy should be protected in Optimal Cutting Temperature Compound (OCT; Tissue-Tek®, Sakura Finetek, USA, Inc., Torrance, CA) or similar freezing compound, snap-frozen, and stored at –80°C for immunofluorescence studies if humoral (vascular) rejection is a clinical concern. Special fixatives for preserving ribonucleic acid (RNA), or to facilitate deoxyribonucleic acid (DNA) extraction, may be used to preserve tissue for molecular diagnostic studies; any such fixative should be pretested on myocardium to ensure it is suitable for routine microscopy.

All the biopsy tissue pieces may be embedded together in one paraffin block. As these are small tissue pieces, expedited processing on an automated tissue processor provides stained slides in approx 4 h from tissue receipt in the pathology lab. Manual processing provides slides in about 2.5 h, but there are high costs in technician time and disruption of the general histology lab schedule. The high quality of the histology makes rapid processing preferable to performing frozen sections for "stat" diagnosis.

Rejection may be a focal process, and, therefore, it is necessary to have multiple sections from at least three levels through the tissue block. Hematoxylin and eosin staining is adequate for the diagnosis of rejection. We have not found any "special" histologic stains, such as a connective tissue stain, to be necessary for grading rejection; unusual histologic findings certainly could warrant special studies. Also, we have not routinely performed stains for "activated" lymphocytes. Distinguishing activated cells likely to damage the graft from "innocent bystander" cells has obvious merit. As noted later, some centers use lymphocyte growth assays to detect activated cells in the graft. Immunohistochemical staining for lymphoid infiltrate subtyping may be useful in the question of Grade 2 rejection vs nodular endocardial infiltrate.

Contraction bands are a common biopsy procedure artifact. The presence of contraction bands in biopsy material must not be interpreted as contraction band necrosis indicative of ischemia and reperfusion injury.

Cellular Rejection Grading

Cellular rejection is classified with an ISHLT grade and with diagnostic terminology. Although the ISHLT grading system includes nomenclature for use in diagnosis, many centers have retained their preexisting terminology and append the ISHLT grade to the diagnosis. One reason for using diagnostic terms different from the ISHLT nomenclature is to avoid confusing patients and physicians who are unfamiliar with transplant recipient management. For example, most centers will not treat Grades 1A, 1B, or 2 rejection; this may be disconcerting to patients or nonspecialist physicians who see a biopsy diagnosis including the word "rejection." The ISHLT terminology appears in parentheses below.

Grade 0 (No acute rejection) is used in the absence of inflammatory infiltrate or myocyte necrosis. Equivocal findings, such as rare interstitial lymphocytes, are generally graded as 0.

Grade 1A (Focal, mild acute rejection) (Fig. 1A) describes the presence of focal perivascular or interstitial infiltrates of lymphocytes. No myocyte necrosis is present.

Grade 1B (Diffuse, mild acute rejection) (Fig. 1B) describes more diffuse perivascular and/or interstitial infiltrates. No myocyte necrosis is present.

Grade 2 (Focal, moderate acute rejection) (Fig. 1C) is a solitary, circumscribed focus of inflammatory infiltrate, which is associated with myocyte damage. The infiltrate is composed of large lymphocytes and may include eosinophils. The infiltrate is associated with clear myocyte damage (necrosis) or occupies space that should be comprised of myocytes. This is a single infiltrate focus; the other biopsied myocardial fragments should be free of any significant infiltrate. The difficulty in distinguishing this lesion from a "nodular endocardial infiltrate with myocardial extension" will be discussed later.

Grade 3A (Multifocal moderate rejection) denotes multifocal inflammatory infiltrates of large lymphocytes, with or without eosinophils, which are space-occupying or associated with myocyte damage. These infiltrates involve one or more endomyocardial fragments.

Grade 3B (Diffuse, borderline severe acute rejection) (Fig. 1D) includes a more diffuse inflammatory infiltrate of large lymphocytes, with or without eosinophils, associated with myocyte damage in several tissue pieces. Interstitial edema is likely to be present, but hemorrhage is not seen.

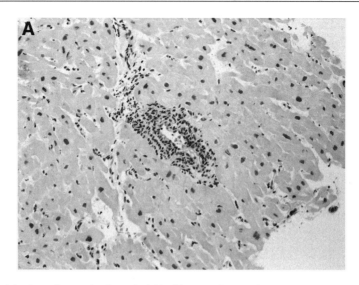

Fig. 1A. A perivascular lymphoid infiltrate (ISHLT Grade 1A). (H&E, ×10)

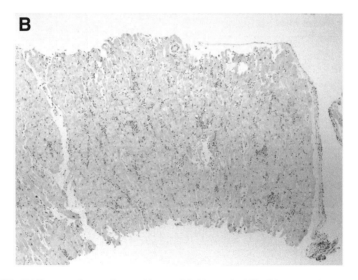

Fig. 1B. Diffuse perivascular and interstitial lymphoid infiltrates (ISHLT Grade 1B). (H&E, ×4)

Grade 4 (Severe acute rejection) includes an intense, polymorphous infiltrate of large lymphocytes, eosinophils and neutrophils, associated with myocyte damage. Edema, hemorrhage, and vasculitis are usually present.

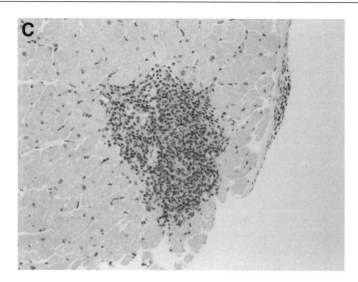

Fig. 1C. A single, dense infiltrate that occupies space that should contain myocytes (ISHLT Grade 2). There is an adjacent small nodular endocardial infiltrate. (H&E, ×10)

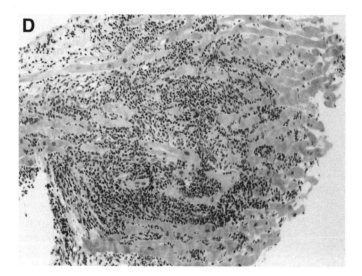

Fig. 1D. Multifocal infiltrates with myocyte damage (ISHLT Grade 3B). (H&E, ×4)

No specific diagnosis denotes "resolving" or "resolved" acute rejection. The biopsy is graded as above; the designation of "resolving rejection, clinically" may be added in parentheses after the grade if there is supporting clinical evidence.

Edema, as noted earlier, is likely to be present in more advanced cellular rejection grades. Interstitial edema may also be present as a manifestation of "leaky" vessels associated with humoral rejection and may occur in apparent isolation. Although not independently graded, the presence of edema is important to note, as it contributes to elevated ventricular filling pressure (2), a hemodynamic finding associated with rejection.

Endocardial infiltrates are not graded; they may be part of the early rejection process or may be related to a previous biopsy site or a nodular endocardial infiltrate. The presence of a vasculitis does not indicate a specific grade or grade modification. However, vasculitis should be described, including the nature of the inflammatory infiltrate and presence and type of necrosis, if any, in the vessel wall. It has been suggested that the presence of vasculitis carries a worse prognosis (3); this may reflect the presence of humoral (vascular) rejection, a particularly aggressive acute cellular rejection, or an additional pathologic process in the patient.

Other histologic changes, which must be distinguished from acute cellular rejection, may also be present in biopsy tissue. These include:

- Nodular endocardial infiltrates (Fig. 2A). These distinctive lesions appeared after the introduction of cyclosporine (CyA) (Neoral, Sandoz, Inc., East Hanover, NJ) immunosuppression and, initially, were termed the "Quilty effect," after the Stanford patient in whom they were first noted. These lesions have never been proved to be a manifestation or harbinger of rejection. Composed of dense infiltrates of cells with admixed capillaries having prominent endothelium, the nodules protrude from the endocardial surface into the chamber. The lesions may also extend irregularly between myocytes into the subjacent myocardium. A tangential cut through this myocardial extension focus, which did not show the relationship of the lesion to the endocardial surface, would histologically resemble a Grade 2 lesion. One study serially sectioned through Grade 2 lesions and found that 91% connected to the endocardial surface and actually were nodular endocardial infiltrates (4). Distinguishing "Quilty" lesions from rejection is one instance in which inflammatory infiltrate immunophenotyping may be useful. Acute cellular rejection is comprised of CD3+ T lymphocytes and macrophages (5). The nodular endocardial infiltrates contain significant numbers of plasma cells and CD20+ B lymphocytes, in addition to T cells and scattered macrophages (6).

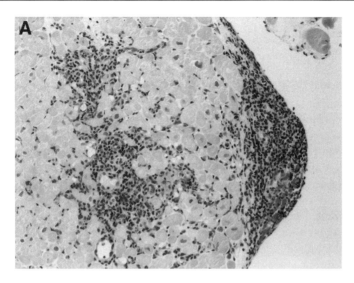

Fig. 2A. A nodular endocardial infiltrate with a focus of myocardial extension that mimics the histology of ISHLT Grade 2. (H&E, ×4)

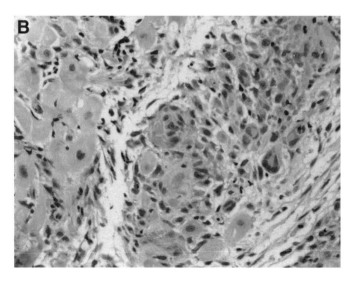

Fig. 2B. Giant-cell myocarditis recurred 190 d posttransplant in the graft of 26-yr-old woman. (H&E, ×20)

- Prior biopsy site. The frequency with which previous biopsy sites are sampled is surprisingly high. A focus of florid damage with extensive inflammation, some fibroblasts, capillaries oriented perpendicular to the endocardial surface, and fibrin on the lumen surface, when other pieces show minimal inflammation, is a typical biopsy site.

- Ischemic damage. In the first biopsies following transplantation, there may be subendocardial myocyte damage with minimal inflammation. Ischemic damage (nuclear karyorrhexis and coagulative necrosis of myocyte cytoplasm) is distinct from acute cellular rejection, in which myocytes maintain nuclear architecture and cross-striations even when engulfed by inflammatory infiltrate.
- Infectious agents. The immunosuppressed transplant recipient is prone to opportunistic infections. These may be *de novo* fungal or viral infections or reactivation of a previous disease such as cytomegalovirus (CMV), toxoplasmosis, or trypanosomiasis (*T. cruzi*). Depending on the organism and the immunosuppression level, there may be little or no inflammatory infiltrate; focal inflammatory infiltrates in heavily immunosuppressed recipients—particularly following an boost immunosuppression to treat rejection—should be carefully studied to exclude opportunistic infection.
- Recurrence of original disease. Sarcoidosis, giant-cell myocarditis (Fig. 2B), and Chagas' disease have recurred in allografts and are likely to have an inflammatory component. Other disease processes less likely to be accompanied by inflammation, but reported to recur in allografts, include amyloidosis, Fabry's disease, and malignancies such as melanoma and cardiac sarcoma.
- Posttransplant lymphoproliferative disease (PTLD). This complication of transplantation will be discussed in more detail below. Distinguishing a polymorphous PTLD infiltrate with large, activated lymphocytes from the large lymphocytes seen in acute rejection is difficult by morphology alone. Immunophenotyping may be helpful, because PTLD is a B-lymphocyte proliferation in the vast majority of cases, whereas rejection is predominantly a T-lymphocyte infiltration. Atypical monomorphic lymphoid infiltrates, which appear malignant by routine histology, are more easily distinguished from rejection.

Cellular Rejection: Clinical Correlations

Not all patients have documented cellular rejection episodes. Approximately 45% of recipients have a Grade 3A rejection in the first posttransplant year; only 10% have hemodynamic compromise. As described in detail in Chapter 7, the clinical response to rejection is graded, considering not only the biopsy, but also hemodynamic studies, immunosuppressive drug levels, and clinical symptoms. Each center determines its own algorithm for dealing with rejection. Included in these protocols is an approach to "biopsy-negative" rejection with hemodynamic compromise. This group includes symptomatic patients with hemodynamic compromise whose biopsies are Grades 0, 1A, 1B or 2—grades not warranting therapy alone.

HUMORAL REJECTION

Hyperacute Rejection

There are rare reports of hyperacute rejection of cardiac allografts by preformed recipient antibodies *(7)*. Hyperacute rejection occurs immediately following, or within hours of, reintroduction of blood flow into the graft. Preformed immunoglobulin (Ig)G and/or IgM antibodies against ABO antigens (expressed on vascular endothelial cells as well as on erythrocytes), human leukocyte antigens (HLAs), and other endothelial cell antigens bind to the donor endothelium. Complement is activated, neutrophils are engaged, and there is resultant endothelial cell destruction with hemorrhage as well as microvascular thrombosis. The heart is swollen, stiff, and hemorrhagic. Histologic sections show aggregated erythrocytes, fibrin thrombi, and neutrophils marginating in small vessels. Thrombi are present in veins. There is extensive edema and hemorrhage in the interstitium. If the patient lives for sufficient time, blood vessels and myocardium may be necrotic.

This rejection form is the primary obstacle to graft survival in xenotransplantation, in which it has been suggested that increased vascular permeability and venous thrombosis are more prominent than microvascular endothelial injury *(8)*. The preformed antibodies are directed against the Gal α 1–3Gal β-4GlcNAc-R epitope abundantly expressed on pig cells *(9)*. Therefore, early xenograft survival strategies are directed against removing the antibody, preventing complement activation, or accelerating complement decay *(10)*.

Humoral (Vascular) Rejection

The *de novo* formation in recipients of antibodies directed against HLAs expressed on graft endothelium is associated with shortened graft survival *(11)*. A histopathologic description of vascular rejection and its clinical correlation was first reported by Hammond et al. *(12,13)*. Their definition is based on the immunohistologic demonstration of linear deposits of complement split products C1q and C3 with IgG, IgM, or IgA on the vascular endothelium of capillaries and arterioles. Although there may be endothelial cell hypertrophy or swelling and vasculitis, these light microscopic changes are not sufficiently sensitive or specific to be diagnostically useful. Subsequent authors have recommended including immunohistochemical staining for fibrinogen and HLA-DR *(14)*.

The occurrence, pathologic features, and clinical relevance of humoral rejection were addressed in subsequent studies *(15–17)* with some concern over diagnostic technique specificity and use *(17)*. Important factors that severely and adversely affect the sensitivity of immune complex detection include (a) the shedding or internalization of deposited Ig from the cell membrane of endothelial cells *(18)* and (b) complement inhibition and destruction by endothelial cells and circulating proteins *(19,20)*. This high turnover and transient presence of antibody and complement bound to vascular endothelium, despite an ongoing humoral response, could be a factor in the poor correlation of immunohistologically-defined humoral rejection with the presence of circulating antidonor HLA antibodies *(21)*.

One technique postulated to have greater sensitivity for vascular rejection detection is staining for C4d covalently bound to vascular endothelium. The C4d fragment is generated by the classical, antibody-induced pathway of complement activation. Consisting of three polypeptide chains linked by disulfide bonds, C4d undergoes proteolysis by activated C1s, releasing a small C4a fragment into the circulation. The residual, larger C4b fragment binds covalently with the activating antibody or with the endothelial cell surface. This bound C4b is broken rapidly into a soluble C4c fragment and a C4d fragment remaining covalently bound to the endothelium. Endothelial C4d deposition is associated with early renal allograft loss *(22)* and poor renal graft function *(23)*, independent of acute cellular rejection, and, also, with a higher risk of cardiac allograft loss *(24)*. However, there are important limitations to C4d staining interpretation.

There is a high incidence of complement activation in patients receiving induction therapy with antibodies (e.g., CD4 chimeric antibody, antithymocyte globulin, or OKT3) *(24,25)*, resulting in a high incidence of vascular deposition of antibody and complement without clinical significance. Also, C4d deposition is more common in multiparous women, and the role of ischemia/reperfusion injury in predisposing to C4d deposition is not fully understood. Whereas C4d persistence on the vascular endothelium makes it a more sensitive assay, when a patient is 'positive' for C4d deposition, the staining persists, limiting the test's usefulness for monitoring therapies aimed at reducing circulating antigraft antibodies.

TRANSPLANT CORONARY ARTERY DISEASE

Beyond 1 yr posttransplantation, malignancy and cardiac allograft vasculopathy (CAV) become important patient and graft survival determinants *(26)*. The incidence of CAV is related to the detection method's sensitivity. Angiographic studies document CAV in up to 45% of heart allograft recipients within 3 yr of transplantation *(27)*; studies using intravascular ultrasound (IVUS) have documented intimal thickening in 58% of recipients at 2 yr *(28)*.

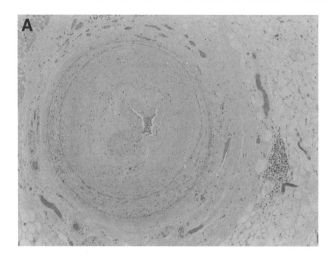

Fig. 3A. Transplant vasculopathy with concentric narrowing of the lumen with a recanalized thrombus and focal thinning of the media. There are focal lymphoid infiltrates in the adjacent epicardial fat. (H&E, ×2)

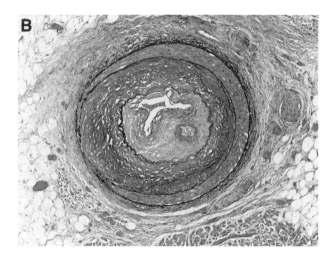

Fig. 3B. An elastic van Gieson stain highlights the intimal proliferation, recanalization, and the focal thinning of the media in an epicardial coronary artery with transplant vasculopathy. (H&E, ×2)

Histology

CAV (Fig. 3A,B) is morphologically distinct from common atherosclerosis: (a) the intimal lesions are concentric rather than eccentric in the lumen, (b) the intimal lesions are diffuse and extensive rather than discrete occlusions, (c) there is, particularly in early lesions, more extensive inflammation with lymphocytes, (d) calcification is rare, (e) the lesions are more likely to extend into small, intramyocardial vessels, and (f) similar, but generally less extensive, lesions may be present in cardiac veins. The process is also distinctive in its accelerated course and lethal occurrence in young children.

The relative contributions of intimal thickening and vessel constriction to vessel lumen loss are detailed with serial IVUS studies. Increase in intimal area is greater in yr 1 than in subsequent years *(29,30)*. After 1 yr, lumen loss is related primarily to constriction of the vessel wall (area circumscribed by the external elastic lamina) *(30)*. Lumen loss resulting from vessel shrinkage is more important in large coronary arteries than in small arteries; intimal proliferation is similar in both large and small vessels *(31)*.

Large- and medium-sized coronary arteries are not sampled by endomyocardial biopsy, but ischemic changes may be seen in myocytes in these biopsies. Rarely, an actual infarct may be sampled. The most common form of reversible ischemic change seen in myocytes is myocytolysis *(32)*. Another rare finding is microvesicular lipid accumulation in chronically ischemic myocytes *(33)*.

Etiology

Both immunologic and nonimmunologic factors have roles in the development of coronary artery disease (CAD) in transplants *(34,35)*. Nonimmunologic factors include warm and cold ischemia before transplantation, donor age, pre-existing vessel disease, and the risk factors for nontransplant atherosclerosis. The mechanisms by which CMV infection is associated with cardiac allograft rejection and arteriopathy involve cytokine release but are incompletely defined . Generally, vasculopathy is accepted as a form of chronic rejection of allografts with an immunologic attack directed primarily against the graft's vascular endothelium *(36)*. The relative roles of T lymphocytes *(37)* and antibodies *(38)* in the genesis of endothelial damage have been hotly debated. Whatever the damage mechanism, the subsequent intimal proliferations likely follow cytokine release, smooth muscle cell migration and proliferation in the intima, macrophage migration into the intima, extracellular matrix synthesis, vessel media thinning (perhaps by smooth muscle cell apoptosis), and alterations in endothelial cell function leading to vessel wall remodeling, as noted earlier. Angiotensin II, and its interaction with its AT1 and AT2 receptors, also plays an important role in CAV and may be critical in the differential involvement of large, epicardial coronary arteries and small, intramyocardial arteries *(39)*.

The relationship of CAV to acute cellular rejection remains unclear in reviews from clinical transplant centers *(40,41)*. A discrepancy between acute rejection and vasculopathy is also noted in at least one experimental transplant model *(42)*. Additionally, it has been clinically observed that incremental improvements in immunosuppression improve patient care and markedly reduce the incidence of fatal acute cellular rejection but do not significantly alter the incidence of CAV as a cause of death *(43)*. It is postulated that CAV primarily results from indirect antigen presentation (donor antigens presented by host antigen-presenting cells), whereas acute cellular rejection relies on direct antigen presentation (donor antigen presented by donor cells). If current immunosuppressives such as CyA are better inhibitors of the direct pathway than the indirect pathway of antigen presentation, cellular rejection could be controlled without significant effect on CAV.

TRANSPLANTED HEART REINNERVATION

Limited sympathetic reinnervation occurs in the majority (75–80%) of heart transplant recipients studied 1 yr or more after transplantation *(44)*. The extent of reinnervation varies; the most frequently reinnervated site is the left ventricular anterior wall. Sympathetic innervation restoration lends improved responses of heart rate and contractile function with exercise *(45)*. There is evidence that parasympathetic reinnervation occurs in a small minority of these patients *(46)*. Although recipients with graft vasculopathy and ischemic damage to the myocardium in the first year posttransplantation may not experience chest pain, angina pectoris is reported by some recipients later in the posttransplant period.

POSTTRANSPLANT LYMPHOPROLIFERATIVE DISORDERS

PTLDs are lymphoid proliferations that develop as a direct consequence of immunosuppression in patients who have undergone organ allograft transplantation. PTLDs are, clinically and pathologically, a heterogeneous group of polyclonal and monoclonal proliferations, predominantly of B-cell type and less often T-cell type. The risk of developing a PTLD varies with the allograft type, immunosuppression intensity and type, the presence or absence of immunity to Epstein–Barr virus (EBV) prior to transplantation, and CMV disease development. The highest incidence of PTLDs (approx 10%) is reported in heart and/or lung recipients, and the lowest incidence (less than 1%) is reported in renal transplant recipients *(26,47)*. Hepatic allograft recipients have an intermediate risk (1–2%). PTLD mortality in solid organ allograft recipients is as high as 50–80% *(48)*.

Pathogenesis

The vast majority of PTLDs (80–90%) are associated with EBV infection and represent EBV-driven proliferations *(49–51)*. This association has been demonstrated by many methods, including Southern blot, polymerase chain reaction, *in situ* hybridization techniques, and Western blot. EBV infection is associated with a variety of human malignancies (e.g., Burkitt's lymphoma, Hodgkin's lymphoma, PTLDs, some T-cell lymphomas, gastric carcinomas, nasopharyngeal carcinoma, and smooth muscle neoplasms), and the role of the viral latent genes in the malignant transformation process has been reviewed *(52,53)*. Most PTLD cases in solid organ transplant recipients are believed to arise from the recipient's B lymphocytes *(54)*, rather than from donor B lymphocytes as seen following bone marrow transplantation. In a minority of cases, lymphoid cells transplanted with the allograft can survive and undergo malignant transformation.

The associated EBV infection may be latent in the recipient or may be acquired posttransplantation in naïve recipients (seronegative for EBV; EBV–)through community contacts or after organ receipt from an EBV+ donor. In either instance, in the absence of an EBV-specific immune response (decreased T-cell immune surveillance), EBV undergoes uncontrolled replication and infects the recipient B lymphocytes. The expansion of multiple, polyclonal, EBV-infected and -immortalized B-lymphocyte clones may correspond to the early and polymorphic PTLD lesions (*see* WHO classification below). The subsequent development of several dominant clones may yield oligoclonal proliferations, and the development of a single dominant clone may yield a monoclonal proliferation. The oligoclonal proliferations may not have undergone malignant transformation but are susceptible to such transformation. It is suggested that mutations in the bcl-6 gene *(55)* might be a useful marker for predicting an aggressive clinical course following transformation *(56)*. With mutations in other proto-oncogenes or in tumor suppressor genes, these proliferations develop into malignant neoplasms. Most of these neoplasms have the monomorphic appearance of malignant lymphoma, but some are histologically polymorphic.

Epidemiology

The key risk factors for PTLD development include lack of specific pretransplantation immunity to EBV (EBV–), high doses of antilymphocyte antibody posttransplantation, and CMV disease development. Pretransplantation EBV seronegativity was the first recognized risk factor *(57)*. It is noted that the risk of developing malignancy posttransplantation is related generally to the overall severity of immunosuppression *(58)*, which is dictated by the type of organ transplanted. The addition of cytolytic agents, such as OKT3, as rejection prophylaxis or for refractory rejection treatment, adds additional risk for developing PTLD *(59)*. Some antilymphocyte agents such as OKT3 not only impair EBV-specific immune surveillance but may also stimulate the production of inflammatory cytokines, such as tumor necrosis factor (TNF), that increase EBV transcription and reactivation *(60)*.

A role for CMV disease in promoting PTLD development has been recognized more recently *(61)*. The CMV-naïve recipients of grafts from CMV+ donors are particularly at risk. This synergy of CMV infection and EBV proliferation may also be mediated by the CMV-induced inflammatory cytokine production.

Diagnosis and Classification

The designation "PTLD" covers a wide spectrum of strikingly heterogeneous, EBV-driven lymphproliferative processes, incorporating hyperplastic, neoplastic, polyclonal, and monoclonal lymphoid proliferations. Therefore, PTLD should not be used as a final pathologic diagnostic term without further subclassification. This lesion subclassification, in a manner accurately predicting the subsequent clinical course, has been a great challenge. Sharp distinction between different categories is not always possible because of significant overlapping of clinical and pathologic features. Various descriptive histological groupings have been advanced *(51,54,62,63)*. Whichever classification system is used at a specific center, the success of interinstitutional collaborative diagnostic and therapeutic trials depends on having some common information on each patient's PTLD *(50)*. Briefly, these include information on histology, lesion EBV status including EBV clonality, B- and T-cell clonality, stage (the Ann Arbor Staging Classification with Cotswald Modification *(64)* used for non-Hodgkin's lymphoma should include information on involvement of the allograft itself, central nervous system involvement, and the presence of symptoms), the presence of other cell types, and cell markers associated with therapy (such as CD20).

Gathering this information from individual specimens has certain practical implications. Excisional biopsy is the preferred method for obtaining diagnostic tissue, and needle core biopsy should be used only when an open biopsy is impractical. Cytology procedures do not yield sufficient tissue for PTLD lesion subclassification. The specimen should be processed promptly, and fresh tissue should be submitted for flow cytometric analysis, if possible. The ancillary diagnostic tests are primarily DNA-based. Identification of EBV early RNA is done by *in situ* hybridization method *(65)*. Identification of this RNA species may be performed on routinely processed, formalin-fixed, paraffin-embedded tissue. It should be noted that polyclonal and monoclonal lesions may develop in multiple sites in one patient and represent clonally distinct tumors (66,67).

The World Health Organization (WHO) has adopted a morphologic PTLD classification in its recently proposed classification of tumors of hematopoietic and lymphoid tissues (68). PTLD categories recognized in the proposed WHO classification are briefly discussed below.

In the early lesion category, there are two possible overlapping lesions: infectious mononucleosis-like PTLD and reactive plasmacytic hyperplasia. Usually, the lymphoid tissue architecture is preserved, with interfollicular area expansion (Fig. 4A). Such lesions are usually polyclonal proliferations and do not have structural alterations in oncogenes or tumor suppressor genes (62). Many lesions have evidence of EBV infection, which may be polyclonal, oligoclonal, or monoclonal (49). Immunosuppressive therapy reduction leads to regression of almost all such lesions (69). Rare patients with a reactive plasmacytic hyperplasia may, subsequently, develop a PTLD with different morphologic and molecular characteristics. The new lesion determines their prognosis.

The polymorphic PTLD category includes polymorphic destructive infiltrates obliterating the normal tissue architecture. The proliferating lymphoid cells may include immunoblasts, plasma cells, and atypical intermediate-sized cells (Fig. 4B,C). Frequently, necrosis is present. These lesions contain monoclonal B-cell proliferations with monotypic surface Ig, or no surface Ig, and clonal Ig heavy- and light-chain gene rearrangements. Most of these lesions have clonal EBV. They may have mutations in bcl-6 but lack gene rearrangements in bcl-6 or other oncogenes or tumor suppressor genes. The clinical course of these lesions is variable. Some regress with a reduction in immunosuppression (50,70). Usually, this is the first therapeutic approach to these lesions. However, other lesions progress despite reduced immunosuppression and the addition of aggressive therapy. Whereas most of the patients have a good prognosis and do not die of PTLD, early identification of the few patients with aggressive lesions, with the hope that early treatment may improve outcome, remains the major challenge for pathologists.

The monomorphic PTLD category includes histologically malignant proliferations identical to the non-Hodgkin's lymphomas and myelomas in nonimmunosuppressed persons. Most of these lesions are diffuse large B-cell lymphomas of the WHO classification (68). Rare Burkitt's and Burkitt's-like lymphoma cases have been reported. Clearly, these lesions are malignant with a monomorphic cell population obliterating normal tissue architecture (Fig. 4D). They are B-cell tumors with clonal

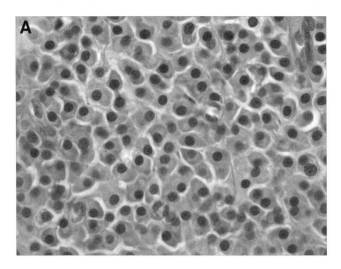

Fig. 4A. Posttransplant lymphoproliferative disorder (PTLD), early lesion, plamacytic hyperplasia. Numerous plasma cells are present. (H&E, ×400)

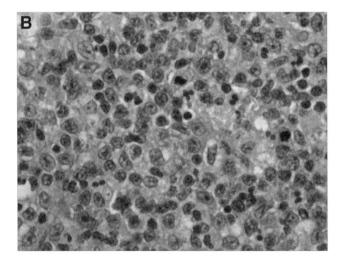

Fig. 4B. PTLD, polymorphic lesion. There is diffuse effacement of the nodal architecture by a polymorphic infiltrate of small, medium, and large trans- formed lymphoid cells. (H&E, ×400)

Ig heavy- and light-chain gene rearrangements. Usually, there is evi- dence of monoclonal EBV infection. The lesions also have structural alterations of one or more proto-oncogenes and/or tumor suppressor genes, most commonly ras, c-myc, or p53 *(62)*. Unlike the early lesions

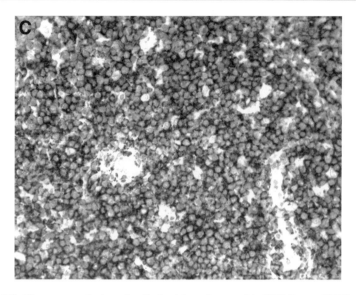

Fig. 4C. The vast majority of cells in this polymorphic PTLD are CD20-positive. (CD20 immunoperoxidase strain, ×200)

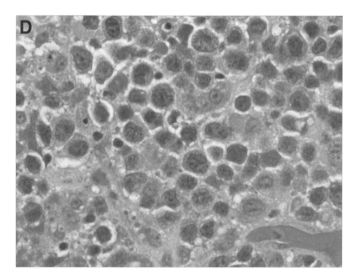

Fig. 4D. PTLD, monomorphic lesion (diffuse large B-cell lymphoma). There is diffuse proliferation of large transformed lymphoid cells. (H&E, ×400)

and the polymorphic PTLD that tend to present with restricted disease, often, these patients present with disseminated (Stage III or IV) disease. These lesions do not regress with immunosuppression reduction and must

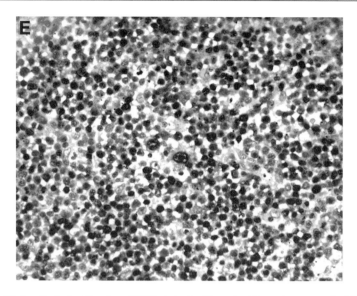

Fig. 4E. *In situ* hybridization (ISH) stain for Epstein–Barr virus encoded RNAs (EBER) showing nuclear staining in many lymphoid cells of variable sizes. (EBER by ISH, ×200)

be treated with combination chemotherapy. Unfortunately, the prognosis is generally poor, and these lymphomas are usually fatal within months.

As noted earlier, the overwhelming majority of PTLDs (80–90%) show EBV infection (Fig. 4E), and, in most, there is evidence of a single EBV infection prior to clonal expansion of the B-cell population *(62,71)*. However, about 10–20% of PTLDs are EBV negative, especially among those occurring at long intervals after organ allograft transplantation *(72)*. It is suggested that the term PTLD be restricted to EBV-positive lesions *(50)* and that late-occurring lymphomas (more than 1 yr after transplant), which are EBV-negative and are identical to lymphomas in immunocompetent subjects should be considered a distinct entity *(73)*. However, it is also noted *(74)* that some of these EBV-negative lesions respond to decreased immunosuppression and EBV-negative positivity should not be an absolute PTLD diagnosis criterion. The classifications noted earlier can also be applied to EBV-negative tumors. Future studies can determine whether the incidence of EBV-negative lymphomas is higher in transplant patients than in the general population, and, if so, they can explain the differences between EBV-positive and EBV-negative PTLD.

T-cell lymphoproliferative disorders following transplantation are rare in the Western world but are reported more frequently in Japan, particularly among renal transplant patients *(75)*. Approximately half of these cases are adult T-cell leukemia/lymphoma with seropositivity for human T-lymphotropic virus (HTLV)-1, and HTLV-1 genome detected in the tumor. Mutations in p53, c-kit, and β-catenin genes are frequently present *(76)*. These T-cell lesions tend to have an aggressive clinical course.

Classical Hodgkin's lymphoma cases have been described in allograft recipients. The diagnosis should be based on both classical morphologic and immunophenotypic features.

Extranodal marginal zone lymphomas of the mucosa-associated lymphoid tissue-type are not considered part of the PTLD spectrum. There is no apparent role for EBV in their pathogenesis, and these lymphomas are not clinically aggressive *(77)*. It remains to be seen whether they occur at an increased frequency in transplant recipients.

OTHER VIRUSES AFFECTING GRAFT SURVIVAL

Viral infection's role in triggering cardiac allograft rejection and graft loss is the subject of debate *(78)*. An association of CMV infection with rejection and vasculopathy has been described *(79)*. The association's pathogenesis is not clear; molecular mimicry between CMV and specific histocompatibility antigens could be a direct link. A stimulation of cytokine release by CMV infection, leading to upregulation of class II antigens on the graft, is an indirect link *(35)*. Adenovirus genome identification in pediatric allograft recipient hearts may predict reduced graft survival resulting from acute rejection, chronic graft dysfunction, or vasculopathy *(80)*.

ALTERNATIVE REJECTION MARKERS

Endomyocardial biopsy's invasive nature and the challenges of performing biopsies in young children have propelled the search for alternative diagnostic rejection markers for rejection of the cardiac allograft. To date, none shows a sensitivity and specificity superior to the biopsy. There has been a full spectrum of innovative and exciting approaches, generally studying peripheral blood or employing noninvasive radiologic, echocardiographic, or electrocardiogram studies. Some approaches are described here.

Peripheral Blood

Elevated plasma levels of C-reactive protein predict cardiac allograft failure and correlate with ISHLT Grade 3 rejection frequency *(79)*. Serum levels of interleukin (IL)-6 and -8 and TNF-α are reported as useful *(80,81)* or not useful *(82)* in acute rejection prediction. Applications of microarray technology ("gene chips") may yield profiles of gene activation in peripheral blood that correlate with acute rejection or immunologic quiescence; this technique's expense and technical limitations must be overcome before the tests can be considered diagnostic. A more productive role for cytokine study may be as an adjunct to the biopsy; intragraft cytokine production may distinguish meaningful lymphoid infiltrates from inactive or resolving infiltrates *(83)*.

Lymphocyte Growth From Biopsies

An adjunct to histologic biopsy studies, lymphocyte growth from biopsies has been used to assess the IL-2 responsiveness of the biopsy cells. One piece of biopsy tissue is placed in culture medium supplemented with IL-2 *(84)*. Presumably, only activated lymphocytes already bearing IL-2 receptors proliferate in response. The study determines whether cells seen histologically in the biopsy are actively engaged in rejection. The authors' center gives patients an oral steroid boost and taper if they have Grade 1B or 2 biopsy histology and have a positive lymphocyte growth assay.

Echocardiographic Data

Noninvasive studies assessing ventricular function or wall motion, or judging the presence of interstitial edema in the graft, could be expected to correlate well with clinical rejection manifestations. Tissue Doppler wall motion imaging detects ventricular dysfunction more sensitively than conventional echocardiography. Using this technique to avoid "unnecessary" scheduled biopsies and to optimize the timing of angiography for transplant CAD detection has been proposed *(85)*.

OTHER PATHOLOGY RESULTING FROM THERAPY

Postoperative complications and morbidity from immunosuppressive agents are addressed in later chapters. Hypertension and renal toxicity are the primary CyA therapy complications; the renal changes have distinctive morphology *(86)*. Additional CyA pathology may be seen as gingival hypertrophy, hirsutism, and hepatotoxicity, including cholestasis and gallstone formation. In up to 5% of patients, CyA and tacrolimus (Prograf, Fujisawa Healthcare, Deerfield, IL), as calcineurin inhibitors, are associated with severe neurologic symptoms including seizures, cerebellar ataxia, psychosis, and leukoencephalopathy *(87)*. The osteoporosis, avascular necrosis, delayed wound healing, hyperlipidemia, hypertension, and obesity generated by corticosteroid therapy make significant contributions to posttransplant morbidity.

REFERENCES

1. Billingham ME, Cary NRB, Hammond ME, et al. A working formulation for the standardization of nomenclature in the diagnosis of heart and lung rejection: Heart Rejection Study Group. J Heart Transplant 1990;9:587–593.
2. Soto PF, Jia CX, Carter YM, et al. Effect of improved myocardial protection on edema and diastolic properties of the rat left ventricle during acute allograft rejection. J Heart Lung Transplant 1998;17:608–616.
3. Herskowitz A, Soule LM, Ueda K, et al. Arteriolar vasculitis on endomyocardial biopsy: a histologic predictor of poor outcome in cyclosporine-treated heart transplant recipients. J Heart Transplant 1987;6:127.
4. Fishbein MC, Bell G, Lones MA, et al. Grade 2 cellular heart rejection: does it exist? J Heart Lung Transplant 1994;13:1051–1057.
5. Marboe CC, Schierman SW, Rose EA, et al. *In situ* lymphocyte typing in cardiac allograft rejection. Transplant Proc 1984;16:1598–1599.
6. Radio SJ, McManus BM, Winters GL, et al. Preferential endocardial residence of B-cells in the "Quilty effect" of human heart allografts: immunohistochemical distinction from rejection. Mod Pathol 1991;4:654.
7. Schuurman HF, Jambroes G, Borlefs JCC, et al. Acute humoral rejection after heart transplantation. Transplantation 1988;46:603.
8. Bustos M, Platt JL. The pathology of cardiac xenografts. J Card Surg 2001;16:357–362.
9. Teranishi K, Manez R, Awwad M, et al. Anti-Gal-α1-3Gal IgM and IgG antibody levels in sera of humans and old world non-human primates. Xenotransplantation 2002;9:148–154.
10. Galili U. The alpha-gal epitope (Gal α 1-3Gal β 1-4GlcNAc-R) in xenotransplantation. Biochemie 2001;83:557–563.
11. Barr ML, Cohen DJ, Benvenisty AI, et al. Effect of anti-HLA antibodies on the long-term survival of heart and kidney allografts. Transplant Proc 1993;25:262–264.
12. Hammond EH, Yowell RL, Nunoda S, et al., Vascular (humoral) rejection in heart transplantation: pathologic observations and clinical implications. J Heart Transplant 1989;8:430.
13. Hammond EH, Hansen JK, Spencer LS, et al. Immunofluorescence of endomyocardial biopsy specimens: methods and interpretation. J Heart Lung Transplant 1993;12:113.
14. Lones MA, Czer LSC, Trento A, et al. Clinical-pathologic features of humoral rejection in cardiac allografts: a study in 81 consecutive patients. J Heart Lung Transplant 1995;14:151.
15. Miller LW, Wesp A, Jamieson SH, et al. Vascular rejection in heart transplant recipients. J Heart Lung Transplant 1993;12:147.
16. Faulk WP, Labarrere CA, Pitts D, et al. Vascular lesions in biopsy specimens devoid of cellular infiltrates: qualitative and quantitative immunocytochemical studies of human cardiac allografts. J Heart Lung Transplant 1993;12:219.
17. Bonnaud EN, Lewis NP, Masek MA, et al. Reliability and usefulness of immunofluorescence in heart transplantation. J Heart Lung Transplant 1995;14:163.
18. Feucht H, Opelz G. The humoral immune response towards HLA-class II determinants in renal transplantation. Kidney Int 1996;50:1464.
19. Cosio FG, Sedmak DD, Mahan JD, et al. Localizaton of decay accelerating factor in normal and diseased kidneys. Kidney Int 1989;36:100.
20. Morgan BP. Complement regulatory molecules: application to therapy and transplantation. Immunol Today 1995;16:257.

21. Cherry R, Nielsen H, Reed E, et al. Vascular (humoral) rejection in human cardiac allograft biopsies: relation to circulating anti-HLA antibodies. J Heart Lung Transplant 1993;11:24.

22. Feucht HE, Schneeberger H, Hillebrand G, et al. Capillary deposition of C4d complement fragment and early renal graft loss. Kidney Int 1993;43:1333.

23. Regele H, Exner M, Watschinger B, et al. Endothelial C4d deposition is associated with inferior kidney allograft outcome independently of cellular rejection. Nephrol Dial Transplant 2001;16:2058–2066.

24. Behr TM, Feucht HE, Richter K, et al. Detection of humoral rejection in human cardiac allografts by assessing the capillary deposition of complent fragment C4d in endomyocardial biopsies. J Heart Lung Transplant 1999;18:904–912.

25. Hammond EH, Wittwer CT, Greenwood J, et al. Relationship of OKT3 sensitization and vascular rejection in cardiac transplant patients receiving OKT3 rejection prophylaxis. Transplantation 1990;50:776.

26. Hosenpud JD, Bennett LE, Keck BM, et al. The registry of the International Society for Heart and Lung Transplantation: 18th Official Report—2001. J Heart Lung Transplant 2001;20:805–815.

27. Julius BK, Attenhofer Jost CH, Sutsch G, et al. Incidence, progression and functional significance of cardiac allograft vasculopathy after heart transplantation. Transplantation 2000;69:847–853.

28. Mills RM, Billett JM, Nichols WW. Endothelial dysfunction early after heart transplantation: assessment with intravascular ultrasound and Doppler. Circulation 1992;86:1171–1174.

29. Pethig K, Klauss V, Heublein B, et al. Progression of cardiac allograft vascular disease as assessed by serial intravascular ultrasound: correlation to immunological and non-immunological factors. Heart 2000;84:494–498.

30. Tsutsui H, Ziada KM, Schoenhagen P, et al. Lumen loss in transplant coronary artery disease is a biphasic process involving early intimal thickening and late constrictive remodeling: results from a 5-year serial intravascular ultrasound study. Circulation 2001;104:653–657.

31. Wong C, Ganz P, Miller L, et al. Role of vascular remodeling in the pathogenesis of early tranplant coronary artery disease: a multicenter prospective intravascular ultrasound study. J Heart Lung Transplant 2001;20:385–392.

32. Pirolo JS, Hutchins GM, Moore GW. Myocyte vacuolization in infarct border zones is reversible. Am J Pathol 1985;121:444–450.

33. Reimer KA, Ideker RE. Myocardial ischemia and infarction: anatomic and biochemical substrates for ischemic cell death and ventricular arrhythmias. Human Pathol 1987;18:462–475.

34. Furukawa Y, Libby P, Stinn JL, et al. Cold ischemia induces isograft arteriopathy, but does not augment allograft arteriopathy in non-immunosuppressed hosts. Am J Pathol 2002;160:1077–1087.

35. Weis M, von Scheidt W. Cardiac allograft vasculopathy: a review. Circulation 1997;96:2069–2077.

36. Marboe CC. Cardiac transplant vasculopathy. In: Hammond EH, ed. Solid Organ Transplantation Pathology. WB Saunders, Philadelphia, PA: 1994, p. 111.

37. Salomon RN, Hughes CCW, Schoen FJ, et al. Human coronary transplantation-associated atherosclerosis: evidence for a chronic immune reaction to activated graft endothelial cells. Am J Pathol 1991;138:791.

38. Itescu S, Tung TC, Burke EM, et al. An immunological algorithm to predict risk of high-grade rejection in cardiac transplant recipients. Lancet 1998;352:263–270.

39. Richter M, Richter H, Skupin M, et al. Do vascular compartments differ in the development of chronic rejection? AT1 blocker candesartan versus ACE blocker enalapril in an experimental heart transplant model. J Heart Lung Transplant 2001;20:1092–1098.
40. Costanzo-Nordin MR. Cardiac allograft vasculopathy: relationship with acute cellular rejection and histocompatibility. J Heart Lung Transplant 1992;11(suppl):S90.
41. Hauptman PJ, Nakagawa T, Tanaka H, et al. Acute rejection: culprit or coincidence in the pathogenesis of cardiac graft vascular disease? J Heart Lung Transplant 1995;14(suppl):S173.
42. Hillebrands JL, Raue HP, Klatter FA, et al. Intrathymic immune modulation prevents acute rejection but not the development of graft atherosclerosis (chronic rejection). Transplantation 2001;71:914–924.
43. Rajasinghe JR, Chen JM, Weinberg AD, et al. Long-term outcomes after cardiac tranplantation: an experience based on different eras of immunosuppressive therapy. Ann Thorac Surg 2001;72:440–449.
44. Wilson RF, Christensen BV, Olivari MT, et al. Evidence for structural sympathetic reinnervation after orthotopic cardiac transplantatin in humans. Circulation 1991;83:1210–1220.
45. Bengel FM, Ueberfuhr P, Schiepel N, et al. Effect of sympathetic reinnervation on cardiac performance after transplantation. New Engl J Med 2001;345:731–738.
46. Uberfuhr P, Frey AW, Reichart B. Vagal reinnervation in the long term after orthotopic heart transplantation. J Heart Lung Transplant 2000;19:946–950.
47. Chadburn A, Cesarman E, Knowles DM. Molecular pathology of the posttransplantation lymphoproliferative disorders. Semin Diagn Pathol 1997;14:15–26.
48. Benkerrou M, Jais JP, Leblond V, et al. Anti-B cell monoclonal antibody treatment of severe posttransplant b lymphoproliferative disorder: prognosis factors and long-term outcome. Blood 1998;92:3137.
49. Knowles DM. Immunodeficiency-associated lymphoproliferative disorders. Mod Pathol 1999;12:200–217.
50. Paya CV, Fung JJ, Nalesnik MA, et al. Epstein–Barr virus-induced posttransplant lymphoproliferative disorders. Transplantation 1999;68:1517–1525.
51. Harris NL, Ferry JA, Swerdlow SH. Posttransplant lymphoproliferative disorders (PTLD): summary of Society for Hematopathology Workshop. Semin Diag Pathol 1997;14:8.
52. Cohen JI. Epstein–Barr virus infection. New Engl J Med 2000;343:481–492.
53. Baumforth KRN, Young LS, Flavell KJ, et al. The Epstein–Barr virus and its association with human cancers. J Clin Pathol: Mol Pathol 1999;52:307–322.
54. Nalesnik MA, Jaffe R, Starzl TE, et al. The pathology of posttransplant lymphoproliferative disorders occurring in the setting of cyclosporine A-prednisone immunosuppression. Am J Pathol 1988;133:173.
55. Ye BH, Cattoretti G, Shen Q, et al. The bcl-6 proto-oncogene controls germinal center formation and Th2-type inflammation. Nat Genetics 1977;16:161–170.
56. Cesarman E, Chadburn A, Liu YF, et al. bcl-6 gene mutations in post-transplantation lymphoproliferative disorders as predictors of response to therapy and clinical outcome. Blood 1998;92:2294–2302.
57. Ho M, Breinig MK, Dummer JS, et al. Epstein–Barr virus infections and DNA hybridization studies inn posttransplantation lymphoma and lymphoproliferative lesions: the role of primary infection. J Infect Dis 1985:152:876.
58. Penn I. Posttransplant malignancy: the role of immunosuppression. Drug Saf 2000;23:101–113.

59. Swinnen LJ, Costanzo-Dordin MR, Fisher SG, et al. Increased incidence of lymphoproliferataive disorder after immunosuppression with the monoclonal antibody OKT3 in cardiac transplant recipients. N Engl J Med 1990;323:1723.

60. Vincenti F, Danovitch GM, Neylan JF, et al. Pentoxifylline does not prevent the cytokine-induced first dose reaction following OKT3—a randomized, double-blind placebo-controlled study. Transplantation 1996;61:573.

61. Manez R, Breinig MC, Linden P, et al. Posttransplant lymphoproliferative disease in primary Epstein–Barr virus infection after liver transplantation: the role of cytomegalovirus disease. J Infect Dis 1997;176:1462.

62. Knowles DM, Cesarman E, Chadburn A, et al. Correlative morphologic and molecular genetic analysis demonstrates three distinct categories of posttransplantation lymphoprolifertive disorders. Blood 1995;85:552.

63. Frizzera G, Hanto DW, Gajl-Peczalska KJ, et al. Polymorphic diffuse B-cell hyperplasias and lymphomas in renal transplant recipients. Cancer Res 1981; 41:4262–4279.

64. Lister TA, Armitage JO. Non-Hodgkin's lymphomas. In: Abeloff MD, Armitage JO, Lichter AS, Niederhuber JE, eds. Clinical Oncology.Churchill Livingstone Inc., New York: 1995, p. 2109.

65. Glickman JN, Howe JG, Steitz JA. Structural analysis of EBER1 and EBER2 ribonucleoprotein particles present in Epstein–Barr virus-infected cells. J Virol 1988;62:902.

66. Cleary ML, Sklar J. Lymphoproliferative disorders in cardiac transplant recipients are multiclonal lymphomas. Lancet 1984;ii:489–493.

67. Chadburn A, Cesarman E, Liu YF, et al. Molecular genetic analysis demonstrates that multiple posttransplantation lymphoproliferative disorders occurring in one anatomic site in a single patient represent distinct primary lymphoid neoplasms. Cancer 1995;75:2747–2756.

68. Pathology and genetics of tumors of hematopoietic and lymphoid tissues. In: Jaffe ES, Harris NL, Stein H, Vardiman JW, eds. World Health Organization Classification of Tumors. IARC Press, Lyon: 2001.

69. Chadburn A, Chen JM, Hsu DT, et al. The morphologic and molecular genetic categories of posttransplantation lymphoproliferative disorders are clinically relevant. Cancer 1998;82:1978–1987.

70. Starzl TE, Nalesnik MA, Porter KA, et al. Reversibility of lymphomas and lymphoproliferative lesions developing under cyclosporin-steroid therapy. Lancet 1984;i:583–587.

71. Cleary ML, Nalesnik MA, Shearer WT, et al. Clonal analysis of transplant-associated lymphoproliferations based on the structure of the genomic termini of the Epstein–Barr virus. Blood 1988;72:49–52.

72. Leblond V, Davi F, Charlotte F, et al. Posttransplant lymphoproliferative disorders not associated with Epstein–Barr virus: a distinct entity? J Clin Oncol 1998;16: 2052–2059.

73. Dotti G, Fiocchi R, Motta T, et al. Epstein–Barr virus-negative lymphoproliferative disorders in long-term survivors after heart, kidney and liver transplant. Transplantation 2000;69:827–833.

74. Nelson BP, Nalesnik MA, Bahler DW, et al. Epstein–Barr virus-negative posttransplant lymphoproliferative disorder: a distinct entity? Am J Surg Path 2000;24:375–385.

75. Hoshida Y, Li T, Dong Z, et al. Lymphoproliferative disorders in renal transplant patients in Japan. Int J Cancer 2001;91:869–875.

76. Hoshida Y, Hongyo T, Nakatsuka S, et al. Gene mutations in lymphoproliferative disorders of T and NK/T cell phenotypes developing in renal transplant patients. Lab Invest 2002;82:257–264.

77. Hsi ED, Singleton TP, Swinnen L, et al. Mucosa-associated lymphoid tissue-type lymphomas occurring in posttransplantation patients. Am J Surg Path 2000; 24:100–106.

78. Avery RK. Viral triggers of cardiac-allograft dysfunction. New Engl J Med 2001;344:1545–1547.

79. Grattan MT, Moreno-Cabral CE, Starnes VA, et al. Cytomegalovirus infection is associated with cardiac allograft rejection and atherosclerosis. JAMA 1989;261: 3561–3566.

80. Shirali GS, Ni J, Chinnock RE, et al. Association of viral genome with graft loss in children after cardiac transplantation. New Engl J Med 2001;344:1498–1503.

81. Eisenberg MS, Chen HJ, Warshofsky MK, et al. Elevated levels of plasma C-reactive protein are associated with decreased graft survival in cardiac transplant recipients. Circulation 2000;102:2100–2104.

82. Kimball PM, Radovancevic B, Isom T, et al. The paradox of cytokine moitoring— predictor of immunologic activity as well as immunologic silence following cardiac transplantation. Transplantation 1996;61:909–915.

83. Abdallah AN, Billes MA, Attia Y, et al. Evaluation of plasma levels of tumour necrosis factor alpha and IL-6 as rejection markers in a cohort of 142 heart-grafted patients followed by endomyocardial biopsy. Eur Heart J 1997;18:1024–1029.

84. George JF, Kirklin JK, Naftel DC, et al. Serial measurements of interleukin-6, interleukin-8, tumor necrosis factor-alpha, and soluble vascular adhesion molecule-

7   Posttransplant Management

Sean P. Pinney, MD

INTRODUCTION

The transition out of the operating room (OR) and into the intensive care unit (ICU) begins the process of caring for the newly transplanted heart. This chapter discusses two distinct aspects of this care: immediate postoperative management, where attention is directed to recovery from the operative procedure, and extended posttransplant care with a focus on immunosuppression, suggested biopsy regimens, and strategies to prevent transplant allograft vasculopathy.

POSTOPERATIVE MANAGEMENT

Hemodynamic Monitoring and Support

The newly transplanted heart faces numerous hemodynamic challenges in the first postoperative days. These include vasodilatory hypotension, allograft dysfunction, right heart failure (RHF), and sinus node dysfunction. To ensure successful allograft function, it is critical that continuous patient monitoring be provided in an ICU staffed by an experienced team that is familiar with transplant patient care. All patients should have a pulmonary artery (PA) catheter and an indwelling arterial

From: *Contemporary Cardiology: Cardiac Transplantation:*
The Columbia University Medical Center/New York-Presbyterian Hospital Manual
Edited by: N. M. Edwards, J. M. Chen, and P. A. Mazzeo © Humana Press Inc., Totowa, NJ

line placed. This allows for adequate monitoring of systemic and PA pressures as well as a left atrial pressure assessment (through wedge pressure measurement).

Adjustments in both positive-inotropic and pressor support can be guided by a continuous cardiac performance assessment. Generally, a slow taper of support begins with vasoconstrictor removal, followed by a reduction in the dose of inotropic drugs. In general, the authors prefer to continue an infusion of dobutamine or milrinone (Primacor, Sanofi Winthrop, New York, NY) for at least 48 h to allow enough time for the sinus node and ventricles to recover from ischemic injury. As long as patients are otherwise hemodynamically stable, they may be moved out of the ICU to a step-down floor with continuous telemetry monitoring and have the medication weaned there.

Respiratory and Ventilatory Management

Although chronic heart failure can produce deleterious changes in the diaphragm and respiratory muscles, most patients can be weaned successfully from the ventilator and extubated within the first 24 h posttransplant. Early extubation is encouraged for all patients to minimize the risk of infection from ventilator-associated pneumonia and obligatory indwelling catheters. In prolonged intubation cases, consideration must be given to performing a tracheostomy. It is our practice to avoid this where possible because of the tracheostomy's proximity to the sternal wound and the increased infection risk in the setting of immunosuppression.

Infection Prevention

Antibiotics are used routinely to prevent surgical wound infections. The usual regimen employs an agent active against Gram-positive cocci, usually a first-generation cephalosporin such as cefazolin. Vancomycin is given to penicillin-sensitive patients. These antibiotics are given only for the first 24 h. Additional nonpharmacologic approaches to minimize perioperative infection risk include strict hand washing, reverse infection control measures, and the prompt removal of indwelling lines and support tubes when deemed appropriate.

Discharge Planning and Patient Education

Discharge planning begins soon after the patient is transferred out of the ICU and onto the floor. There, the patient begins a cardiac rehabilitation program under the care of specially trained physical therapists. This also allows time for transplant team members to meet with patients and their families; they are given personal instruction about their medications including indications, dosing regimens, and potential side effects.

Our nurses also provide in-depth counseling about the lifestyle changes that are required following heart transplantation, including the need to adopt a heart-healthy diet that is low in saturated fat and salt. Patients are advised to limit caloric intake and are strongly encouraged to begin a daily exercise program to promote physical and mental well-being. By the time patients are discharged, they should have a clear understanding of their medical regimen, follow-up appointments, and, most importantly, how to contact the transplant program should questions or an emergency arise.

The first biopsy is planned for postoperative d 7. A biopsy result of International Society for Heart and Lung Transplantation (ISHLT) grade 0 or 1A is required before the patient is suitable for discharge. Low-grade or moderate rejection (ISHLT 1B or 2) usually is treated with intensification of the immunosuppression regimen. Patients with compromised hemodynamics remain in the hospital and receive intravenous therapy. Those with more severe rejection grades, irrespective of hemodynamics, receive either intravenous methylprednisolone or an appropriate rescue agent. When patients have a therapeutic level of a calcineurin inhibitor and demonstrate compensated hemodynamics, they are released from the hospital.

POSTOPERATIVE COMPLICATIONS

Vasodilatory Hypotension

Vasodilatory hypotension is frequently encountered following heart transplant operations. One mechanism underlying this loss of vascular tone includes the common preoperative use of angiotensin-converting enzyme (ACE) inhibitors, amiodarone, and vasodilatory inotropic drugs (inodilators) such as milrinone *(1)*. Sometimes, vasodilation is the manifestation of a systemic inflammatory response following cardiopulmonary bypass with membrane oxygenation resulting from inflammatory cytokine activation *(2)*. Vasodilation may also result from a baroreflex-mediated depletion of arginine vasopressin (AVP) *(3,4)*. Although most patients with congestive heart failure, especially those in cardiogenic shock, have elevated levels of endogenous AVP, low AVP levels have been documented in patients with decompensated heart failure *(5)*. It is suggested that excess preoperative, baroreflex-mediated release of vasopressin could expedite the depletion of endogenous AVP stores in response to an acute stimulus (such as cardiopulmonary bypass) and, thereby, precipitate vasodilatory hypotension *(6)*.

Vasopressor catecholamines, such as norepinephrine, are the mainstay of postcardiotomy vasodilation treatment, but the effectiveness of these drugs is limited both by the frequency of catecholamine resistance and by significant toxicity at higher doses. In several studies, AVP infusion at doses ranging from 2 to 6 U/h had a dramatic effect in patients with postcardiotomy shock following cardiac transplant surgery or left ventricular assist device (LVAD) implantation *(7,8)*. In those studies, patients receiving norepinephrine who had persistent refractory hypotension (defined as a mean arterial pressure less than 60 mmHg) experienced an increase in systemic blood pressure after receiving vasopressin that was great enough to reduce, and eventually terminate, norepinephrine infusion. The increase in systemic pressure was not produced at the expense of constriction of other vascular beds; indeed, no increase in PA pressure was demonstrated, thereby supporting the belief that there is an absence of vasopressin receptors in the pulmonary vascular bed. These qualities make vasopressin particularly useful in the transplant population, in which RHF and pre-existing pulmonary hypertension can be exacerbated by catecholamine-induced pulmonary vascular constriction.

Treatment with vasopressin also obviates the need for an indwelling left atrial catheter, which was advocated as a means of facilitating vasopressor catecholamine infusion directly into the systemic circulation and bypassing the pulmonary vascular bed. Vasopressin does not compromise renal function. Unlike catecholamine receptors, which are concentrated primarily in the afferent arteriole and produce a decline in filtration fraction when stimulated, vasopressin receptors are concentrated on the efferent arteriole *(9)* and, therefore, increase filtration fraction and spare renal perfusion when stimulated. The end result is that vasopressin helps preserve, and in some cases increase, the volume of urine output.

Acute Allograft Dysfunction

Acute postoperative allograft dysfunction is a significant clinical problem that accounts for 30% of early posttransplant deaths *(10)*. The causes of acute allograft dysfunction include ischemia-reperfusion injury, problems with preservation, prolonged ischemic time (particularly in excess of 4 h), and unrecognized or underappreciated donor heart dysfunction. Myocardial dysfunction occurs, to some degree, in all brain-dead organ donors and is so severe in approx 20% of cases that it precludes organ donation *(11)*. Whereas contraction band necrosis is seen in the hearts of brain-dead donors, a recent study suggested that the acute myocardial dysfunction in these patients arises from increased activity of inhibitory G proteins that impair myocardial contractility *(12)*. Hyperacute rejection (perhaps the most feared cause of postoperative allograft dysfunction) is a risk in patients with an elevated panel reactive antibody pretransplant because of the presence of preformed antibodies to human leukocyte antigens (HLA); however, prospective cross-matching virtually eliminates this possibility.

Allograft dysfunction may be detected by several modalities, beginning with intraoperative transesophageal echocardiography (TEE). A need for multiple inotropic agents to wean the patient from cardiopulmonary bypass, or an early decline in PA saturation or thermodilution cardiac output in the ICU, also suggests allograft dysfunction.

Electrocardiograms (EKGs) should be obtained in all patients arriving in the ICU and should be repeated daily. A loss of QRS voltage may be a harbinger of acute rejection. Widespread ST-segment elevation may be seen in a pattern suggestive of acute pericarditis; however, localized ST-segment elevation may be an indication of focal injury. Air embolism down the right coronary artery may produce ST-segment elevation in the inferior leads with other indicators of right ventricular dysfunction. Typically, these findings are transient and usually resolve over a few hours without any negative sequelae. Rarely, ST-segment elevation is a sign of infarction from donor-transmitted coronary artery disease (CAD) or a manifestation of severe rejection.

Dobutamine or milrinone infusions are almost always sufficient treatment for lesser degrees of allograft dysfunction. Some patients require a slower taper of these drugs after discharge from the ICU, but most donor hearts recover without substantial long-term sequelae. More severe degrees of dysfunction from either poor preservation or acute rejection require mechanical support with the use of intra-aortic balloon counterpulsation, placed in the OR, to facilitate weaning from cardiopulmonary bypass. Finally, in rare instances, the implantation of a LVAD or biventricular assist device is necessary to provide full support until recovery from preservation injury occurs. Patients who can successfully be weaned from the device have a survival rate similar to the general of transplant recipient population *(13)*. Patients who fail to wean from these devices have a uniformly fatal outcome; often, they succumb to multisystem organ failure and generally are not acceptable retransplantation candidates.

Right Heart Failure

RHF is a frequent complication of cardiac transplantation. The thin-walled right ventricle (RV) is particularly vulnerable to both ischemic and reperfusion injury (14). Poor preservation may also occur because of the difficulties of perfusing the RV with preservation solution. Many transplant recipients have pre-existing pulmonary hypertension. When faced with such afterload mismatch, the donor heart may strain and acutely fail. Inotrope infusions support the failing RV, which may require as long as 2–4 wk to adapt. Multiple blood product infusions, including packed red blood cells and fresh frozen plasma, may exacerbate an already fully loaded RV. In the face of this additional preload, ventricular function may deteriorate, and thromboxane release may worsen pulmonary hypertension. Transplantation of a smaller donor heart into a larger recipient, so-called donor–recipient mismatch, predisposes to RV dysfunction more than to left ventricle (LV) dysfunction.

RHF should be suspected when the central venous pressure (CVP) is elevated and the cardiac output is low. Transthoracic echocardiography may not offer adequate RV visualization in postoperative patients because of an inability to obtain sufficient echocardiographic windows or position the patient properly; thus, TEE is usually preferred in intubated patients.

Recipients with pulmonary hypertension and low cardiac outputs may be treated with inhaled nitric oxide to lower pulmonary pressures and unload the RV (15). Inotropic support with milrinone is preferred to dobutamine, because the former is more effective in dilating the pulmonary vascular bed. Attempts to remove fluid should be made with diuretic agents or continuous veno-venous hemofiltration (CVVH) to reduce RV preload. A Swan–Ganz catheter is particularly helpful to guide fluid management and accurately measure CVP and RV hemodynamics.

Atrial and Ventricular Arrhythmias

Sinus bradycardia is the most commonly encountered arrhythmia after heart transplant surgery. Realizing that the denervated heart has a resting rate of 90–115 beats per minute (bpm), rates slower than this are inappropriately low and arise commonly because of sinoatrial (SA) node ischemia or preoperative use of animodarone. The use of bicaval anastamoses significantly reduces the incidence of sinus node dysfunction, likely from reduced trauma to the SA node. In the past, isoproterenol was used commonly to maintain heart rate, but it is rarely, if ever, used now, having been replaced by temporary epicardial pacing.

We recommend pacing at 100 bpm, especially in patients with allograft dysfunction. Pacing wires should remain in place until all chronotropic agents are weaned off to ensure that sinus node dysfunction is not present.

Atrial arrhythmias are seen uncommonly in transplant patients, but the presence of atrial fibrillation or atrial flutter may be a harbinger of acute allograft rejection *(16)*. Rarely, ventricular tachyarrhythmias are seen. Unlike atrial arrhythmias, which are suggestive of rejection, ventricular arrhythmias are usually a marker of myocardial ischemia and CAD (although they may also be present in the setting of severe rejection). Transplantation of donor hearts with pre-existing conduction abnormalities has occurred. In one report, three donor hearts were discovered, posttransplant, to have underlying conduction system disease, including one with AV nodal re-entrant tachycardia, one with Wolf–Parkinson–White syndrome, and one with atrial flutter *(17)*. All were successfully treated with catheter ablation.

Postoperative Renal Failure

Renal dysfunction is a frequent perioperative complication occurring in almost half of all heart transplant recipients. Postoperative renal failure is usually a consequence of ischemic injury resulting from aortic cross-clamping, thromboemboli, or perioperative hypotension. Renal failure may lengthen hospital stay and increase posttransplant mortality. In our experience with older recipients, those who experienced a postoperative rise in creatinine above 2.5 mg/dL had an increased incidence of sternal wound infection, longer ventilatory support times, and prolonged ICU and hospital stays *(18)*.

Because of pre-existing heart failure, many patients are volume-overloaded at the time of heart transplantation. Blood product infusions during the operation only add to this volume load. Often, most patients "auto-diurese" once the kidneys enjoy a normal cardiac output and begin to regulate volume status. Others, particularly those with underlying renal dysfunction, require intermittent treatment with a loop diuretic to remove excess fluid volume. The introduction of calcineurin inhibitors and the addition of corticosteroids may result in additional fluid reabsorption in the early postoperative period, further necessitating diuretic use. Those patients with reduced urine outputs may not be able to match their obligatory inputs while they receive inotropes, pressors, and blood products. These patients require mechanical renal replacement therapy. In this situation, CVVH allows for removal of large volumes of fluid and may facilitate renal recovery.

The presence of a rising creatinine can delay cyclosporine (CyA) administration; CyA is a vasoconstrictor and nephrotoxic drug. Induction therapy with daclizumab can safely allow the delayed introduction of CyA a few days after heart transplantation. For many, this extra time allows renal function to recover enough to tolerate the initiation of CyA. For those patients in whom prompt renal recovery appears unlikely, cytolytic therapy with OKT3 needs to be given. Because of the risk of cytokine release and capillary leak syndrome, such patients must remain euvolemic, even if this requires CVVH.

Unfortunately, many heart transplant recipients, particularly those who are hypertensive, have an impaired ability to effectively regulate salt and water balance after transplant. These patients have a blunted diuretic and natriuretic response to volume expansion that may be mediated by a failure to suppress fluid regulatory hormones such as atrial natriuretic peptide and angiotensin II *(19)*. In these patients, salt-sensitive hypertension can be treated with loop diuretics and may be ameliorated by treatment with an ACE inhibitor *(20)*.

EXTENDED POSTTRANSPLANT MANAGEMENT

Routine Immunosuppression

The introduction of CyA in the 1980s revolutionized transplantation by greatly reducing the incidence of acute rejection and improving survival. CyA remains the cornerstone of a three-drug immunosuppressive regimen, but the development of newer drugs allows for some flexibility and individualization of therapy. Like most, our regimen includes a calcineurin inhibitor (CyA or tacrolimus) in combination with an antimetabolite (mycophenolate mofetil [MMF] or azathioprine) and prednisone. Occasionally, rapamycin is administered in combination with a lower dose of a calcineurin inhibitor, as the combination may have a renal-sparing effect. Immunospuppression begins preoperatively with the oral administration of azathioprine (4 mg/kg), followed by methylprednisolone (500 mg) in the OR, usually after the patient is weaned from cardiopulmonary bypass. An overview of the most commonly prescribed immunosuppressive drugs and a typical schedule for maintenance immunosuppression used at Columbia–Presbyterian are presented in Tables 1 and 2, respectively.

Induction therapy with monoclonal or polyclonal antibodies has met with varied success in preventing acute rejection episodes. Allograft rejection only appears to be delayed by their use, and the generalized immunosuppression they induce inscreases posttransplant complication

Table 1
Immunosuppressive Drugs

Drug	Mechanism of action	Dose	Side effects
Azathioprine (Imuran)	Inhibit purine synthesis	2 mg/kg/d (titrated to WBC of 5000/cc)	Bone marrow suppression; hepatotoxicity; nausea; diarrhea; leukopenia
Mycophenolate mofetil (Cell cept)	Inhibit purine synthesis	1500 mg bid	Nausea; diarrhea; leukopenia
Corticosteroids	Inhibit macrophage migration factor; inhibit processing and display of Ag; inhibit IL-1 release and synthesis of IL-1 and 2	0–100 mg/d	Diabetes; osteoporosis; obesity; dyslipidemia
Cyclosporine (Neoral, Sandimmune)	Inhibits IL-2 production by blocking the calcineurin pathway	6 mg/kg/d administered bid (titrated to a trough blood level)	Nephrotoxicity; headache; tremor; hyperkalemia; photosensitivity; gingival hyperplasia
Tacolimus (Prograf)	Binds to FKBP-12 and interferes with IL-2 production	0.15–0.3 mg/kg/d administered bid (titrated to trough blood level)	Nephrotoxicity; hyperkalemia; headache; tremor
Rapamycin, sirolimus (Rapamune)	Binds to FKBP-12 and inhibits cell cycle progression	6 mg loading dose; 2–4 mg/d	Thrombocytopenia; hypertriglyceridemia
ATGAM	Induces lymphocyte depletion	10–20 mg/kg IV	Thrombocytopenia: leukopenia; fever; serum sickness; allergic reaction

continued

Table 1 (*Continued*)
Immunosuppressive Drugs

Drug	Mechanism of action	Dose	Side effects
OKT3	CD3 receptor blockade	5 mg/d IV	Cytokine release syndrome; fever; myalgia; aseptic meningitis; antibody formation
Basiliximab	IL-2 receptor blockade	20 mg prior to transplant and on d 4	None
Daclizumab (Zenapax)	IL-2 receptor blockade	1 mg/kg on d 1 and every 2 wk for 5 doses	None

Abbreviations: IL, interleukin; WBC, white blood cell; bid, twice daily; IV, intravenous; ATGAM, antithymocyte globulin; FKBP-12, FK-binding protein-12.

Table 2
Maintenance Immunosuppression

Week	1	2	3	4	5	6	7	8	12	16–24	25–52	>52
Daclizumab (1 mg/kg)	+		+		+		+					
Prednisone (mg/d)	50	30	25	20		15		10	7.5	5	Taper as tolerated	
Mycophenolate mofetil (mg/d)								3000				
Cyclosporine level (ng/mL)	300–350							250–350			150–250	100–150
Tacrolimus level (ng/mL)	15–20							12–15			8–12	5–10

risks, including opportunistic infection and the development of posttransplant lymphoproliferative disorder (PTLD). Daclizumab (Zenapax, Hoffman-LaRoche, Nutley, NJ) is a humanized monoclonal antibody that binds to activated interleukin (IL)-2 receptors. It is administered on postoperative d 1 and at 2-wk intervals for a total of five doses. It is given intravenously (1 mg/kg) over 15 min without the need for premedication.

Daclizumab's use as induction therapy for cardiac allograft recipients was tested in a single-center study conducted at Columbia–Presbyterian *(21)*. Daclizumab reduced both the severity and frequency of cardiac allograft rejection during the induction period and increased the time to a first rejection episode. Its administration was not associated with any short-term adverse reactions such as allergy, cytokine release, or myalgias. Similarly, there was no increase in the rates of infection or cancer in daclizumab-treated patients. Although this study was not powered to detect a survival difference, a multicenter trial will be completed soon and will provide further information regarding the safety and efficacy of daclizumab. Studies with basiliximab (Simulect, Novartis, East Hanover, NJ), another IL-2 monoclonal antibody, are ongoing.

In addition to receiving daclizumab, patients on postoperative d 1 begin to receive tapering doses of intravenous methylprednisolone and MMF (1500 mg) twice daily (bid). Oral prednisone is substituted for methylprednisolone when the patient is extubated and tolerating clear liquids, and MMF can be given orally at this time.

CyA is the most frequently used immunosuppressive agent at most cardiac transplant centers. Its major immunosuppressive effect is to inhibit the production of IL-2 and other cytokines by activated lymphocytes. CyA binds to cyclophilin in the cytoplasm of T lymphocytes, and this complex then binds to and inhibits calcineurin, a calcium calmodulin-dependent phosphatase responsible for intracellular calcium signaling. Interruption of this signal prevents IL-2 gene transcription and, therefore, IL-2 production. CyA affects T helper and cytotoxic T cells but has little or no effect on suppressor T cells. The drug is metabolized by cytochrome P450 3A4, located in the liver and along the gastrointestinal tract. Approximately 5–10% of the parent compound is excreted unchanged in the urine. CyA has a half-life of 19 h.

Different formulations of CyA are supplied for both intravenous and oral administration. When given intravenously, CyA is mixed in a 1:1 concentration in either normal saline or 5% dextrose and infused continuously. CyA (Sandimmune, Novartis, East Hanover, NJ) for oral use is provided in liquid (100 mg/mL) and capsule form and is administered two or three times daily. Neoral (Novartis, East Hanover, NJ) is a

Table 3
Target Whole Blood CyA[a] Levels

Time posttransplant	CyA[a] level (ng/mL)
0–1 mo	300–350
1–6 mo	250–350
6–12 mo	150–250
> 12 mo	100–150

[a]Cyclosporine

microemulsion formulation of CyA that has improved absorption and bioavailability and is given in two daily doses; it is the preferred formulation at the authors' center.

The method by which CyA is administered to patients varies at different transplant centers. Some choose to begin a continuous CyA infusion immediately after transplant. This method allows for the prompt initiation of potent immunosuppression, with an ability to titrate the dose based on whole blood levels, but must be tempered by renal function. A typical continuous infusion begins at 0.5–1.0 mg/h and is adjusted accordingly. When converting to oral CyA, approximately three times the total daily intravenous dose is given.

Other providers adopt a different approach toward initiating CyA, delaying the drug's initiation a couple of days. This is accomplished by using induction therapy, such as with daclizumab. In such a scenario, one can administer CyA on postoperative d 2 or 3, when renal function has recovered and the patient can begin enteral nutrition. In the early posttransplant period, CyA is administered to achieve a trough whole blood level of 300–350 ng/mL (usually in the range of 3–8 mg/kg/d). Target levels decrease with time as rejection risk begins to taper. The levels the authors aim for are 250–350 in the first 6 mo, 150–250 in mo 6–12, and 100–150 long-term (see Table 3).

CyA produces many side effects, including nephrotoxicity, hypertension, hypertrichosis, gingival hyperplasia, tremor, and seizures. Serum levels of CyA are affected by many medications (see Table 4). Those that elevate serum levels are drugs that inhibit its metabolism through the cytochrome P450 system, such as erythromycin, fluconazole, and amiodarone. Diltiazem is prescribed at many centers, because it not only treats the hypertension that is present in as many as 80% of CyA-treated patients but also helps raise CyA levels so that the required daily Neoral or Sandimmune dose is lowered, thereby saving money. Drugs that

Table 4
Common Drug Interactions With CyA[a]

Increase CyA[a] levels	Decrease CyA[a] levels
Diltiazem	Ethanol
Amiodarone	Phenobarbital
Ciprofloxacin	Phenytoin
Ketoconazole	Rifampin
Fluconazole	Isoniazid
Erythromycin	Cholestyramine
Verapamil	Carbamazepine
Cimetidine	
Nicardipine	
Metoclopromide	

[a]Cyclosporine

induce hepatic enzymes (e.g., ethanol, phenytoin, phenobarbital, and rifampin) increase the CyA clearance and lower serum levels.

Tacrolimus (FK-506, Prograf, Fujisawa, Deerfield, IL) is a newer immunosuppressive drug that was introduced in the late 1980s as a replacement for CyA in liver transplant recipients. Like CyA, tacrolimus is a calcineurin inhibitor that blocks IL-2 production. Unlike CyA, which binds to cyclophilin, tacrolimus binds to FKBP-12, which, in turn, blocks calcineurin-dependent calcium signaling. Studies and clinical experience demonstrate tacrolimus to be an effective substitute for CyA when treating refractory rejection *(22)*. Other small studies support its initial use in lieu of CyA *(23,24)*. The major advantage of tacrolimus over CyA is the lesser degree of hypertension and hyperlipidemia. Some prescribers prefer its use in women for cosmetic reasons, because it produces less hirsutism and gingival hyperplasia. Although tacrolimus is associated with a worsening of glycemic control, later studies have not supported this finding. As with CyA, the major side effect is nephrotoxicity, the mechanism of which is not fully known.

Tacrolimus is supplied both for intravenous and oral administration. When given intravenously, an initial dose of 0.01–0.05 mg/kg/d is infused continuously and adjusted to achieve a level around 15–20 ng/mL. Tacrolimus is administered orally bid, with typical maintenance doses ranging from 2 to 8 mg bid. Doses are adjusted to achieve the trough levels listed in Table 5.

The second of a three-drug regimen usually consists of an anti-proliferative drug such as MMF (Cellcept, Hoffman-LaRoche, Nutley,

Table 5
Target Trough Tacrolimus Levels

Time posttransplant	Tacrolimus level (ng/mL)
0–1 mo	15–20
1–6 mo	12–15
6–12 mo	8–12
> 12 mo	5–10

NJ) or azathioprine (Imuran, Faro, Houston, TX). In our center, MMF has essentially replaced azathioprine as the drug of choice. This decision is supported by the results of a large multicenter clinical trial that randomized 650 patients to receive standard immunosuppressive therapy with CyA and corticosteroids in addition to either MMF or azathioprine *(25)*. In that trial, the group receiving MMF experienced a significant reduction in both mortality and hemodynamically significant rejection in yr 1 of follow-up, as well as a trend toward a lesser incidence of severe (grade 3A or greater) rejection. Opportunistic infections were seen more commonly in patients receiving MMF, but most of these infections resulted from either herpes simplex virus (HSV) or herpes zoster and were not life-threatening.

MMF is a prodrug that is rapidly hydrolyzed to mycophenolic acid (MPA) following ingestion. MPA is a selective, noncompetitive, reversible inhibitor of inosine monophosphate dehydrogenase, an enzyme involved in the *de novo* pathway of purine biosynthesis. Unlike other marrow-derived and parenchymal cells that use the hypoxanthine-guanine phosporibosyl transferase (salvage) pathway, activated lymphocytes rely predominantly on the *de novo* pathway to recycle purine nucleotides. By selectively targeting lymphocyte proliferation, MPA is less likely to produce neutropenia and anemia than is azathioprine, which affects the proliferation of all dividing cells. The most frequently encountered side effect of MPA is gastrointestinal upset, which is sometimes ameliorated by reducing the dose.

MMF is administered commonly at a fixed dose of 1.0 or 1.5 g bid. This dosing fails to consider MPA's significant interpatient pharmacokinetic variability. Recent studies demonstrate a significant relationship between MPA area under the concentration-time curve (AUC) and the risk for rejection and, in some studies, the risk for hematologic side effects *(26,27)*. The ability to measure MPA levels routinely could help clinicians optimize MMF dosing, but this is hindered by the lack of a widely available assay and the need to draw multiple samples over time

Table 6
Corticosteroid Taper-1

Time	Methylprednisolone	Prednisone
Intraoperatively	500 mg IV once	—
POD 0	125 mg IV q 8 h	—
POD 1	40 mg IV bid	50 mg PO bid
POD 2	36 mg IV bid	45 mg PO bid
POD 3	32 mg IV bid	40 mg PO bid
POD 4	28 mg IV bid	35 mg PO bid
POD 5	24 mg IV bid	30 mg PO bid
POD 6	20 mg IV bid	25 mg PO bid
POD 7	16 mg IV bid	20 mg PO bid
POD 8–14	12 mg IV bid	15 mg PO bid

Abbreviations: POD, postoperative day; IV, intravenous; PO, by mouth; bid, twice daily; q, every.

to determine the AUC. Unfortunately, predose trough MPA levels and free MPA levels, both of which would be easier to obtain, are noisier and correlate poorly with MPA AUC values *(27)*.

Corticosteroids have been used in clinical transplantation since the first organ transplants in the 1960s. Their effects on the immune system are complex but relate mostly to their ability to decrease cytokine production including IL-1, IL-2, tumor necrosis factor-α and interferon-α. Innumerable dosing strategies exist for corticosteroid use. At the authors' center, methylprednisolone is first administered as a 500 mg IV bolus as the patient is weaned from cardiopulmonary bypass. Three additional 125 mg IV doses are given in postoperative d 1 before a standardized taper begins (*see* Table 6). Oral prednisone is substituted for methylprednisolone when the patient is able to take oral medications.

Corticosteroids have numerous troublesome side effects: they worsen glycemic control, increase serum lipids, and stimulate appetite, allowing some patients to become obese. They have profound effects on bone absorption that can result in osteoporosis and a susceptibility to fractures. Avascular necrosis of the hips and shoulders from steroid use necessitates joint replacement surgery in some patients. Other debilitating side effects include cataract formation, colonic perforation, and, especially with higher doses, mood disorders such as psychosis. Motivated to limit these toxicities, many centers attempt to wean patients entirely off corticosteroids after 6–12 mo (*see* Table 7). Historically, fewer than 20% of patients can be maintained on a steroid-free regimen,

Table 7
Corticosteroid Taper-2

Time posttransplant	Prednisone dose (mg)
2 wk	15 mg bid
3 wk	12.5 mg bid
4 wk	10 mg bid
1.5 mo	7.5 mg bid
2 mo	5 mg bid
3 mo	7.5 mg qd
4 mo	5 mg qd
5 mo	4 mg qd
6 mo	3 mg qd
8 mo	2 mg qd
10 mo	1 mg qd
12 mo	0

Note: The steroid taper is slowed in those patients with severe rejection, multiple moderate rejection episodes, or a rejection episode with hemodynamic compromise. Despite attempts to withdraw all corticosteroids, most patients require low-dose prednisone indefinitely.

Abbreviations: bid, twice daily; qd, daily.

as most experience recurrent rejection. We feel that it is acceptable for those patients who remain clinically stable and rejection free to remain off corticosteroids.

Rapamycin (sirolimus, Rapamune, Wyeth-Ayerst, Philadelphia, PA) is a newer immunosuppressive drug that has the unique feature of being a potent inhibitor of vascular smooth muscle cell proliferation and migration. In both animal models and clinical trials, rapamycin-coated stents have prevented in-stent restenosis *(28)*. Based on these inhibitory properties, rapamycin appears to be an ideal drug to treat and prevent transplant coronary artery disease (TCAD), which continues to limit the long-term survival of heart transplant recipients. Preliminary results from a multicenter trial using everolimus (SDZ-RAD, Novartis, East Hanover, NJ), a derivative of rapamycin, in *de novo* heart transplant recipients demonstrate a reduction in both allograft rejection and intimal thickening of the coronary arteries in the first year of follow-up *(29)*. In a single-center study involving patients with established TCAD, rapamycin slowed disease progression and reduced the clinical endpoints of death, myocardial infarction, and need for revascularization *(30)*. In that trial, rapamycin had no effect on the production of anti-HLA antibodies, leading the authors to conclude that rapamycin's beneficial effect on stabilizing transplant vasculopathy is attributable more to its antiproliferative properties than its immunosuppressant effects.

Rapamycin has a mechanism of action that is distinct from the calcineurin inhibitors. Unlike CyA and tacrolimus, rapamycin does not inhibit IL-2 production from antigen-induced T-cell activation; rather, it prevents cellular proliferation in response to allo-antigens. Rapamycin binds to FK506-binding protein 12 (FKBP12), and, in turn, this dimeric molecule inhibits the mammalian target of rapamycin (mTOR) and upregulates the cyclin-dependent kinase inhibitor p27^{kip1}, thereby inhibiting cell-cycle progression at the G1-S phase *(28)*. Because rapamycin inhibits the cell cycle through a mechanism distinct from the calcineurin inhibitors, when combined, these drug classes work synergistically.

Generally, rapamycin is reserved for one of two clinical situations: (a) for the treatment of patients with established TCAD and (b) for those with advanced renal insufficiency induced by calcineurin inhibitors. In the first scenario, rapamycin is given as a loading dose of 6 mg and continued at 2–5 mg/d to achieve trough levels of 5–10 ng/mL. Higher levels (up to 15–20 ng/mL) are sometimes recommended when used within the first 6 mo of transplant. When adding rapamycin, it is important to reduce the CyA dose by half and to discontinue azathioprine or MMF. Rapamycin should be given several hours after CyA to reduce additive nephrotoxicity risk. Alternatively, rapamycin may be substituted for calcineurin inhibitors to limit nephrotoxicity. However, rapamycin should be used cautiously in acute renal failure, because it can impair recovery from acute tubular necrosis and induce apoptosis in renal tubular cells *(31)*. Side effects that are commonly seen with rapamycin include hyperlipidemia, thrombocytopenia, fluid retention, and an increased susceptibility to infection.

Detection and Treatment of Allograft Rejection

Acute heart rejection is a major cause of posttransplant morbidity and mortality. Despite the effectiveness of current immunosuppressive strategies, greater than 60% of patients experience at least one rejection episode within the first year of transplantation, with approx 5% of these rejection episodes accompanied by severe hemodynamic compromise *(32)*. Factors associated with an increased rejection risk include young recipient age, female donor, and female recipient *(33)*. A greater number of rejection episodes in the first year also increases recurrent rejection

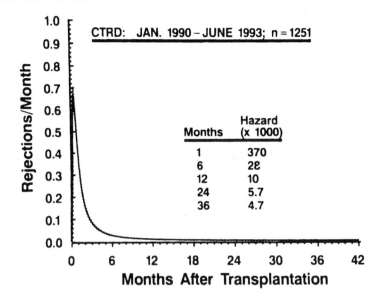

Fig. 1. Hazard function for initial rejection episode after heart transplantation. The greatest risk for experiencing a first rejection episode is in the first 2 mo following transplantation, then decreases rapidly by the end of yr 1, but never becomes zero. Reproduced with permission from ref. *34.*

risk*(34).* The chance of experiencing a first rejection episode, expressed as a hazard ratio, is highest in the first 1–2 mo after transplant, then decreases rapidly by the end of yr 1 but never becomes zero (Fig. 1) *(34).* Also, the cumulative risk of rejection is greatest within 1 yr and increases asymptotically over time without plateauing (Fig. 2) *(34).*

The clinical manifestations of rejection can be subtle, and patients frequently remain entirely asymptomatic. Constitutional symptoms including fever, malaise, and lethargy may be seen but are nonspecific. When rejection is associated with a compromise in cardiac allograft function, an S3 or S4 gallop may be auscultated and the neck veins may be distended. Echocardiography can help document diminished ventricular function. As noted previously, the new onset of atrial arrhythmias—particularly atrial fibrillation or flutter—often correlates with rejection episodes, whereas ventricular arrhythmias do not unless accompanied by severe hemodynamic compromise *(16).* Other clues to the presence of rejection include a reduction in QRS voltage on the EKG (perhaps as a result of myocardial edema) and the new ability to control hypertension that was previously refractory to medical therapy.

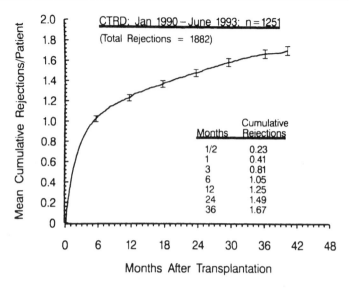

Fig. 2. Cumulative frequency distribution of the mean rejection episodes per patient after heart transplantation. Vertical bars represent the 70% confidence limits. Reproduced with permission from ref. *34*.

Table 8
Columbia–Presbyterian Biopsy Schedule

Time posttransplant	Frequency
1 mo	Weekly
2 mo	Biweekly
3–6 mo	Monthly
7–12 mo	Every 2 mo
12–18 mo	Every 3 mo
≥ 19 mo	Every 6–12 mo

Because most rejection episodes are clinically silent, endomyocardial biopsy is essential to detect acute allograft rejection. Despite its invasiveness, endomyocardial biopsy can be performed safely with minimal patient discomfort. The biopsy schedule followed by the authors' center attempts to match the frequency of biopsies with the rejection risk (*see* Table 8). As such, biopsies are performed more frequently in the first weeks and months after transplant, becoming no more frequent than once or twice annually later after transplant. Biopsy specimens are graded according to the standardized scale adopted by the ISHLT (*see* Table 9) (*35*).

Table 9
Standardized ISHLT[a] Cardiac Biopsy Grading Scale (35)

Grade	Description
0	No rejection
1A	Focal perivascular or interstitial infiltrate without necrosis
1B	Diffuse but sparse infiltrate without necrosis
2	One focus only with aggressive infiltration and/or focal myocyte damage
3A	Multifocal aggressive infiltrates and/or myocyte damage
3B	Diffuse inflammatory process with necrosis
4	Diffuse aggressive polymorphous infiltrate, with or without edema, hemorrhage, or vasculitis; with necrosis

[a]International Society for Heart and Lung Transplantation

Specific treatment algorithms for acute allograft rejection differ among centers but usually consist of the administration of oral or intravenous corticosteroids tailored according to the rejection's severity, its impact on hemodynamics, and the time from transplant. The treatment algorithm followed by most cardiologists at Columbia–Presbyterian is listed in Table 10 and illustrated in Fig. 3.

Grade 0 and 1A rejection do not require treatment, whereas most 1B and 2 biopsies can be treated with an intensification of the immunosuppression regimen (an increase in the dose of the calcineurin inhibitor or MMF) or with oral prednisone starting at 100 mg/d followed by a taper over 7–10 d to the baseline dose. Symptomatic rejection with evidence of hemodynamic compromise is usually treated with intravenous methlyprednisolone followed by an oral prednisone taper. Repeat biopsy in both instances is performed in 7–10 d.

Moderately severe rejection (Grade 3A) may be treated out of hospital with high-dose oral or intravenous steroids, provided patients are asymptomatic, have normal resting hemodynamics, and are greater than 3 mo post-transplant. Symptomatic patients with 3A rejection are treated in hospital with intravenous methylprednisolone (1000 mg/d for 3 d) followed by a prednisone taper. Repeat biopsy is performed in 1 wk. Severe rejections (ISHLT grade 3B or 4) with cytolytic therapy consisting of either OKT3 or ATGAM. In-patient admission and close attention is mandatory, as hemodynamic compromise and circulatory collapse progresses rapidly and may require intensive hemodynamic monitoring and support.

Table 10
Algorithm for the Initial Treatment of Acute Allograft Rejection

ISHLT biopsy grade	Time post-transplant	Sypmtomatic or impaired hemodynamics[a]	Treatment
Grade 0 or 1A	—	—	No treatment
Grade 1B	< 3 mo	Absent	Optimize immunosuppressive therapy[b]
		Present	Intravenous methylprednisolone[c]
	> 3 mo	Absent	Optimize immunosuppressive therapy[b]
		Present	PO prednisone[d]
Grade 2	< 3 mo	Absent	PO prednisone[d]
		Present	Intravenous methylprednisolone[c]
	> 3 mo	Absent	Optimize immunosuppressive therapy[b] or PO prednisone[d]
		Present	Intravenous methylprednisolone[c]
Grade 3A	< 3 mo	Absent	Intravenous methylprednisolone[c]
		Present	Intravenous methylprednisolone[c]; if severely compromised hemodynamics, begin OKT3 or ATGAM.
	> 3mo	Absent	PO prednisone[d]
		Present	Intravenous methylprednisolone[c]; if severely compromised hemodynamics, begin OKT3 or ATGAM.
Grade 3B and 4	—	—	Admit for OKT3. If volume overloaded or if anti-OKT3 antibodies present, then begin ATGAM. Consider early initiation of plasmapheresis if severely compromised hemodynamics are present.

[a]PA saturation < 50% or low cardiac output with elevated filling pressures

[b]Increase calcineurin inhibitor if levels are subtherapeutic; increase mycophenolate mofetil to maximum of 1500 mg bid

[c]Intravenous methylprednisolone 1000 mg/d × 3 d followed by 100 mg/d prednisone with 10 mg/d taper to baseline dose

[d]Oral steroid taper e.g., prednisone 100 mg/d × 3 d with 10 mg/d taper to baseline dose

Abbreviations: PO, by mouth; ATGAM, antithymocyte globulin; PA, pulmonary artery; bid, twice daily.

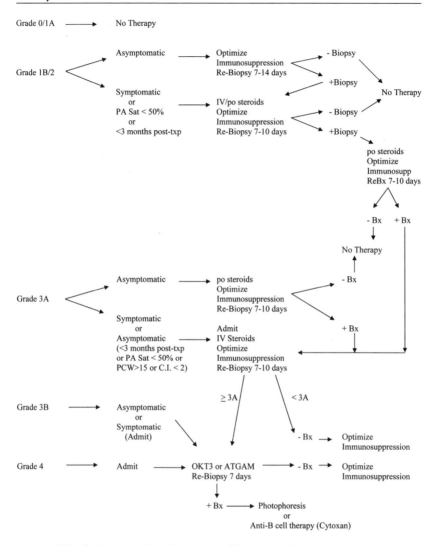

Fig. 3. An algorithm for acute cellular rejection management.

Humoral or antibody-mediated rejection occurs when donor-specific antibodies attack the transplanted allograft. As opposed to T-cell-mediated rejection, humoral (vascular) rejection is a B-cell-mediated process that occurs earlier after transplant and is associated with a higher rate of graft loss, development of transplant vasculopathy, and decreased long-term survival (36). Light microscopy with hematoxylin and eosin staining is insufficient for detecting humoral rejection. Instead, immunofluorescent staining is required to identify the endothelial deposits of immunoglobulin, complement, and fibrinogen necessary to make the diagnosis.

Because humoral rejection is a B-cell-mediated process, T-cell-directed immune suppression is not effective therapy. Currently, standard humoral rejection treatment includes high-dose corticosteroids, antithymocyte globulin, cyclophosphamide, and plasmapheresis *(37)*. More recently, anti-CD20 monoclonal antibody (rituximab, Genentech, San Francisco, CA), a chimeric humanized antibody directed against the pan-B-cell surface molecule CD20, has been used with some anecdotal success. Ultimately, rituximab may provide long-term benefits by eliminating "memory" B cells and preventing the adverse late sequelae of humoral rejection *(38)*.

Antimicrobial Prophylaxis

Transplant recipients on immunosuppressive therapy are susceptible to infections from a broad range of ordinary and opportunistic pathogens. Prevention strategies aimed at reducing or eliminating the risk of life-threatening infection take into account two principal factors: (a) the intensity of potential pathogen exposure and (b) the combined effect of all factors that contribute to a recipient's susceptibility to infection, the "net state of immunosuppression" (*see* Table 11) *(39)*. Also taken into consideration is the well-recognized time-related nature of infection (Figs. 4 and 5).

This timetable is divided into three distinct segments: early (1 mo after transplant), intermediate (1–6 mo), and late (greater than 6 mo). Patients in the first month are most susceptible to infection from donor-transmitted pathogens as well as nosocomial bacterial and fungal infections. Although immunosuppressive therapy is most intense early after transplant, opportunistic infections are not commonly seen until after this first month.

During mo 1 through 6, opportunistic infection from *Pneumocystis carinii*, *Aspergillus*, *Cryptococcus* and *Nocardia* may develop. Infection symptoms may be minimal, and fever may be suppressed by corticosteroid therapy. A high index of suspicion combined with a careful physical examination and chest radiography are critical for disease detection. The sustained level of maximal immune suppression in mo 1–6 places patients at particular risk for infection from reactivation of viruses such as cytomegalovirus (CMV), Epstein–Barr Virus (EBV), HSV, and hepatitis B (HBV) and hepatitis C viruses. Infection risk declines after the sixth month as the dose of corticosteroids and calcineurin inhibitors are decreased, although an increased susceptibility to common respiratory viruses and bacterial pathogens may persist.

Table 11
Factors Affecting the Net State
of Immunosuppression in Transplant Recipients

Immunosuppressive therapy: dose, duration, and temporal sequence
Underlying immune deficiency: autoimmune disease, functional immune deficits
Integrity of the mucocutaneous barrier: catheters, epithelial surfaces
Devitalized tissue, fluid collections
Neutropenia, lymphopenia
Metabolic conditions
    Uremia
    Malnutrition
    Diabetes
    Alcoholism with cirrhosis
Infection with immunomodulating viruses
    Cytomegalovirus
    Epstein–Barr virus
    Hepatitis B and C virus
    Human immunodeficiency virus

Reproduced with permission from ref. *39*.

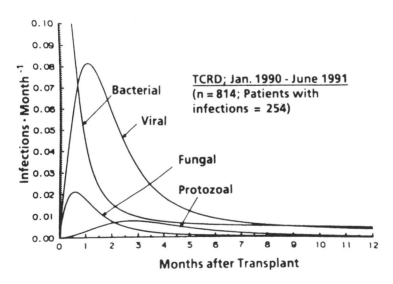

Fig. 4. Hazard function for first infection from the different classes of microorganisms. Reproduced with permission from ref. *39a*.

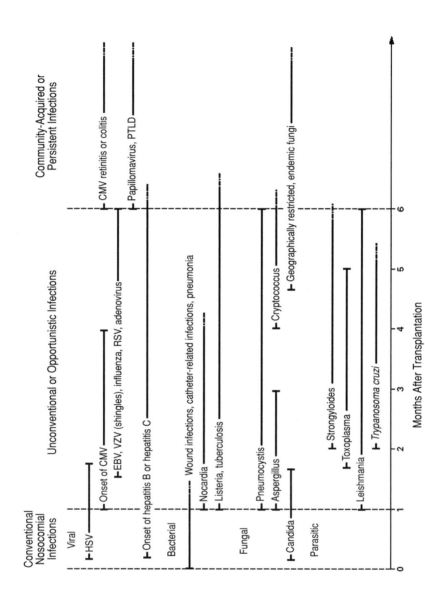

Fig. 5. The time-related nature of infection in the transplant recipient. Reproduced with permission from ref. 39.

148

Approximately 10% of patients experience chronic or persistent infection from viruses such as CMV, HBV, and EBV *(39)*. Chronic viral infection may contribute to the development of certain malignancies. EBV infection is associated with PTLD development, particularly among patients treated with cytolytic OKT3 therapy, whereas chronic papillomavirus infection may cause squamous-cell carcinoma. Another 5–10% of patients experience recurrent allograft rejection and receive augmented corticosteroid therapy or other intensive immunosuppressive regimens that can render them susceptible to recurrent infection, especially from organisms such as *Pneumocystis carinii, Aspergillus,* and *Cryptococcus.* Ongoing prophylactic trimethoprim-sulfamethoxazole (TMP/SMX) use should be considered for these patients. Patients should avoid contact with animal droppings and never change cat litter, as this is a known vector for the spread of toxoplasmosis.

Infection from CMV occurs from latent virus reactivation or direct donor transmission. The greatest risk of developing CMV disease arises in seronegative recipients who lack CMV antibodies and receive an organ from a seropositive donor; the infection risk in this instance exceeds 50% *(40)*. Among seropositive recipients, the incidence of CMV illness in the first 120 d following transplantation has been as high as 46% *(41)*. Clinical manifestations of CMV infection commonly include constitutional symptoms of fever, malaise, and a flu-like syndrome. When shed in the gastrointestinal tract, CMV classically produces profuse, watery diarrhea, occasionally associated with hepatic enzyme elevation. Pulmonary infection produces dyspnea and a nonproductive cough that is associated with pulmonary interstitial infiltrates. Other infection forms include pancreatitis, retinitis, and encephalitis. CMV diagnosis is best made by the detection of viremia with polymerase chain reaction (PCR) or from the identification of virus in pathologic specimens (e.g., gastric or colonic biopsy). Leukopenia, thrombocytopenia, and atypical lymphocytosis are seen frequently as well. Virus recovery from the buffy coat of a spun serum sample is possible but is a less sensitive test than PCR.

CMV has numerous indirect effects on the immune system and transplanted allograft. CMV suppresses antigen-specific cytotoxic T-lymphocyte function and causes a change in the proportion of T-cell subsets *(42)*. As a result, CMV infection increases the susceptibility to infection with other opportunistic pathogens such as *Pneumocystis carinii, Aspergillus fumigatus,* and *Candida albicans (42)*. CMV infection is associated with the development of LV dysfunction *(43)* and an increased incidence of graft atherosclerosis *(44)*. Endothelial cells infected by CMV produce adhesion molecules, such as ICAM-1 *(45)*, and inflammatory cytokines that, in turn, upregulate the expression of MHC class II antigens and accelerate the pathogenesis of transplant vasculopathy *(39)*. Finally, there exists a reciprocal relationship between CMV and allograft rejection whereby viral infection may precipitate allograft rejection, and rejection episodes, with their associated inflammation and immunotherapies, increase viral replication and the likelihood of CMV infection *(39)*.

CMV disease treatment is best accomplished with a 2-wk course of intravenous ganciclovir. Patients intolerant or hypersensitive to ganciclovir may be treated with foscarnet (Foscavir, Astra Zeneca, Wilmington, DE). As a general rule, intravenous ganciclovir should be continued until patients become afebrile with resolution of their symptoms accompanied by elimination of PCR-documented viremia.

Prophylactic strategies to prevent the onset of CMV disease are designed to match a patient's individual risk. Seronegative patients receiving a heart from a seropositive donor are at greatest risk early after transplant. Intravenous ganciclovir (5 mg/kg bid) adjusted for creatinine clearance is administered within the first few postoperative days. Valganciclovir (Valcyte, Hoffman-LaRoche, Nutley, NJ), a newly approved oral formulation of ganciclovir, replaces intravenous ganciclovir when patients are tolerating oral medicines; this continues for 6 mo. Usual maintenance doses are 900 mg/d in patients with preserved renal function and 450 mg in those with GFR 20–50 mL/min. Seropositive patients receiving a seronegative organ should also receive valganciclovir prophylaxis for 6 mo, but half the dose may be sufficient. Patients with recurrent disease should be considered for life-long prophylaxis.

Pneumocystis carinii is an opportunistic fungus that produces pulmonary infection in immunosuppressed individuals. The infection risk appears to be directly related to the degree of immunosuppression, with the greatest risk encountered in the first 6 mo, around the time of a steroid pulse for rejection, and following cytolytic OKT3 therapy. Symptoms of fever, nonproductive cough, and dyspnea predominate and are occasionally accompanied by headache and confusion. Although several different patterns are described in chest radiographs, classical Pneumocystis carinii pneumonia (PCP) produces interstitial infiltrates in a "bat-wing" distribution. Blood gas analysis may reveal hypoxemia and a widened A-a gradient. Frequently, serum lactate dehydrogenase is elevated. Definitive diagnosis is made by silver staining of the organisms in respiratory specimens from expectorated sputum or bronchoalveolar lavage. Treatment is with intravenous TMP/SMX. Sulfa-allergic patients receive intravenous pentamidine. A single-strength tablet containing 80 mg of TMP and 400 mg SMX given daily throughout the first year is extraordinarily effective for primary PCP prevention. Patients with sulfa allergies receive either dapsone or atovaquone (Mepron, Glaxo-SmithKline, Research Triangle, NC). It is generally recommended that patients more than 1 yr from transplant receive a short course of TMP/SMX prophylactically around the time of any intensification of immunosuppression when being treated for allograft rejection.

Toxoplasma gondii is an intracellular parasite that produces myocarditis and can lead to acute heart failure and death in transplant recipients. Seropositive recipients have protective antibodies and are at low risk of acquiring donor-transmitted toxoplasmosis or for experiencing disease reactivation. However, seronegative recipients of a seropositive donor heart are at risk for acute disease and usually receive prophylaxis with pyrimethamine 50 mg/d for 6 wk to prevent donor-transmitted infection. Folinic acid (leukovorin) (5 mg bid) is co-administered to prevent hepatotoxicity. Prophylaxis against PCP with TMP/SMX also provides further protection against toxoplasmosis.

Invasive fungi such as *Candida albicans*, *Aspergillus fumigatus*, and *Cryptococcus neoformans* produce life-threatening infection in immunocompromised transplant recipients. The most commonly encountered fungal infection is mucosal candidiasis, which can be entirely prevented by daily nystatin swish and swallow (Mycostatin, Bristol-Myers Squibb, Princeton, NJ) for the first 3 mo posttransplant. Vaginal candidiasis (yeast infection) can be successfully eradicated with topical nystatin or with a short course of fluconazole (Diflucan, Pfizer, New York, NY), though fluconazole raises the serum CyA level. Often, prophylactic nystatin is re-administered during intensification of immunosuppressive therapy or with steroid pulses, as temporary immune system suppression makes one susceptible to mucosal candidiasis. Pulmonary aspergillosis is a dreaded infection in transplant recipients associated with significant mortality risk even for patients receiving intravenous Amphotericin-B. Prophylaxis with aerosolized Amphotericin-B is provided to all patients during any hospitalization within 1 yr of transplantation. Avoiding construction sites is recommended to reduce the chance of acquiring pulmonary disease.

Varicella-zoster virus reactivates in the setting of immunosuppression, causing painful shingles episodes. Treatment with acyclovir can shorten the course of infection, but analgesics are often required to control herpetic neuralgia. Transplant patients are counseled to avoid direct contact with other individuals with shingles. They should also avoid sharing bed sheets and dinner utensils while vesicles are present because live virus is present until the lesions are covered by a crust. Because aerosolized spread does not occur, they do not have to isolate themselves from people with shingles.

Reactivation of *Mycobacterium tuberculosis* is an infrequently observed occurrence that can produce isolated pulmonary disease or may disseminate. To eliminate this risk, all potential transplant recipients must have a purified protein derivative test placed with anergic controls prior to listing. Patients with a positive test result require treatment with isoniazid to eradicate the organism.

Prevention of posttransplant infection is dependent on the efforts of both patients and physicians. Strict hand washing is a simple and effective strategy that prevents pathogen transmission. All physicians caring for patients should be reminded of the necessity of hand washing after patient contact. When examining patients early after transplant, it is the author's habit to wear gloves as a form of "reverse isolation" to minimize the chance of spreading antibiotic-resistant pathogen strains commonly encountered in ICUs and hospital wards. Patients are encouraged to wear a surgical mask when visiting the hospital and during times of close contact with strangers where airborne spread of respiratory viruses is possible (e.g., on an airplane). They should avoid people with colds and children who have received live virus vaccines. In general, patients are discouraged from spending time in damp basements or from participating in home renovation to prevent exposure to various forms of mold and fungi that might aerosolize. Although many opportunistic pathogens live in the soil, gardening is possible for patients more than 6 mo posttransplant, provided they wear rubber gloves and a mask and wash their hands after digging in the soil. All fresh fruits and vegetables should be washed thoroughly.

Transplant Vasculopathy Prevention

The development of TCAD limits the long-term success of cardiac transplantation. In a multicenter study of 2609 heart transplantation recipients, 42% had evidence of graft vasculopathy on angiography by 5 yr after transplantation *(46)*. Both immunologic and nonimmunologic endothelial damage may initiate pathological remodeling of the transplanted coronary arteries, resulting in graft vasculopathy (Fig. 6). Presently, no known therapy entirely prevents development or progression of this disease, although several strategies minimize this risk. These include strict blood pressure control administration of lipid-lowering statin drugs and prevention of rejection and CMV infection.

Because 80% of patients develop hypertension, blood pressure control is mandatory to reduce the incidence of vascular disease. Calcium

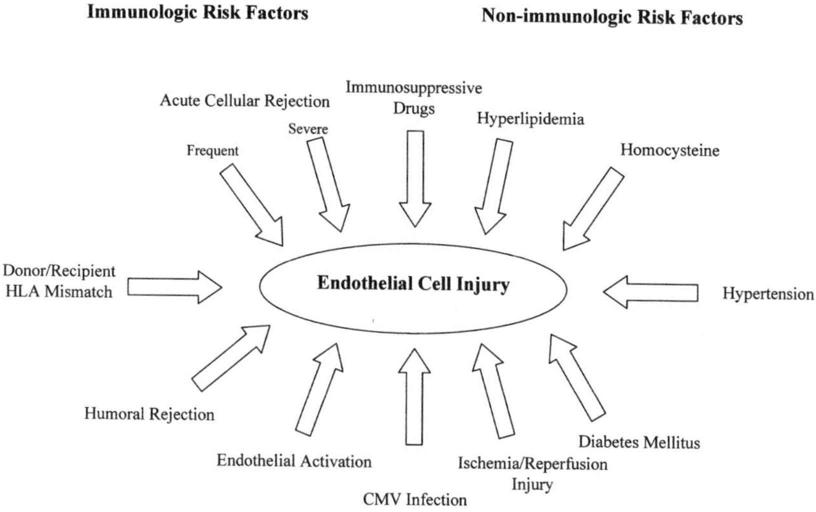

Immunologic Risk Factors   **Non-immunologic Risk Factors**

Fig. 6. Both immunologic and nonimmunologic factors produce endothelial cell injury and lead to the pathogenesis of transplant allograft vasculopathy.

channel blockers, such as diltiazem and nifedipine, limit intimal thickness, as detected by intravascular ultrasound. Although it is unclear whether calcium channel blockers have anything other than an indirect effect on vascular endothelium, through their effects in lowering blood pressure, many centers continue to prescribe diltiazem to all heart transplant recipients. ACE inhibitors do have anti-atherothrombotic effects. In the Heart Outcomes Prevention Evaluation (HOPE) trial, ramipril (Altace, Monarch, Bristol, TN) significantly reduced the incidence of myocardial infarction and stroke and slowed diabetes progression *(47)*. Although no clinical trial has tested ACE inhibitors or angiotensin receptor blockers (ARB) in cardiac transplant recipients, there is reason to believe that, by preserving endothelial function, these drugs could reduce the incidence of transplant vasculopathy. However, limiting their widespread use is the additive renal insufficiency risk when these drugs are combined with calcineurin inhibitors. Patients with preserved renal function and hypertension, especially those with concomitant diabetes, should receive either an ACE inhibitor or ARB.

Hyperlipidemia is encountered frequently after heart transplantation and is exacerbated by the need for corticosteroid treatment. HMG-CoA reductase inhibitors (statins) appear to have benefits in transplant patients beyond simply lowering cholesterol. When tested in a randomized clinical trial, pravastatin (Pravachol, Bristol-Myers Squibb, Princeton, NJ) lowered cholesterol levels, reduced the incidence of transplant vasculopathy, and improved survival in study patients when compared to control patients *(48)*. In another clinical trial, early use of simvastatin (Zocor, Merck, West Point, PA) resulted in significantly better 8-yr survival rates and a lower incidence of transplant vasculopathy *(49)*. Among other beneficial effects, statins have immunomodulatory properties. Specifically, statin-treated patients experienced fewer severe rejection episodes in clinical trials *(49)*. This may result from the fact that, in the presence of CyA, statins directly inhibit natural killer cell activity *(50)*.

Although no therapy exists to reverse transplant vasculopathy, the novel immunosuppressive drug rapamycin appears to stabilize the disease. In a recent single-center study conducted at Columbia–Presbyterian, rapamycin effectively slowed graft vasculopathy progression in patients with documented moderate to severe TCAD *(30)*. The incidence of clinically significant cardiac events, defined as death, myocardial infarction, or the need for revascularization, was reduced in the rapamycin group compared to the control group. A semiquantitative catheterization score remained unchanged in the rapamycin group, whereas it worsened in controls. Production of anti-HLA class I and II antibodies was not reduced with rapamycin, suggesting that its mechanism of action is not mediated by B-cell suppression but by its antiproliferative effects. Recently published data from a multicenter trial using everolimus also showed a reduction in intimal thickness at 1 yr in the everolimus-treated patients *(29)*. Further study with these promising drugs needs to be conducted to determine whether these observations translate into a long-term survival benefit. Until that time, the only definitive treatment for transplant vasculopathy remains retransplantation.

CONCLUSION: REHABILITATION AND RETURN TO PHYSICAL ACTIVITY

The goal of cardiac transplantation is not simply to extend life but to restore productivity to all transplant recipients. Despite this attempt, less than 30% of transplant recipients return to full-time work *(51)*. One reason for this is the increasing recipient age over the past decade. However, other obstacles prevent not only the return to work but the return to full functional capacity. Patients with advanced heart failure prior to transplantation experience severe deconditioning and muscle atrophy requiring intensive physical therapy to regain full function. Hindering this recovery is chronic corticosteroid therapy, which may produce proximal muscle weakness in addition to central obesity. The denervated heart also limits full cardiovascular performance, because it produces a slightly diminished maximal cardiac output. This is particularly evident in size-mismatched recipients. Despite these limitations, 80–85% of heart transplant recipients enjoy a physically active lifestyle and an improvement in quality of life, especially when compared to their pretransplant state *(51)*.

REFERENCES

1. Mets B, Michler RE, Delphin ED, et al. Refractory vasodilation after cardiopulmonary bypass for heart transplantation in recipients on combined amiodarone and angiotensin-converting enzyme inhibitor therapy: a role for vasopressin administration. J Cardiothorac Vasc Anesth 1998;12:326–329.
2. Morales DLS, Gregg D, Helman DN, et al. Arginine vasopressin in the treatment of 50 patients with postcardiotomy vasodilatory shock. Ann Thorac Surg 2000;69: 102–106.
3. Landry DW, Levin HR, Gallant EM, et al. Vasopressin deficiency contributes to the vasodilation of septic shock. Circulation 1997;95:1122–1125.
4. Landry DW, Oliver JA. The pathogenesis of vasodilatory shock. N Engl J Med 2001;345:588–595.
5. Anand IS, Ferrari R, Kalra GS, et al. Edema of cardiac origin. Circulation 1989;80:299–305.
6. Robertson GL. The regulation of vasopressin function in health and disease. Rec Prog Horm Res 1977;33:333–386.
7. Argenziano M, Chen JM, Cullinane S, et al. Arginine vasopressin in the management of vasodilatory hypotension after cardiac transplantation. J Heart Lung Transplant 1999;18:814–817.
8. Argenziano M, Choudhri AF, Oz MC, et al. A prospective randomized trial of arginine vasopressin in the treatment of vasodilatory shock after left ventricular assist device placement. Circulation 1997;96(suppl 9):II.286–II.280.
9. Edwards RM, Rinza W, Kinter LB. Renal microvascular effects of vasopressin and vasopressin antagonist. Am J Physiol 1989;256(2 pt 2):F274–F278.
10. Hosenpud JD, Bennett LE, Berkeley MK, et al. The registry of the International Society for Heart and Lung Transplantation: 15th official report—1998. J Heart Lung Transplant 1998;17:656–668.
11. Hosenpud JD, Novick RJ, Breen TJ, et al. The registry of the International Society for Heart and Lung Transplantation: 12th official report—1995. J Heart Lung Transplant 1995;14:805–815.
12. Owen VJ, Burton PBJ, Michel MC, et al. Myocardial dysfunction in donor hearts: a possible etiology. Circulation 1999;99:2565–2570.
13. Kavarna MN, Sinha P, Eng M, et al. Mechanical support for the failing cardiac allograft: a single-center experience. J Heart Lung Transplant 2003;22:542–547.
14. Mankad P, Yacoub M. Influence of basal release of nitric oxide on systolic and diastolic function of both ventricles. J Thorac Cardiovasc Surg 1997;113:770–776.
15. Ardehali A, Hughes K, Sadeghi A, et al. Inhaled nitric oxide for pulmonary hypertension after heart transplantation. Transplantation 2001;72:638–641.
16. Cui G, Tung T, Kobashigawa J, et al. Increased incidence of atrial flutter associated with the rejection of heart transplantation. Am J Cardiol 2001;88:280–284.
17. Magnano AR, Garan H. Catheter ablation of supraventricular tachycardia in the transplanted heart: a case series and literature review. Pacing Clin Electrophysiol 2003;26:1878–1886.

18. Chen JM, Hammond KM, Kherani AR, et al. Is the alternate waiting list too high risk? The Columbia–Presbyterian experience. J Heart Lung Transplant 2003; 1S:S175.

19. Braith RW, Mills RM Jr., Wilcox CS, Davis GL, Wood CE. Breakdown of blood pressure and body fluid homeostasis in heart transplant recipients. J Am Coll Cardiol 1996;27:375–383.

20. Braith RW, Mills RM, Wilcox CS, et al. High-dose angiotensin-converting enzyme inhibition restores body fluid homeostasis in heart-transplant recipients. J Am Coll Cardiol 2003;41:426–432.

21. Beniaminovitz A, Itescu S, Lietz K, et al. Prevention of rejection in cardiac transplantation by blockade of the interleukin-2 receptor with a monoclonal antibody. N Engl J Med 2000;342:613–619.

22. Chan MCY, Kwok BW, Shiba B, et al. Conversion of cyclosporine to tacrolimus for refractory or persistent myocardial rejection. Transplant Proc 2002;34: 1850–1852.

23. Taylor DO, Barr ML, Radovancevic B, et al. A randomized, multicenter comparison of tacrolimus and cyclosporine immunosuppressive regimens in cardiac transplantation: decreased hyperlipidemia and hypertension with tacrolimus. J Heart Lung Transplant 1999;18:336–345.

24. Reichart B, Meiser B, Vigano M, et al. European multicenter tacrolimus (FK506) heart pilot study: one-year results. J Heart Lung Transplant 1998;17:775–781.

25. Kobashigawa J, Miller L, Renlund D, et al. A randomized active-controlled trial of mycophenolate mofetil in heart transplant recipients. Transplantation 1998; 66:507–515.

26. DeNofrio D, Loh E, Kao A, et al. Mycophenolic acid concentrations are associated with cardiac allograft rejection. J Heart Lung Transplant 2000;19:1071–1076.

27. Shaw LM, Pawinski T, Korecka M, et al. Monitoring of mycophenolic acid in clinical transplantation. Ther Drug Monit 2002;24:68–73.

28. Marx S, Marks A. Bench to bedside: the development of rapamycin and its application to stent restenosis. Circulation 2001;104:852–855.

29. Eisen HJ, Tuzcu EM, Dorent R, et al. Efficacy and safety of everolimus as part of a triple immunosuppressive regimen in de novo cardiac transplant recipients: 12 month results. N Engl J Med 2003;349:847–858.

30. Mancini DM, Pinney SP, Burkhoff D, et al. Use of rapamycin slows progression of cardiac transplantation vasculopathy. Circulation 2003;108:48–53.

31. Lieberthal W, Fuhro R, Andry CC, et al. Rapamycin inhibits recovery from acute renal failure: role of cell-cycle arrest and apoptosis of tubular cells. Am J Physiol Renal Physiol 2001;281:F693–F706.

32. Mills RM, Naftel DC, Kirklin JK, et al. Heart transplant rejection with hemodynamic compromise: a multiinstituional study of the role of endomyocardial cellular infiltrate. J Heart Lung Transplant 1997;16:813–821.

33. Kobashigawa JA, Kirklin JK, Naftel DC, et al. Pretransplant risk factors for acute rejection after heart transplantation: a multiinstitutional study. J Heart Lung Transplant 1993;12:355–366.

34. Kubo SH, Naftel DC, Mills RM Jr., et al. Risk factors for late recurrent rejection after heart transplantation: a multi-institutional, multivariable analysis. J Heart Lung Transplant 1995;14:409–418.

35. Billingham ME, Cary NR, Hammond ME, et al. A working formulation for the standardization of nomenclature in the diagnosis of heart and lung rejection: heart rejection study group. J Heart Transplant 1990;9:587–593.

36. Olsen SL, Wagoner LE, Hammond EH, et al. Vascular rejection in heart transplantation: clinical correlation, treatment options, and future considerations. J Heart Lung Transplant 1993;12:S135–S142.

37. Grauhan O, Knosalla C, Ewert R, et al. Plasmapheresis and cyclophosphamide in the treatment of humoral rejection after heart transplantation. J Heart Lung Transplant 2001;20:316–321.

38. Aranda JM Jr., Scornik JC, Normann SJ, et al. Anti-CD20 monoclonal antibody (rituximab) therapy for acute cardiac humoral rejection: a case report. Transplantation 2002;73:907–910.

39. Fishman JA, Rubin RH. Infection in organ-transplant recipients. N Engl J Med 1998;338:1741–1751.

39a. Miller LW, Naftel DC, Bourge RC, et al. Infection after heart transplantation: a multiinstitutional study. J Heart Lung Transplant 1993;13:381–393.

40. Rubin RH. Infection in the organ transplant recipient. In: Rubin RH, Young LS, eds. Clinical approach to infection in the compromised host. 3rd ed. New York: Plenum Publishing, 1994:629–705.

41. Merigan TC, Renlund DG, Keay S, et al. A controlled trial of ganciclovir to prevent cytomegalovirus disease after heart transplantation. N Engl J Med 1992;326: 1182–1186.

42. Sia IG, Patel R. New strategies for prevention and therapy of cytomegalovirus infection and disease in solid-organ transplant recipients. Clin Microbiol Rev 2000;13:83–121.

43. McNamara D, DiSalvo T, Mathier M, et al. Left ventricular dysfunction after heart transplantation: incidence and role of enhanced immunosuppression. J Heart Lung Transplant 1996;15:506–515.

44. Valantine HA, Gao SZ, Menon SG, et al. Impact of prophylactic immediate posttransplant ganciclovir on development of transplant atherosclerosis : a post hoc analysis of a randomized, placebo-controlled study. Circulation 1999;100: 61–66.

45. Craigen JL, Grundy JE. Cytomegalovirus induced up-regulation of LFA-3 (CD58) and ICAM-1 (CD54) is a direct viral effect that is not prevented by ganciclovir or fosacarnet treatment. Transplantation 1996;62:1102–1108.

46. Costanzo M, Naftel D, Pritzker M, et al. Heart transplant coronary artery disease detected by coronary angiography: a multi-institutional study of preoperative donor and recipient risk factors. J Heart Lung Transplant 1998;17:744–753.

47. Yusuf S, Sleight P, Pogue J, et al. Effects of an angiotensin-converting-enzyme inhibitor, ramipril, on cardiovascular events in high-risk patients. N Engl J Med 2000;342:145–153.

48. Kobashigawa JA, Katznelson S, Laks H, et al. Effect of pravastatin on outcomes after cardiac transplantation. N Engl J Med 1995;333:621–627.

49. Wenke K, Meiser B, Thiery J, et al. Simvastatin initiated early after heart transplantation: 8-year prospective experience. Circulation 2003;107:93–97.

50. Katznelson S, Huang XM, Chia D, et al. The inhibitor effects of pravastatin on natural killer T-cell activity in vivo in cytotoxic T-lymphocyte activity in vitro. J Heart Lung Transplant 1998;259:414–419.

51. Data on file, International Society for Heart and Lung Transplantation, June 2003.

8 Immunosuppression for Cardiac Transplantation

Ranjit John, MD,
Mario C. Deng, MD,
and Silviu Itescu, MD

CONTENTS

INTRODUCTION

Cardiac transplantation has long been the gold standard for the treatment of end-stage heart disease *(1)*. After the first human-to-human heart transplant in 1967, the initial flurry of activity surrounding heart transplantation quickly diminished because of poor results, primarily stemming from an inability to control cardiac allograft rejection without subjecting patients to the risk of overwhelming sepsis. However, among the major advances made in the following decade were the use of endomyocardial biopsy techniques for diagnosing and monitoring rejection and the use of rabbit antithymocyte globulin and, subsequently, cyclosporine (CyA). Many immunosuppressive protocols used for car-

From: *Contemporary Cardiology: Cardiac Transplantation:*
The Columbia University Medical Center/New York-Presbyterian Hospital Manual
Edited by: N. M. Edwards, J. M. Chen, and P. A. Mazzeo © Humana Press Inc., Totowa, NJ

diac transplantation were based on protocols already in place for clinical renal transplantation. This chapter discusses the current status of immunosuppression in cardiac transplantation and reviews novel modalities of immunosuppression as well as immunosuppressive management of the sensitized cardiac allograft recipient.

EARLY POSTTRANSPLANT PERIOD

Role of Induction Therapy

Induction therapy is greatly important to ensure that acute rejection risk is minimized; in the past, standard regimens have included induction agents. However, using induction phase agents in heart transplantation is controversial.

Acute rejection episodes adversely affect short-term survival following cardiac transplantation. Rejection occurs most frequently during the first 3 mo after transplantation, with the incidence decreasing exponentially thereafter. Repeated or severe episodes of allograft rejection may lead to cardiac allograft vasculopathy development, which, in these patients, is the main cause of death after the first year. Using induction therapy in the perioperative period has been advocated to decrease the frequency and severity of early acute rejection. The success obtained with these nonselective agents has varied *(2–4)*.

The main induction agents are the polyclonal antilymphocyte and antithymocyte globulins and, more recently, the murine monoclonal antibody (MAb) OKT3. Randomized trials evaluating relative efficacy and tolerance of these potential agents failed to show a significant difference in survival among these agents. Further, several trials that studied the relative efficacy of the polyclonal antilymphocyte preparations against the MAb OKT3 failed to demonstrate an improved efficacy of the MAb. Although these agents have been effective in terminating acute allograft rejection and in treating refractory rejection, results of comparative studies of outcomes with and without monoclonal induction therapy have varied, with most studies demonstrating an effect on rejection that is maintained only while antibody therapy is ongoing. Without repeated administration, these agents only delay the time to a first rejection episode and do not decrease the overall frequency or severity of rejection.

More importantly, their use is associated with increased complication risk—both short-term (infections) and long-term (lymphoproliferative disorders). A large, multicenter analysis reported that the use of antilymphocyte antibody therapy, specifically OKT3, is associated with an increased incidence of nonfatal cytomegalovirus (CMV) infections.

Swinnen et al. reported a high incidence of posttransplant lympho-proliferative disease (PTLD) in patients receiving perioperative or res-cue OKT3 *(3)*. However, other large series using OKT3 did not report as high an incidence of PTLD, thereby suggesting that PTLD risk is more likely dependent on the overall immunosuppression degree, rather than on the use of a specific agent *(5,6)*. A side effect specific to OKT3 is the development of a "flu-like syndrome" characterized by fever, chills, and mild hypotension, typically seen with the first dose *(7)*.

Because antilymphocyte antibodies are produced in nonhuman spe-cies, their use is associated with the sensitization phenomenon, leading to decreased efficacy with repeated use, as well as the possibility of serum sickness. Sensitization development is linked with an increased acute vascular rejection risk. Although this association is not reported by other centers using OKT3 prophylaxis, immune-complex disease devel-opment, inadequate immunosuppression resulting from decreased OKT3 levels, or OKT3 sensitization are believed to be markers for patients at higher risk for humoral rejection.

Despite the lack of consistent data supporting the routine use of induc-tion therapy with antilymphocyte antibody agents, the therapy has a clear role in select situations. Specifically, patients with early postopera-tive renal or hepatic dysfunction may benefit by avoiding CyA therapy while using these induction agents. Antilymphocyte antibody therapy provides effective immunosuppression for at least 10–14 d without CyA or tacrolimus therapy. Also, patients with overwhelming postoperative bacterial infections or diabetics with severe postoperative hyperglyce-mia may benefit from the comparatively low doses of corticosteroids required during antilymphocyte induction therapy.

Despite the extensive use of induction therapy using antilymphocyte antibodies in solid organ transplantation, the exact role of these agents is unclear. There is no doubt that their routine use is unwarranted, as the generalized immunosuppression that they induce increases infection and malignancy risks. Until recently, the agents were ideal in the early post-operative period in patients with renal or hepatic dysfunction in whom CyA could not be used. With the recent success achieved by interleukin (IL)-2 receptor blockade in these situations, the role of antilymphocyte agents may be relegated to salvage therapy.

IL-2 Receptor Inhibition

The high-affinity IL-2 receptor is composed of three noncovalently bound chains: a 55 kd α chain (also referred to as CD25 or Tac), a 75 kd β chain, and a 64kd γ chain. This receptor is present on nearly all acti-vated T cells but not on resting T cells. In vivo activation of the high-affinity IL-2 receptor by IL-2 promotes the clonal expansion of the activated T-cell population (8,9). Various rodent MAbs directed against the receptor's α chain have been used in animals and humans to achieve selective immunosuppression by targeting only T-cell clones responding to the allograft (10,11). Chimerization or humanization of these MAbs has resulted in antibodies with a predominantly human framework that retain the antigen specificity of the original rodent MAbs. A fully humanized anti-IL-2R MAb (daclizumab) and a chimeric anti-IL-2R MAb (basiliximab) have undergone successful Phase III trials demonstrating their efficacy in the immunoprophylaxis of patients undergoing renal transplantation (11–13).

DACLIZUMAB

Daclizumab™ is a molecularly engineered human immunoglobulin (Ig)G1 MAb that binds but does not activate the high-affinity IL-2 receptor. Because it consists of 90% human Ig sequences, daclizumab has low immunogenicity; its serum half-life is 21 d.

Flaventi et al. studied the administration of daclizumab to cadaveric renal transplantation recipients and showed decreases in the number of allograft rejection episodes and an increase in the time to a first rejection episode without a concomitant increase in the incidence of infection or cancer (13).

Beniaminovitz et al. showed that, as compared with conventional triple-drug immunosuppressive therapy, induction with daclizumab decreased rejection frequency, prolonged the time to a first rejection episode in the first 3 mo after cardiac transplantation, and decreased overall rejection severity. In this study, treatment with daclizumab significantly reduced the frequency and severity of rejection in the treatment period, but, after the cessation of therapy, rejection frequency increased to a level similar to the control group (8).

This finding suggests that daclizumab has an immunomodulatory effect similar to other MAb-based therapies (i.e., it induces clonal anergy rather than clonal deletion). However, daclizumab has several advantages over other induction agents. Given its unique composition, its use is not functionally immunogenic. Its effective serum half-life is 21 d; thus, five doses provide saturation for at least 3 mo, which covers the period of highest cardiac allograft rejection incidence. Moreover, lack of immunogenicity makes prolonged courses possible and may permit repeated use of this agent for more than 3 mo. Furthermore, rejection that occurred after daclizumab therapy cessation was preceded by the development of circulating anti-human lymphocyte antigen (HLA) antibodies. Therefore, careful immunologic screening may identify patients who require prolonged, higher-dose, or repeated daclizumab therapy.

Also, daclizumab therapy produced a marked reduction in anti-HLA antibody formation that sustained even after therapy stopped. This suggests that the drug prominently affects the indirect recognition pathway. The indirect pathway of CD4 T-cell activation plays an important part in acute and chronic rejection development. Whereas primary rejection is accompanied by recognition by the recipient's T cells of a dominant HLA-DR allopeptide presented by self-antigen-presenting cells, recurrent rejection episodes and transplant-related coronary artery disease (CAD) development appear to result from the activation of antigen-specific B cells by soluble HLA-DR molecules. Because the development of anti-HLA IgG antibodies to the graft is associated with the development of cellular rejection and graft atherosclerosis, effective inhibition by IL-2 receptor blockade may favorably influence both transplant-related CAD development and long-term survival *(14)*.

Daclizumab's short-term safety profile appears superior to that of other therapies based on MAbs or polyclonal antibodies. Daclizumab administration is not associated with any detectable signs of cytokine release syndrome or allergic responses. Furthermore, when compared to the control group, the incidence of infection or cancer was not higher in the daclizumab group *(8)*.

BASILIXIMAB

The chimeric anti-CD25 MAb basiliximab has been studied as an immunoprophylactic agent against acute rejection in patients undergoing renal transplantation. Patients treated with this agent had a significant reduction in acute rejection and did not have an increased incidence of infections or malignancy. In keeping with the chimeric structure, the half-life of basiliximab was approx 7 d, considerably shorter than human IgG or daclizumab *(15,16)*.

Daclizumab appears to be an effective adjuvant immunomodulating agent in cardiac allograft recipients. It has advantages over conventional induction therapy because it is more selective and can be used for prolonged, and potentially repeated, periods. Studies with larger cohorts are needed to further examine short-term and long-term survival benefits for patients following cardiac transplantation and determine the optimal dosing daclizumab schedules. Also, further studies using basiliximab in cardiac transplantation are needed to determine its efficacy and safety profile.

Commonly Used Immunosuppressive Agents

AZATHIOPRINE

Available for more than 35 yr, azathioprine remains useful as an immunosuppressive agent. Following administration, azathioprine is converted into 6-mercaptopurine, with subsequent transformation into a series of intracellularly active metabolites. These inhibit an early step in *de novo* purine synthesis and several steps in the purine salvage pathway. The net effect is cellular purine store depletion, thus inhibiting deoxyribonucleic acid (DNA) and ribonucleic acid synthesis, the impact of which is most marked on actively dividing lymphocytes responding to antigenic stimulation *(17)*.

In current immunosuppressive protocols, azathioprine is used as part of a triple-therapy regimen with prednisone and CyA or tacrolimus. As this chapter later discusses, improved mycophenolate mofetil (MMF) efficacy led the authors, as well as other centers, to replace azathioprine with MMF.

CYCLOSPORINE

Over the past two decades, CyA has been the most important factor associated with improved outcomes after cardiac transplantation. A review of the first decade of heart transplantation experience revealed a total of 379 cardiac allograft recipients worldwide; actuarial survival rates in this cohort at 1 yr and 5 yr were 56 and 31%, respectively; the main causes of death were acute rejection and immunosuppression side effects. With the introduction and widespread use of CyA over the following decade, survival rates dramatically improved to 85 and 75% at 1 and 5 yr, respectively *(18)*. Sarris et al. from Stanford University, reported on a group of 496 patients who underwent cardiac transplantation since the introduction of CyA (between 1980 and 1993) with 82, 61, and 41% survival at 1, 5, and 10 yr, respectively *(19)*. Olivari et al., from the University of Minnesota, reported outstanding results in a group of patients receiving cardiac transplants between 1983 and 1988; 1- and 5-yr survivals were 92 and 78%, respectively *(20)*. Several studies showed that CyA-based regimens were associated with significant prolongation in survival after cardiac transplantation *(21–23)*.

The binding of IL-2 to the IL-2 receptors on the T-lymphocyte surface is a key stimulant in promoting lymphocyte proliferation and activation. CyA first binds to a cytosolic protein, cyclophilin (CyP), at the cellular level. The CyA–CyP complex then binds to calcineurin and subsequently blocks IL-2 transcription.

The major adverse effects of CyA are nephrotoxicity, hypertension, neurotoxocity, and hyperlipidemia; less common side effects include hirsutism, gingival hyperplasia, and liver dysfunction. CyA nephrotoxicity manifests as acute or chronic renal dysfunction. It is important to note numerous drugs commonly used in transplant patients, such as aminoglycosides, amphotericin B, and ketoconazole, can potentiate the nephrotoxicity induced by CyA. More than half the patients receiving CyA require treatment for hypertension within the first year following transplantation. Corticosteroids also potentiate CyA side effects, such as hypertension, hyperlipidemia, and hirsutism *(17)*. To lessen these side effects, steroid weaning is practiced, as discussed later in this chapter.

The pharmacokinetics and pharmacodynamics of CyA are complex. Frequent serum level monitoring is essential to minimize adverse effects. One major limitation of the original oil-based CyA formulation (Sandimmune) is its variable and unpredictable bioavailability. The introduction of Neoral in the mid-1990s was a major advance; Neoral is a microemulsion formula of CyA that has greater bioavailability and more predictable pharmacokinetics than Sandimmune *(24,25)*. The OLN 351 study, involving 380 recipients at 24 centers, compared the safety and efficacy of these two CyA preparations in a double-blind, randomized trial. The study's results showed fewer Neoral patients needing antilymphocyte therapy to treat rejection, fewer rejection episodes among female patients receiving Neoral, fewer infections in the Neoral group, and equivalent tolerability of the two formulations *(26)*.

Although CyA remains the cornerstone of maintenance immunosuppression, the availability of newer agents certainly reduced previous dependence on CyA. Immunosuppressive protocols avoiding CyA altogether have developed with good success. Use of newer agents in combination with CyA may further decrease rejection incidence or may enable lower, better-tolerated CyA doses to be administered. At the authors' center, CyA is currently the core immunosuppressant of choice in the majority of transplant patients.

MYCOPHENOLATE MOFETIL

MMF, which is rapidly hydrolyzed to mycophenolic acid after ingestion, is a selective, noncompetitive, reversible inhibitor of onosine monophosphate dehydrogenase, a key enzyme in the *de novo* guanine nucleotide synthesis. Unlike other marrow-derived cells and parenchymal cells that use the hypoxanthine–guanine phosphoribosyl transferase (salvage) pathway, activated lymphocytes rely predominantly on the *de novo* pathway for purine synthesis. This functional selectivity allows lymphocyte proliferation to be specifically targeted with less anticipated effect on erythropoiesis and neutrophil production than with azathioprine *(27)*.

Early studies in human heart transplant recipients demonstrated that MMF, when substituted for azathioprine in standard triple-therapy regimens, is well tolerated and more efficacious than azathioprine *(28–30)*. In a large, double-blind, randomized multicenter study comparing MMF to azathioprine (with CyA and prednisone) in 650 patients, Kobashigawa et al. showed that the MMF group had a significant reduction in mortality as well as a reduction in the requirement for rejection treatment. Also, there was a trend for MMF patients to have fewer 3A rejections. The lower mortality in the MMF group seemed to result mostly from a decrease in deaths related to immunosuppression use (rejection and infection). However, there was an increase in the incidence of opportunistic viral infections in the MMF group *(31)*.

Others have shown that MMF is superior to azathioprine for prevention of B-cell activation and production of anti-HLA antibodies, perhaps explaining its superior efficacy as an antirejection agent *(32–34)*. By decreasing B-cell proliferation, MMF may have a beneficial effect on transplant coronary artery disease (TCAD) development.

Since 1996, our center has substituted MMF for azathioprine as part of a triple-drug immunosuppression regimen with CyA and prednisone. Initially, successful MMF use in cardiac transplant patients has been based on its efficacy in refractory rejection management in patients treated by CyA, azathioprine, and prednisone; MMF replaces azathioprine in these patients for maintenance immunosuppression.

TACROLIMUS

Tacrolimus (Prograf, Fujisawa Healthcare, Deerfield, IL) is a macrolide antibiotic that inhibits T-cell activation and proliferation and inhibits other cytokine production *(36)*. The product of *Streptomyces tsurubaensis* fermentation, tacrolimus was discovered in 1984 and first used in clinical studies in 1988 at the University of Pittsburgh. Tacrolimus use in heart transplantation began at the same institution in the early 1990s, initially as "rescue therapy" and later as primary therapy *(37)*. Recently, Taylor et al. reviewed the guidelines for tacrolimus use in cardiac transplant recipients *(36)*.

The initial trial comparing tacrolimus with CyA in clinical heart transplantation demonstrated that patients receiving tacrolimus had a lower hypertension risk and required a lower steroid dose. Although the mean serum creatinine concentration was higher at 1 yr in the tacrolimus group, this difference disappeared after 2 yr. This study concluded that an intermediate-term analysis indicated that tacrolimus compares favorably with CyA as a primary immunosuppressant in cardiac transplant recipients *(37)*.

An improved understanding of the efficacy and pharmacokinetics of tacrolimus came from European and US multicenter trials *(38,39)*. Patient survival and the probability of freedom from rejection were similar between the two treatment groups in both trials. In the European trial, the overall infection rates, impaired renal function, and glucose intolerance did not differ significantly between the tacrolimus and CyA groups. However, tacrolimus-treated patients possessed an advantage with regard to a reduced requirement for antihypertensive therapy. Similarly, in the US trial, there were no differences in infection rates, renal function, hyperglycemia, or hyperkalemia during the first year of treatment. Comparable to those in the European trial, more CyA-treated patients in the US trial developed new-onset hypertension requiring treatment. Also, the incidence of elevated cholesterol and triglycerides was higher in CyA-treated patients. The conclusion from these trials was that tacrolimus-based immunosuppression is effective for rejection prophylaxis after cardiac transplantation and, when compared to CyA treatment, may be associated with less hypertension and hyperlipidemia and comparable renal function and infection risk.

In addition, whereas these comparative clinical trials suggest similar efficacy between the two therapies, it is suggested that some patient groups may benefit from tacrolimus, rather than CyA, as primary immunosuppressive therapy after cardiac transplant *(40)*. Unlike with CyA, hirsutism and gingival hyperplasia occur infrequently with tacrolimus; thus, tacrolimus-based therapy may improve compliance and quality of life in female and pediatric transplant recipients. It should be noted that alopecia is documented with tacrolimus use, but it is known to improve with dose reductions. The decreased incidence of hypertension and hyperlipidemia with tacrolimus makes it preferable to CyA in patients with refractory hypertension or hyperlipidemia.

A final indication for tacrolimus has been as a rescue immunosuppressant in cardiac transplant recipients receiving CyA who have refractory rejection or intolerance to immunosuppression (severe side effects) *(41)*. Baran et al. reported on their experience with tacrolimus monotherapy in cardiac transplant recipients, showing that tacrolimus use alone after steroid weaning provides effective immunosuppression with low rejection incidence, infection, and TCAD *(42)*.

Because tacrolimus is metabolized using the same cytochrome P450 enzyme system as CyA, drug interactions are essentially the same. Thus, drugs that induce this system may increase the metabolism of tacrolimus, thereby decreasing its blood levels. Conversely, drugs that inhibit the P450 system decrease the metabolism of tacrolimus, thereby increasing its blood levels. Some studies have indicated a higher incidence of nephrotoxicity with tacrolimus as compared to CyA.

Current data clearly show that tacrolimus has efficacy comparable to CyA with decreased incidence of hypertension and hyperlipidemia. It may be safely combined as part of a triple-drug immunosuppression regimen. Our experience with tacrolimus at Columbia–Presbyterian is limited. Ongoing experience with tacrolimus in cardiac transplant recipients will refine current recommendations for its use.

Immunosuppressive Regimens

Since 1983, all patients undergoing transplantation at Columbia–Presbyterian have received CyA-based immunosuppression. Current dosing for standard triple-therapy immunosuppression consists of the following:

- CyA: a preoperative dose (3–6 mg/kg) followed by intravenous CyA (1–2 mg/kg/24 h) until oral intake is tolerated. Daily oral doses (3–6 mg/kg) are adjusted so that serum levels are maintained at 300–350 ng/mL. After 6–12 mo, CyA dosing is reduced to maintain serum levels between 100 and 150 ng/mL.
- Azathioprine: administered in a preoperative oral dose (4 mg/kg) followed by daily doses of 2 mg/kg IV until the patient can tolerate oral medications, at which point azathioprine is changed to MMF, starting at a dose of 1000 mg, twice daily (since 1996).
- Intravenous methylprednisolone: 500mg administered during the operation and followed in the postoperative period by 125 mg every 8 h for three doses. Prednisone is then instituted at a daily oral dose of 1 mg/kg and gradually tapered over 4 mo to 0.1 mg/kg/d. In some patients, the authors make an attempt to wean off prednisone completely. Daclizumab is administered to certain transplant recipients.

At other centers, the standard regimen used in cardiac transplant patients is a combination of CyA with azathioprine or MMF in addition to prednisone. With this regimen, MMF is used more commonly because of the lower incidence of acute rejection. In recent years, some centers started using tacrolimus in place of CyA as part of a triple-drug regimen, along with azathioprine or MMF in addition to prednisone.

LONG-TERM POSTTRANSPLANT CONSIDERATIONS
Steroid Withdrawal

Steroids are used routinely in almost all immunosuppressive protocols after cardiac transplantation. The metabolic side effects of steroids are well known and lead to significant morbidity and mortality in the posttransplant period. Since the first report by Yacoub et al., growing evidence suggests that steroids may not be a requirement for post-transplant immunosuppression *(43)*. Despite these data, almost 90% and 70% of patients continue to receive prednisone at 1 yr and 3 yr posttransplant, respectively.

A recent review of more than 1800 patients from a combined registry outlined the morbid complications that patients suffer within the first year after transplantation. Many of these complications are known side effects of prednisone, including hypertension (16%), diabetes mellitus (16%), hyperlipidemia (26%), bone disease (5%), and cataracts (2%) *(44)*. Therefore, it is obvious that avoiding of steroids may decrease morbidity and mortality after heart transplantation *(45)*. Two general approaches are used to institute prednisone-free immunosuppression: early and late withdrawal.

EARLY WITHDRAWAL

Withdrawal of prednisone during mo 1 posttransplant has resulted in long-term success of steroid withdrawal in 50–80% of patients. In these studies, antilymphocyte antibody induction therapy appears to increase the likelihood of successful steroid withdrawal. Several centers reported their results with immunosuppressive regimens that did not include steroids in the early posttransplant period *(46)*. Studies reporting high success rates of 80% used specific enrollment criteria, such as excluding patients with recurrent acute rejections or those of female gender.

In a series of nonrandomized patients, Katz et al. showed that 61% of patients could be treated without steroids immediately posttransplant; these patients had similar survival, infection, and rejection rates, but a lower incidence of diabetes when compared to patients with triple-drug immunosuppression. Keogh et al. reported a 5-yr follow-up on over 100 patients prospectively randomized to triple-drug therapy or double-drug therapy with CyA and azathioprine *(47)*. Patients with significant renal dysfunction or recurrent acute rejection (more than three episodes) were converted to maintenance steroids. Only 47% of patients required conversion to triple-drug therapy. There was no difference in actuarial survival between the two patient groups. Rejection in the first 3 mo was lower with triple-drug therapy, but did not differ between the two groups beyond 3 mo. However, patients on triple-drug therapy had higher serum cholesterol as well as an increased requirement for antihypertensive medication.

Clearly, these studies demonstrate that steroid-free maintenance immunosuppression is possible in at least 50% of patients, is as safe as triple-drug therapy, and may reduce some long-term steroid complications.

LATE WITHDRAWAL

Owing to the majority of acute rejection episodes occurring in the first 3 mo posttransplant, steroid withdrawal often begins after this time period, resulting in long-term success in about 80% of patients *(48)*. Generally, there is no need for conventional induction agents when late steroid withdrawal is employed. Using center-specific indications for steroid withdrawal, Taylor et al. reported successful steroid discontinuation in 30% of patients *(49)*. Both early- and long-term mortality were significantly lower in patients in whom successful early withdrawal from steroids was achieved. Also, there was a trend toward decreased TCAD in those in whom steroids were weaned. Olivari et al. found that the degree of posttransplantation weight gain, number of lipid abnormalities, and incidence of hypertension were not modified by steroid tapering, whereas the incidence of cataracts and compression fractures and the degree of bone loss were significantly reduced *(50)*.

Successful weaning from steroids may be limited to an immunologically privileged patient subgroup. Kobashigawa et al. reported higher success rates from steroid withdrawal in patients with two or three HLA-DR matches *(51)*. Felkel et al. revealed that being a black recipient is a negative predictive factor for both successful steroid withdrawal and survival, after adjusting for potential predictors for survival *(52)*. This raises the question of whether avoiding steroid toxicity or being immunologically privileged by a favorable donor–recipient match is contributory to the improved survival reported.

We believe that there is a role for steroid weaning after the first 6 mo following cardiac transplantation. In most patients, steroids should be administered during the period of greatest rejection risk, namely the first 3–6 mo, with a determined attempt to wean it subsequently. There is significant room for improvement in this area of immunosuppression, based on recent data from the International Society of Heart and Lung Transplantation database revealing that 70% of patients are maintained on long-term prednisone treatment *(53)*.

NOVEL MODALITIES OF IMMUNOSUPPRESSION

Rapamycin

Rapamycin (Rapamune, Wyeth–Ayerst Laboratories, Madison, NJ), a microbial product isolated form the actinomycete *Streptomyces hygroscopicus*, was discovered initially as an antifungal agent in the mid-1970s *(54)*. The advent of tacrolimus and the recognition of structural similarities between these two drugs led research groups to study rapamycin's immunosuppressive properties. Similar to tacrolimus, the drug contains the same tricarbonyl region including an amide, a ketone, and a hemiketal, but a triene segment in rapamycin differentiates the two drugs. A new derivative of rapamycin, SDZ-RAD, has been developed with similar in vivo potency.

In contrast to CyA or tacrolimus, rapamycin does not affect calcineurin activity or lymphokine gene transcription. It selectively inhibits proteins that are associated with cell cycle phase G1 as well as ribosomal proteins that result in cell cycle prolongation at G1/S interphase. In addition, rapamycin inhibits IL-2-induced binding of transcription factors in the proliferating cell nuclear antigen promoter, thus inhibiting progression to DNA synthesis and the S phase.

The consequences of these actions make rapamycin a unique immunosuppressive agent. Although its net effects make it a less potent cytokine synthesis inhibitor than CyA, rapamycin inhibits immune functions such as B-cell Ig synthesis, antibody-dependent cellular cytotoxicity, and killer cell activity. Also important is its ability to exert an antiproliferative effect, thereby suggesting a potential benefit of rapamycin in chronic rejection and TCAD. Morris et al. showed that rapamycin can reverse established allograft vascular disease in a rat cardiac allograft model as well as a monkey aortic allograft model (55,56).

The efficacy of rapamycin as an immunosuppressive agent is shown in several animal models of transplantation. Clinical trials using rapamycin have been performed mainly in kidney transplant patients with efficacious antirejection effects; it has also been used as rescue therapy for refractory rejection. These trials suggest that rapamycin, used in conjunction with CyA-based regimens, has a synergistic effect on rejection (57). Studies evaluating the role of rapamycin in cardiac transplant patients are ongoing and offer the prospects of significant improvements in transplant immunosuppression in the form of further reduced acute rejection, lesser immunosuppressant-induced toxicity, and a lower incidence of TCAD.

Photopheresis

Photopheresis is a leukopheresis-based immunomodulatory therapy form in which lymphocytes treated with 8-methoxypsoralen are irradiated with ultraviolet-A ex vivo and reinfused into the patient (58). Photopheresis is effective in a number of nontransplant disease states, such as cutaneous T-cell lymphoma, scleroderma, pemphigus vulgaris, systemic lupus erythematosus, and rheumatoid arthritis; these conditions are mediated partially by expanded populations of unregulated effector T cells.

Early experimental work included a primate cardiac transplantation model, in which photochemotherapy in conjunction with CyA and steroids suppressed the cellular immune response and the formation of cytotoxic antibodies against the transplanted antigens *(59,60)*. This led to initial clinical studies that showed that the low toxicity and potential efficacy of photopheresis could lead to a role for this modality in the prevention and treatment of cardiac transplant rejection *(61)*.

In a nonrandomized study by Barr et al. for the Photopheresis Transplant Study Group, 60 consecutive cardiac transplant patients randomly received standard triple-drug immunosuppression (CyA, azathioprine, steroids) alone or in combination with photopheresis. The photopheresis group received a total of 24 photopheresis treatments, each pair of treatments given consecutively on 2 d , during the first 6 mo after transplantation. The study concluded that the addition of photopheresis to a triple-drug regimen significantly decreased cardiac rejection risk. However, there was no significant difference in the time to a first rejection episode, incidence of rejection associated with hemodynamic compromise, or survival at 6 and 12 mo. There were no differences in the infection rates or types, although CMV DNA was detected less frequently in the photopheresis group *(62)*.

In another randomized single-center study, Barr et al. reported that the addition of prophylactic photopheresis to standard CyA-based triple-drug immunosuppression significantly decreased coronary artery intimal thickness at 1- and 2-yr follow-up. Further, the photopheresis group had a significant reduction in panel reactive antibody (PRA) levels within the first 6 mo posttransplant. These results are exciting, and further studies are needed to assess whether the application of photopheresis to cardiac allograft recipients will result in a sustained decrease in intimal hyperplasia progression and whether this translates into improved graft and patient survival *(63)*.

PRETRANSPLANT AND POSTTRANSPLANT MANAGEMENT OF THE SENSITIZED PATIENT

To identify patients at risk for donor-specific alloreactivity, cardiac transplantation candidates are screened for antibodies that are reactive with lymphocytes from a panel of volunteers representative of the major HLA allotypes; these antibodies are collectively referred to as PRAs. Patients with high PRA levels are considered sensitized to various alloantigens and require donor-specific T-cell cross-matches before transplantation to exclude the presence of lymphocytotoxic IgG

Table 1
Influence of Preformed Anti-HLA Antibodies
in Cardiac Allograft Recipients at Risk for Sensitization (n = 88)
on Cumulative Annual Rejection Frequency Posttransplantation[a]

	Cumulative annual rejection frequency (no. of 3A or 3B rejections/yr)		
Preformed antibody type	Positive	Negative	p value
IgG anti-HLA class II	1.29	0.48	0.02
IgG anti-HLA class I	0.611	0.291	0.09
IgM anti-HLA class II	0.468	0.328	0.88

[a]Cumulative high-grade (3A/3B) rejections were modeled by the method of Wei, Lin, and Weissfeld (13), computing robust variance estimates allowing for the dependence among multiple event times.

antibodies against donor class I HLAs, which can cause early graft failure resulting from complement-mediated humoral rejection (64,65).

Because a positive donor-specific T-cell cross-match is a contraindication to transplantation, sensitized candidates have longer waiting times and higher mortality rates while waiting for organs (see Table 1) (66,67). In addition, the presence of preformed anti-HLA antibodies predicts poorer long-term outcome, including an increased number of cellular rejections, earlier TCAD onset, and decreased long-term graft survival compared with nonsensitized patients treated with standard triple-drug immunosuppressive regimens. These complications seem primarily related to the presence of preformed antibodies against allogeneic HLA class II molecules and may reflect an underlying state of CD4 T-cell allosensitization to class II antigens (68–71).

The proportion of highly sensitized patients on cardiac transplant waiting lists has increased as a result of widespread use of left ventricular assist devices (LVADs) and more patients undergoing retransplantation (72). Whereas alloreactivity in retransplant candidates, blood product recipients, and multiparous women is a result of repeated B- and T-cell exposure to alloantigens, the high frequency of alloreactivity in LVAD recipients seems to result additionally from polyclonal B-cell activation. This activation is attributable to selective loss of Th1-type cells through activation-induced cell death and unopposed production of Th2-type cytokines (73,74). Interventions in sensitized recipients have focused on therapies aimed predominantly at Ig depletion and B-cell suppression (75–80).

Pretransplant Management

Recent studies suggest that pooled human intravenous Ig is an effective modality to reduce allosensitization *(81,82)*. Postulated mechanisms include the presence in intravenous Ig of anti-idiotypic antibodies *882,83)*, antibodies against membrane-associated immunologic molecules such as CD4 or CD5 *(84,85)*, or soluble forms of HLA molecules *(86,87)*. The authors investigated the effects of intravenous Ig on serum reactivity to HLA class I molecules in LVAD recipients and compared these effects to those obtained with plasmapheresis, an alternative modality for alloreactive antibody reduction *(66)*. They first evaluated the efficacy of monthly intravenous Ig courses at 2 g/kg, together with monthly infusions of intravenous cyclophosphamide (0.5–1.0 g/m^2), in reduction of reactivity of circulating IgG antibodies for allogeneic HLA class I molecules. Within 1 wk following intravenous Ig infusion in four divided daily doses, the reactivity of circulating IgG antibodies for allogeneic HLA class I molecules decreased by a mean of 33% (range: 14–52%) (p = <0.01). This was the maximal level of alloreactivity reduction during the 4 wk after intravenous Ig infusion, with the efficacy of intravenous Ig progressively decreasing by the end of the wk 4 to a mean reduction in alloreactivity of 8% ±7%.

Then, we compared the effects of intravenous Ig (2 g/kg) with plasmapheresis on reduction of reactivity of circulating IgG antibodies with allogeneic HLA class I molecules in LVAD recipients. Reactivity of circulating IgG antibodies with allogeneic HLA class I molecules did not significantly reduce within the first 2 wk after initiation of plasmapheresis. Maximal reduction in alloreactivity, 38% ± 11%, occurred by the wk 4 of plasmapheresis. These results showed that intravenous Ig has an earlier onset of action and greater efficacy in reducing IgG anti-HLA alloreactivity as compared with plasmapheresis.

We also investigated whether treatment with intravenous Ig (2 g/kg) together with intravenous cyclophosphamide (0.5–1.0 g/m^2) to reduce alloreactivity in sensitized recipients would impact waiting time to transplantation. The first three highly sensitized LVAD recipients to receive desensitization therapy had been waiting for cardiac transplantation for a mean of 303 ± 25 d prior to the onset of therapy, as a result of repeated positive donor-specific cross-matches (mean: 33; range: 24–43). Following initiation of intravenous Ig/cyclophosphamide therapy, with or without additional immunodepletion using plasmapheresis, all patients obtained negative donor-specific cross-matches and were successfully transplanted in a mean time of 99 ± 8 d.

On the basis of these results, a formal protocol was established to initiate monthly courses of intravenous Ig therapy (2g/kg) with intravenous cyclophosphamide following initial allosensitization detection. Whereas the mean wait time to cardiac transplantation was 7.1 mo (range: 0.2–17.9) in patients with IgG antibodies against HLA class I molecules, this significantly decreased to 3.3 mo (range 0.3–6.2) in sensitized recipients receiving one or two courses of intravenous Ig (2 g/kg) ($p < 0.05$). No patient in either group was transplanted across a positive donor-specific IgG T-cell cross-match. This duration was similar to the waiting time to transplantation of 3.1 mo (range: 0.3–10.7) in 27 unsensitized patients.

Posttransplant Management

The posttransplant induction of immunologic allograft rejection markers has been compared in sensitized cardiac allograft recipients who were treated with CyA/steroid-based triple-drug immunosuppressive regimens incorporating intravenous cyclophosphamide pulses or oral MMF. In comparison with MMF, treatment for 4–6 mo with intravenous pulses of cyclophosphamide protected against IL-2-receptor-positive T-cell outgrowth from biopsy sites during the first posttransplant year ($p < 0.01$), as well as the posttransplant induction of IgG antibodies against HLA class II, but not class I, antibodies (defined as an increase by more than 10% above pretransplant values).

Immunosuppression using intravenous pulses of cyclophosphamide, as compared to MMF, in sensitized recipients for 4–6 mo posttransplantation significantly prolonged the rejection-free interval (*see* Table 2). Overall, only 4 of 26 (15%) cyclophosphamide-treated patients developed one or more high-grade rejections within the first posttransplant year, compared with 22 of 48 (46%) patients treated with MMF ($p = 0.009$). Cyclophosphamide treatment had the same effect on sensitized recipients with either preformed IgG anti-HLA class I antibodies ($p = 0.02$) or class II antibodies ($p = 0.04$). Moreover, treatment with cyclophosphamide reduced the cumulative annual rejection frequency by 63%, from 0.94 rejections per year for sensitized patients treated with MMF to 0.35 rejections per year ($p = 0.03$).

By Cox Proportional Hazard modeling for multivariable analysis, the only significant protective factor against high-grade cellular rejection development in sensitized patients was treatment with cyclophosphamide (*see* Table 3). In comparison with cyclophosphamide, MMF treatment conferred a 3.7-fold higher rejection risk ($p = 0.009$) *(87)*.

Table 2
Intravenous Pulse Therapy With Cyclophosphamide Is Superior to Mycophenolate Mofetil for Reduction of Cumulative Annual Rejection Frequency in Sensitized Cardiac Allograft Recipients[a]

Preformed antibody type	Cumulative annual rejection frequency (no. of 3A or 3B rejections/yr)		
	Intravenous cyclophosphamide	Mycophenolate mofetil	p value
gG anti-HLA (total)	1.29	0.48	0.02
IgG anti-HLA class II	0.611	0.291	0.09
IgG anti-HLA class I	0.468	0.328	0.88

[a]Cumulative high-grade (3A/3B) rejections were modeled by the method of Wei, Lin, and Weissfeld (13), computing robust variance estimates allowing for the dependence among multiple event times.

Table 3
By Multivariable Analysis, Using the Cox Proportional Hazards Model,
Treatment of Sensitized Cardiac Allograft Recipients With Mycophenolate
Mofetil (n = 48) Portends a Significantly Higher Risk for Cellular Rejection
Than Intravenous Cyclophosphamide (n = 26)

Variable	Coefficient ± SE	p value	Risk ratio	95% CI
Mycophenolate mofetil	1.035 ± 0.4393	0.0184	3.7	(1.19, 6.66)
Cyclophosphamide	0.908 ± 0.5295	0.0863	1.0	(0.88, 7.00)

Treatment with intravenous cyclophosphamide is extremely safe. The incidence of CMV disease (defined as clinical disease together with virologic culture confirmation) was lower in cyclophosphamide-treated patients (3 of 26, 12%) than in those treated with MMF (10 of 54, 19%). No other viral, bacterial, or fungal infections were seen in patients treated with cyclophosphamide. Intravenous pulse therapy with cyclophosphamide was frequently (in greater than 80% of cases) accompanied by transient nausea and vomiting, which responded to antiemetic therapy. Mesna was coadministered with cyclophosphamide and may have contributed to the absence of any hemorrhagic cystitis cases. No malignancies developed after 540 mo of follow-up (range of follow-up per patient: 6–38). Intravenous Ig therapy was associated with clinical manifestations of immune complex disease in 4 of 27 (15%) monthly courses, as evidenced by fevers, arthralgias, and maculopapular rashes. Reversible renal insufficiency (defined as greater than a 50% increase in serum creatinine level) occurred in four cases, all of which resolved spontaneously over the ensuing 3 wk postinfusion.

These results demonstrate that intravenous pulse cyclophosphamide therapy, together with pretransplantation intravenous Ig as part of a CyA/steroid-based regimen in sensitized cardiac allograft recipients, is extremely effective and safe for decreasing recipient serum and cellular alloreactivity, shortening transplant waiting time, and reducing allograft rejection.

It is likely that the principal component of our immunomodulatory regimen responsible for pretransplant reduction in anti-HLA alloreactivity is intravenous Ig. Although intravenous Ig stimulates the production of IgM anti-idiotypic-blocking antibodies to HLA in recipient serum, this immunomodulatory mechanism is unlikely to account for the rapid, transient, and nonsustained clinical effect on reduction in anti-HLA alloreactivity observed when using intravenous Ig in sensitized cardiac transplant patients. In contrast, our combined intravenous Ig/

intravenous cyclophosphamide regimen has a prolonged inhibitory effect on CD4 T-cell activation, as defined by sustained prevention of both T-cell-mediated allograft rejection and induction of anti-HLA class II antibodies after transplantation. This immunomodulatory effect suggests that the principal regimental component responsible for these effects is cyclophosphamide.

Presently,we advocate that all patients at risk for sensitization before transplantation be screened specifically for the presence of antibodies against both HLA class I and II antibodies. On the basis of our results, immunosuppressive therapy for sensitized patients should commence before transplantation. Initiation of an immunosuppressive protocol using intravenous cyclophosphamide pulses before and after transplantation is a safe and effective modality for reducing donor-specific B- and T-cell alloreactivity *(88)*.

TRANSPLANT TOLERANCE

Despite the dramatic improvement of early graft survival after CyA introduction, late-graft loss resulting from transplant CAD and the major consequences of long-term immunosuppression, such as infection and malignancy, remain obstacles to longer allograft recipient survival. The development of tolerance to the allograft would avoid these problems *(89)*. Tolerance is defined as the lack of detrimental immune reactivity to the donor antigen (allograft) with normal immune reactivity to other antigens occurring in the absence of ongoing immunosuppression *(90)*. Despite the discovery of the immunological tolerance phenomenon by Billingham, Brent, and Medawar almost 50 yr ago, true immunological tolerance remains the "holy grail" of transplantation *(91)*. In that experiment, naturally immunocompromised recipient neonatal animals injected with replicating donor-strain hematopoietic lymphoid cells became lymphoid-cell chimeras and subsequently exhibited tolerance to donor-specific grafts as adults.

Increasing clinical and experimental evidence that transplantation tolerance is an achievable goal is mounting. The beneficial effect of blood transfusions on kidney allograft survival raises the possibility of inducing nonspecific hyporesponsiveness by infusing foreign cells *(92)*. Salvatierra et al. showed that donor-specific blood transfusions improve survival of kidney transplants coming from the same donor, thus suggesting that donor-derived cells could play a role in improving graft acceptance *(93)*. The observation that liver transplant recipients can maintain graft survival despite immunosuppression discontinuance is reported *(94)*. Further, long-term allograft acceptance in nonhuman primates was obtained using strategies with reduced toxicity such as costimulation blockade or induction of mixed chimerism *(89)*.

Chimerism is the condition in which donor cells engraft without further immunosuppressive therapy; there are two major types of chimerism. Microchimerism exists when only a low percentage of cells (less than 1%) are of donor origin. This phenomenon was well described by Starzl et al., who identified cells of donor origin in various tissues in functionally tolerant liver transplant patients *(95)*. However, macro-chimerism exists when all cells are of donor origin (full chimerism) or there is co-existence of cells of both donor and recipient origin (mixed chimerism, greater than 1% but less than 100% of cells of donor origin).

Donor hematopoietic stem cell transplantation (HSCT) has been used successfully in numerous experimental settings to induce donor-specific tolerance. However, other cells have also been used for tolerance induction. These include dendritic cells, regulatory T cells, and embryonic stem cells. Ideally, attempts to induce tolerance using cell therapy should precede solid organ transplantation. It is suggested, in HSCT for mixed chimerism induction, that the time interval between stem cell and organ transplantation should be approx 4–6 wk to allow hematopoiesis recovery before transplant surgery *(89,96)*. However, several questions need to be answered before clinical trial initiation. These include the cell type to be infused, infusion route and timing, and, finally, the need for a conditioning regimen or associated immunosuppressive therapy in addition to the infusion of donor derived cells.

CONCLUSION

Immunosuppression is rapidly changing because of the increasing number of drugs and biological agents making the transition from the laboratory to clinical trials. Future immunosuppressive protocols will likely be individually tailored, multidrug regimens using less toxic doses of nonoverlapping, synergistic, and alloimmune-specific agents. The final hope for the future is that specific inhibition of antigen recognition, T-cell costimulation, and accessory molecule function will induce long-term acceptance of a transplanted organ without the complications of "broad-spectrum" immunosuppression.

REFERENCES

1. John R, Rajasinghe HA, Chen JM, et al. Impact of current management practices on early and late mortality in over 500 consecutive heart transplant recipients. Ann Surg 2000;232:302–311.

 2. Kirklin JK, Naftel DC, Levine TB, et al. Cytomegalovirus after heart transplanta-
    tion. Risk factors for infection and death: a multi-institutional study. The Cardiac
    Transplant Research Database Group. J Heart Lung Transplant 1994;13:394–404.
 3. Swinnen LJ, Costanzo-Nordin MR, Fisher SJ, et al. Increased incidence of
    lymphoproliferative disorder after immunosuppression with the monoclonal anti-
    body OKT3 in cardiac-transplant recipients. N Engl J Med 1990;323:1723–1728.
 4. Johnson MR, Mullen GM, O'Sullivan EJ, et al. Risk/Benefit ration of perioperative
    OKT3 in cardiac transplantation. Am J Cardiol 1994;74:261–266.
 5. O'Connell JB, Bristow MR, Hammond EH, et al. Antimurine antibody to OKT3 in
    cardiac transplantation: implications for prophylaxis and retreatment of rejection.
    Transplant Proc 1991;23:1157–1159.
 6. Taylor DO, Kfoury AG, Pisani B, et al. Anti-lymphocyte-antibody prophylaxis:
    review of the adult experience in heart transplantation. Transplant Proc 1997;
    29:13S–15S.
 7. Ma H, Hammond EH, Taylor DO, et al. Transplantation 1996;62:205.
 8. Beniaminovitz A, Itescu S, Lietz K, et al. Prevention of the rejection in cardiac
    transplantation by blockade of the interleukin-2 receptor with a monoclonal anti-
    body. N Engl J Med 2000;342:613–619.
 9. Taniguchi T, Minami Y. The IL-2/IL-2 receptor system: a current overview. Cell
    1993;73:5–8.
10. Reed MH, Shapiro ME, Strom TB, et al. Prolongation of primate renal allograft
    survival by anti-Tac, an anti-human IL-2 receptor monoclonal antibody. Transplan-
    tation 1989;47:55–59.
11. Kirkman RL, Shapiro ME, Carpenter CB, et al. A randomized prospective trial of
    anti-Tac monoclonal antibody in human renal transplantation. Transplantation
    1991;51:107–113.
12. Vincenti F. Daclizumab in solid organ transplantation. Biodrugs 1999;11:333–341.
13. Vincenti F, Kirkman R, Light S, et al. Interleukin-2 receptor blockade with
    daclizumab to prevent acute rejection in renal transplantation. N Engl J Med
    1998;338:161–165
14. Lietz K, John R, Beniaminovitz A, et al. A randomized study of interleukin-2 recep-
    tor blockade in cardiac transplantation: influence of HLA-DR locus incompatibility
    on treatment efficacy. Transplantation, in press.
15. Nashan B, Moore R, Amlot P, et al. Randomized trial of basiliximab versus placebo
    for control of acute cellular rejection in renal allograft recipients. Lancet
    1997;350:1193–1198.
16. Kahan BD, Rajagopalan PR, Hall M, et al. Reduction of the occurrence of acute
    cellular rejection among renal allograft recipients treated with basiliximab, a
    chimeric anti-interleukin-2 receptor monoclonal antibody. Transplantation
    1999;67:276–284.
17. Costanzo MR. New immunosuppressive drugs in heart transplantation. Curr Control
    Trials Cardiovasc Med 2001;2:45–53.
18. Cheung A, Menkis AH. Cyclosporine heart transplantation. Transplant Proc
    1998;30:1881–1884.
19. Sarris GE, Moore KA, Schroeder JS, et al. Cardiac Transplantation: the Stanford
    experience in the cyclosporine era. J Thorac Cardiovasc Surg 1994;108:240–251.
20. Olivari MT, Kubo SH, Braunlin EA, et al. Five-year experience with triple-drug
    immunosuppressive therapy in cardiac transplantation. Circulation 1990;82;
    IV 276–IV280.

21. DeCampli WM, Luikart H, Hunt S, et al. Characteristics of patients surviving more than 10 years after cardiac transplantation. J Thorac Cardiovasc Surg 1995;109: 1103–1114.

22. John R, Rajasinghe HA, S Itescu, et al. Factors affecting long term survival (>10 years) after cardiac transplantation in the cyclosporine era. J Am Coll Cardiol 2001;37:189–194.

23. John R, Rajasinghe HA, Chen JM, et al. Long-term outcomes following cardiac transplantation: an experience based on different eras of immunosuppression. Ann Thorac Surg 2001;72:440–449.

24. Valentine H. Neoral use in the cardiac transplant recipient. Transplant Proc 2000;32:27S–44S.

25. Kahan BD, Welsh M, Schoenburg L, et al. Variable absorption of cyclosporine: a biological risk factor for chronic renal allograft rejection. Transplantation 1996;62:599–606.

26. Eisen HJ, Hobbs RE, Davis SF, et al. Safety, tolerability and efficacy of cyclosporine microemulsion in heart transplant recipients: a randomized, multicenter, double-blind comparison with the oil-based formulation of cyclosporine—results at six months after transplantation. Transplantation 1999;68:663–671.

27. Allison AC, Eugui EM. Immunosuppressive and other effects of mycophenolic acid and an ester prodrug, mycophenolate mofetil. Immuno Rev 1993;136:5.

28. Ensley RD, Bristow MR, Olsen SL, et al. The use of mycophenolate mofetil (RS-61443) in human heart transplant recipients. Transplantation 1993;13:571.

29. Renlund DG, Gopinathan SK, Kfoury AG, et al. Mycophenolate mofetil (MMF) in heart transplantation: rejection prevention and treatment. Clin Transplant 1996;10:13.

30. Kobashigawa JA. Mycophenolate mofetil in cardiac transplantaion. Curr Opin Cardiol 1998;13:117–121.

31. Kobashigawa JA, Miller L, Renlund D, et al. A randomized active-controlled trial of mycophenolate mofetil in heart transplant recipients. Transplantation 1998; 66:507–515.

32. Lietz K, John R, Schuster M, et al. Mycophenolate mofetil educes anti-HLA antibody production and cellular rejection in heart transplant recipients. Transplant Proc 2002;34:1828–1829.

33. Weigel G, Griesmacher A, Karimi A, et al. Effect of mycophenolate mofetil on lymphocyte activation in heart transplant recipients. J Heart Lung Transplant 2002;21:1074–1079.

34. Rose ML, Smith J, Dureau G, et al. Mycophenolate mofetil decreases antibody production after cardiac transplantation. J Heart Lung Transplant 2002;21: 282–285.

35. Kino T, Hataraka H, Miyata S, et al. FK 506, a novel immunosuppression isolated from a streptomyces: immunosuppressive effect of FK 506 in vitro. J Antibiotics 1987;40:1256–1260.

36. Taylor DO, Barr ML, Meiser BM, et al. Suggested guidelines for the use of tacrolimus in cardiac transplant recipients. J Heart Lung Transplant 2001;20: 734–738.

37. Pham SM, Kormos RL, Hattler BG, et al. A prospective trial of tacrolimus (FK 506) in clinical heart transplantation: intermediate-term results. J Thorac Cardiovasc Surg 1996;111:764–772.

38. Reichart BR, Meiser BM, Vigano M, et al. European multi-center tacrolimus (FK 506) heart pilot study: one-year results—European Multicenter Heart Study Group. J Heart Lung Transplant 1998;17:775–781.

39. Taylor DO, Barr ML, Radovancevic B, et al. Randomized, multicenter, comparison of tacrolimus and cyclosporine immunosuppressive regimens in cardiac transplantation: decreased hyperlipidemia and hypertension with tacrolimus. J Heart Lung Transplant 1999;18:336–345.

40. Meiser BM, Pfeiffer M, Schmidt D, et al. Combination therapy with tacrolimus and mycophenolate mofetil following cardiac transplantation: importance of mycophenolic acid therapeutic drug monitoring. J Heart Lung Transplant 1999;18:143–149.

41. Mentzer RM Jr., Jahania MS, Lasley RD. Tacrolimus as a rescue immunosuppressant after heart and lung transplantation. The US Multicenter FK506 Study Group. Transplantation 1998;65:109–113.

42. Baran DA, Segura L, Kushwaha S, et al. Tacrolimus monotherapy in adult cardiac transplant receipients: intermediate-term results. J Heart Lung Transplant 2001;20:59–70.

43. Yacoub MA, Khaghani P, Mitchell A. The use of cyclosporine, azathioprine, and antithymocyte globulin with or without low dose steroids for immunosuppression of cardiac transplant patients. Transplant Proc 1985;17:221–222.

44. Brann WM, Bennett LE, Keck BM, et al. Morbidity, functional status, and immunosuppressive therapy after heart transplantation: an analysis of the joint International Society for Heart and Lung Transplantation/United Network for Organ Sharing thoracic registry. J Heart Lung Transplant 1998;17:374–382.

45. Esmore DS, Spratt PM, Keogh AM, et al. Cyclosporine and azathioprine immunosuppression without maintenance steroids: a randomized prospective trial. J Heart Lung Transplant 1989;8:194–199.

46. Oaks TE, Wannenberg T, Close SA, et al. Steroid-free maintenance immunosuppression after heart transplantion. Ann Thorac Surg 72:102–106.

47. Keogh A, Macdonald P, Mundy J, et al. Five-year follow up of a randomized double-drug versus triple drug therapy immunosuppressive trial after heart transplantation. J Heart Lung Transplant 1992;11:550–555.

48. Kobashigawa JA, Stevenson LW, Brownfield ED, et al. Initial success of steroid weaning late after heart transplantation. J Heart Lung Transplant 1992;11:428–430.

49. Taylor DO, Bristow MR, O'Connell JB, et al. Improved long-term survival after heart transplantation predicted by successful early withdrawal from maintenance corticosteroid therapy. J Heart Lung Transplant 1996;15:1039–1046.

50. Olivari MT, Jessen ME, Baldwin BJ, et al. Triple-drug immunosuppression with steroid discontinuation by six months after heart transplantation. J Heart Lung Transplant 1995;14:127–135.

51. Kobashigawa JA, Stevenson LW, Brownfield ED, et al. Corticosteroid weaning late after heart transplantation: relation to HLA-DR mismatching and long-term metabolic effects. J Heart Lung Transplant 1995;14:963–967.

52. Felkel TO, Smith AL, Reichenspurner HC, et al. Survival and incidence of acute rejection in heart transplant recipients undergoing successful withdrawal from steroid therapy. J Heart Lung Transplant 2002;21:530–539.

53. Hosenpud JD, Bennett LE, Keck BM, et al. The registry of the International Society for Heart and Lung Transplantation: 17th official report—2000. J Heart Lung Transplant 2000;19:909–931.

54. Gummert JF, Ikonen T, Morris RE. Newer immunosuppressive drugs: a review. J A Soc Nephrol 1999;10:1366–1380.

55. Poston RS, Billingham M, Hoyt EJ, et al. Rapamycin reverses chronic graft vascular disease in a novel cardiac allograft model. Circulation 1999;1000:67–74.

56. Ikonen TS, Gummert JF, Honda Y, et al. Sirolimus (rapamycin) blood levels correlate with prevention of graft vascular disease (GVD) in monkey aortic transplants as monitored by graft ultrasound. J Heart Lung Transplant 1999;18:72.

57. Groth CG, Backman L, Morales JL, et al. Sirolimus(rapamycin)-based therapy in human renal transplantation: similar efficacy and different toxicity compared with cyclosporine. Transplantation 1999;67:1036–1042.

58. Barr ML. Photopheresis in transplantation: future research and directions. Transplant Proc 1998;30:2248–2250.

59. Pepino P, Berger CL, Fuzesi L, et al. Primate cardiac allo- and xenotransplantation: modulation of the immune response to chemotherapy. Eur Sur Res 1989;21: 105–113.

60. Rose E, Barr M, Xu H, et al. Photochemotherapy in human heart transplant recipients at high risk for fatal rejection. J Heart Lung Transplant 1992;11:746–750.

61. Costanzo-Nordin MR, Hubell EA, O'Sullivan EJ, et al. Photopheresis versus corticosteroids in the therapy of heart transplant rejection. Preliminary clinical report. Circulation 1992;86:II242–II250.

62. Barr ML, Meiser BM, Roberts RF, et al. Photopheresis for the prevention of rejection in cardiac transplantation. Photopheresis Transplantation Study Group. N Engl J Med 1998;339:1744–1751.

63. Barr ML, Baker CJ, Schenkel FA, et al. Prophylactic photopheresis and chronic rejection: effects on graft intimal hyperplasia in cardiac transplantation. Clin Transplant 2000;14:162–166.

64. Smith JD, Danskine AJ, Laylor RM, et al. The effect of panel reactive antibodies and the donor specific crossmatch on graft survival after heart and heart-lung transplantation. Transplant Immunol 1993;1(1):60–65.

65. Ratkovec RM, Hammond EH, O'Connell JB, et al. Outcome of cardiac transplant recipients with a positive donor-specific crossmatch—preliminary results with plasmapheresis. Transplantation 1992;54(4):651–655.

66. John R, Lietz K, Burke E, et al. Intravenous immunoglobulin reduces anti-HLA alloreactivity and shortens waiting time to cardiac transplantation in highly sensitized left ventricular assist device recipients. Circulation. 1999;100:II.229–II.235.

67. Itescu S, Tung T, Burke E, et al. Preformed IgG antibodies against major histocompatibility class II antigens are major risk factors for high-grade cellular rejection in recipients of heart transplantation. Circulation 1998;98:786–793.

68. Liu Z, Colovai AI, Tugulea S, et al. Indirect recognition of donor HLA-DR peptides in organ allograft rejection. J Clin Invest 1996;98:1150–1157.

69. Tugulea S, Ciubotariu R, Colovai AI, et al. New strategies for early diagnosis of heart allograft rejection. Transplantation 1997;64:842–847.

70. Ciubotariu R, Liu Z, Itescu S, et al. Persistent allopeptide reactivity and epitope spreading in chronic rejection of organ allografts. J Clin Invest 1997;101:398–405.

71. Vanderlugt CJ, Miller SD. Epitope spreading. Curr Opin Immunol 1996;8:831–836.

72. John R, Chen JM, Weinberg A, et al. Long-term survival after cardiac retransplantation: a twenty-year single center experience. J Thorac Cardiovasc Surg 1999;117:543–555.

73. Mamula MJ, Janeway CA Jr. Do B cells drive the diversification of immune responses? Immunol Today 1993;14:151–154.

74. Reed EF, Hong B, Ho E, et al. Monitoring of soluble HLA alloantigens and anti-HLA antibodies identifies heart allograft recipients at risk of transplant associated coronary artery disease. Transplantation 1996;61:556–572.

75. John R, Lietz K, Naka Y, et al. Immunologic sensitization in recipients of left ventricular assist devices. J Thorac Cardiovasc Surg 2003;125:578–591.

76. Glotz D, Haymann J, Sansonetti N, et al. Suppression of HLA-specific alloanti-bodies by high-dose intravenous immunoglobulins (IVIg). Transplantation 1993;56:335–337.
77. Tyan TB, Li VA, Czer L, et al. Intravenous immunoglobulin suppression of HLA alloantibody in highly sensitized transplant candidates and transplantation with a histoincompatible organ. Transplantation 1994;57:553–562.
78. Peraldi M, Akposso K, Haymann J, et al. Long-term benefit of intravenous immunoglobulins in cadaveric kidney retransplantation. Transplantation 1996; 62:1670–1673.
79. McIntyre JA, Higgins N, Britton R, et al. Utilization of intravenous immunoglobu-lin to ameliorate alloantibodies in a highly sensitized patient with a cardiac assist device awaiting cardiac transplantation. Transplantation 1996;62:691–693.
80. De Marco T, Damon LE, Colombe B, et al. Successful immunomodulation with intravenous immunoglobulin and cyclophosphamide in an alloimmunized heart transplant recipient. J Heart Lung Transplant 1997;16:360–365.
81. Dwyer JM. Manipulating the immune system with immune globulin. N Engl J Med 1992;326:107–116.
82. Dietrich G, Algiman M, Sultan Y, et al. Origin of anti-idiotypic activity against anti-factor VIII autoantibodies in pools of normal human immunoglobulin G (IVIg). Blood 1992;79:2946–2951.
83. Rossi F, Kazatchkine MD. Antiidiotypes against autoantibodies in pooled normal human polyspecific Ig. J Immunol 1989;143:4104–4109.
84. Hurez V, Kaveri SV, Mouhoub A, et al. Anti-CD4 activity of normal human immu-noglobulins for therapeutic use (IVIg). Therapeut Immunol 1993;1:269–278.
85. Vassilev T, Gelin C, Kaveri SV, et al. Antibodies to the CD5 molecule in normal human immunoglobulins for therapeutic use (IVIg). Clin Exp Immunol 1993; 92:369–372.
86. Blasczyk R, Westhoff U, Grossewilde H. Soluble CD4, CD8, and HLA molecules in commercial immunoglobulin preparations. Lancet 1993;341:789–790.
87. Lam L, Whitsett CF, McNicholl JM, et al. Immunologically active proteins in intra-venous immunoglobulin. Lancet 1993;342:678.
88. Itescu S, Burke E, Lietz K, et al. Intravenous pulse administration of cyclophospha-mide is an effective and safe treatment for sensitized cardiac allograft recipients. Circulation 2002;105:1214–1219.
89. Toungouz M, Donckier V, Goldman M. Tolerance induction in clinical transplan-tation: the pending questions. Transplantation 2003;75:58S–60S.
90. Taylor DO. Immunosuppressive therapies after heart transplantation: best, better, and beyond. Curr Opin Cardiol 2000;15:108–114.
91. Billingham RE, Brent L, Medawar PB. "Actively acquired tolerance" of foreign cells. Nature 1953;172:603–606.
92. Opelz G, Mickey MR, Sengar DPS, et al. Effect of blood transfusions on subsequent kidney transplants. Transplant Proc 1973;5:253.
93. Salvatierra O, Vincenti F, Amend W, et al. Deliberate donor-specific blood trans-fusions prior to living related renal transplantation: a new approach. Ann Surg 1982;192:543.
94. Mazariegos GV, Reyes J, Marino IR, et al. Weaning of immunosuppression in liver transplant recipients. Transplantation 1997;63:243.
95. Starzl TE, Demetris AJ, Trucco M, et al. Cell migration and chimerism after whole organ transplantation: the basis of graft acceptance. Hepatology 1993;17:1127.
96. Rifle G, Mousson C. Donor-derived hematopoietic cells in organ transplantation: a major step toward allograft tolerance. Transplantation 2003;75:3S–7S.

9 Long-Term Outcomes With Transplantation

Mario C. Deng, MD

INTRODUCTION

For patients with truly refractory end-stage cardiomyopathy in the current era, the overall long-term survival after cardiac transplantation is superior to that achieved with maximal medical therapy alone. However, whether long-term nonsurvival outcomes after transplant (because of the complex, and sometimes subtle, morbidities of permanent immunosuppression) are similarly enhanced remains a matter of contention. This chapter seeks to define these complications and strategies for their management, from early postoperative considerations to the enduring challenges of lifestyle issues and compliance.

From: *Contemporary Cardiology: Cardiac Transplantation:*
The Columbia University Medical Center/New York-Presbyterian Hospital Manual
Edited by: N. M. Edwards, J. M. Chen, and P. A. Mazzeo © Humana Press Inc., Totowa, NJ

WAITING LIST MORTALITY AND SURVIVAL STATISTICS

The appropriate identification of heart transplant candidates is based on expected gains in the survival and quality of life of patients with advanced heart failure, compared to the gains that might be derived from all other organ-conserving medical and surgical treatment options. Traditional selection criteria are articulated in expert consensus guidelines *(1,2)*; however, these guidelines are increasingly controversial, because the assumption of a survival benefit across the entire advanced heart failure spectrum may no longer be valid in the era of improved medical and surgical therapies for end-stage heart disease.

Two opposing trends bring these former assumptions into question. First, medical therapy improvements, as well as new surgical alternatives to transplantation, have demonstrated significantly improved patient survival when compared to the survival of historical medically managed controls. In contrast, outcomes after cardiac transplantation have not improved as much, partly because of the listing of more critically ill patients, use of so-called marginal donor hearts from an extended donor pool *(3)*, and the initiation of new heart transplantation centers with an inevitable learning phase *(4)*.

The death rates of advanced heart failure patients on the United Network for Organ Sharing waiting list have decreased dramatically over time, from 432.2 per 1000 patient years in 1990 to 172.4 per 1000 patient years in 1999. Despite this fact, waiting list mortality remains hierarchical by medical necessity: for patients with advanced medical urgency status (Status 1A), the death rate per 1000 in 1999 was 581.9, as compared with 204.7 for medical urgency status (Status 1B) and 130.7 for regular urgency status (Status 2) registrants (www.unos.org).

In contrast to these outcomes, the 1-yr posttransplant survival rates for patients transplanted between 1995 and 2000 were 81.4%, 86.2%, and 87.7% for Status 1A, 1B, and 2, respectively. Thus, patient survival posttransplant, unlike waiting list mortality, does not appear to be entirely hierarchical—high-dose inotrope-dependent patients, once transplanted, appear to do almost as well posttransplant as patients who waited for transplantation at home on oral medications only. In other words, the survival benefit from cardiac transplantation is greatest for those patients who are at highest risk of dying from advanced heart failure without transplantation *(5)*.

These findings are corroborated by those of the Comparative Outcomes & Clinical Profiles In Transplantation study by the German Transplantation Society and Eurotransplant International Foundation (www.eurotransplant.org) *(6)*. In that study, patients with a predicted high risk of dying according to the heart failure survival score (HFSS) *(7)* experienced not only the highest risk of dying on the waiting list (32%, 20%, and 20% for high-, medium-, and low-risk patients, respectively; $p = 0.0003$) but also the greatest survival benefit from transplantation.

NONREJECTION CLINICAL COMPLICATIONS
Infections

Opportunistic infections after transplantation continue to constitute a management challenge *(see* Table 1). The variety and timing of these infectious processes is significantly dependent on the geography and demographics of the transplant center and the time interval since transplantation. In a review of 620 consecutive patients transplanted at Stanford University between 1980 and 1996, 1073 infectious episodes represented not only the second most common cause of early mortality but also the most common cause of late mortality. Of these infectious episodes, 468 (43.6%) were caused by bacteria, 447 (41.7%) by viruses, 109 (10.2%) by fungi, 43 (4.0%) by *Pneumocystis carinii*, and 6 (0.6%) by protozoa. The largest number of these infections occurred in the lungs (301, 28.1%). Over the time period studied, there was a significant reduction in infection incidence and an increase in the time interval from transplant to presentation, likely related to improved chemoprophylaxis for cytomegalovirus (CMV) infections *(8)*.

Of the various infectious processes, CMV remains the most important process chronically affecting heart transplant recipients. In CMV disease prevention, those at risk of primary disease (donor seropositive, recipient seronegative) should receive CMV prophylaxis *(9)*. *Legionella pneumophila* may also cause pneumonia of variable severity after cardiac transplantation; chlorination and heating of water are important preventive measures. Specific cultures in outbreak situations should be considered to identify less common *Legionella pneumophila* serotypes, and nonpneumophila *Legionella* species *(10)*, *Pneumocystis carinii* pneumonia *(11)*, tuberculosis *(12)*, toxoplasmosis *(13)*, pulmonary aspergillosis *(14)*, and other fungal infections *(15,16)* constitute additional challenges for the immunocompromised heart transplant recipient.

Renal Dysfunction

Posttransplant renal dysfunction has emerged gradually over the past decade as one of the most significant long-term permanent immunosuppression morbidities. This dysfunction often begins pretransplantation

Table 1
Management of Opportunistic Infections After Cardiac Transplantation

Organism	Test	Treatment
CMV	IE–Gene, PCR, IgM	(Val)-gancyclovir, if severe consider CMV antibodies
Herpes simplex virus	IgM	Acyclovir
Varicella-zoster virus	IgM	Acyclovir
Hepatitis B virus	IgM	Lamivudine
Legionella	Urine antigen, X-ray	Erythromycin
Mycobacterium tuberculosis	Ziehl–Neelson	Rifampicin, isoniacid, myambutol
Nocardia asteroides	Brain CT	TMP/SFX
Pneumocystis carinii	X-ray	TMP/SFX
Toxoplasma gondii	X-ray, IFT, CBR, IgA, IgM	Pyrimethamine + sulfadiazine, folic acid
Candida albicans	Direct	Fluconazole, itroconazole
Aspergillus fumigatus	X-ray	Itroconazole, amphotericin B, flucytosine
Cryptococcus neoformans	Brain CT	Itroconazole, amphotericin B, flucytosine, or fluconazole
Listeria monocytogenes		CNS: ampicillin + gentamycin

Abbreviations: CMV, cytomegalovirus; PCR, polymerase chain reaction; Ig, immunoglobulin; CT, computed tomography; TMP/SFX, trimethoprine/sulfamethoxazole; CNS, central nervous system; IFT, immunofluorescence testing; CBR, complement binding reaction.

and may represent ongoing acute tubular necrosis (ATN) owing to the chronic low-output heart failure state. Intraoperatively, the low-flow nonpulsatile duration of cardiopulmonary bypass contributes to this prerenal azotemia, which may ultimately present difficult problems with perioperative fluid management. Superimposed on this background of intermediate renal dysfunction is the well-described immunosuppressant nephrotoxicity. Indeed, calcineurin inhibitor use as primary immunosuppressants in cardiac transplantation is associated with considerable end-stage renal disease and dialysis risks. Accordingly, the chronic progressive tubulointerstitial fibrosis/arteriopathy induced by the calcineurin inhibitors cyclosporine (CyA) (Neoral, Sandoz Inc., East Hanover, NJ) and tacrolimus (Prograf, Fujisawa Healthcare, Deerfield, IL) has become one of the essential criteria by which immunosuppressive agents are evaluated.

Exposure to calcineurin inhibitors may result in a biphasic decrease in renal function. The initial acute renal failure may occur as early as a few weeks or months after therapy initiation and is thought to result from vasoconstriction of renal arterioles, with associated hypertension, hyperkalemia, tubular acidosis, sodium reabsorption, reduction in the glomerular filtration rate, and oliguria. Acutely, these changes are thought to be dose-related, while, chronically, this nephropathy (and later potential progression to dialysis) may, in fact, occur independently of acute renal dysfunction, dosage, or blood concentration. In the pediatric heart transplant population particularly, decline in renal function posttransplantation correlates primarily with early CyA exposure; this dysfunction persists even when CyA doses are subsequently reduced *(17)*.

Conversion to tacrolimus in individual cases can result in a prompt and significant improvement in serum creatinine concentrations, and this strategy may be effective in reducing CyA-associated renal failure in this setting *(18)*. However, tacrolimus is not without its own nephrotoxicity; therefore, rapamycin (Rapamune, Wyeth-Ayerst Laboratories, Madison, NJ) has been employed recently as "rescue" immunosuppression in those patients for whom persistent acute renal failure limits CyA or tacrolimus use.

Other efficacious adjuncts for immunosuppression during the perioperative period for those in renal failure include antithymocyte globulin and the murine anti-CD3 monoclonal antibody OKT3. However, the cytokine release syndrome associated with OKT3 can also contribute to the pathogenesis of transient ATN and, therefore, to renal dysfunction following transplantation *(19,20)*.

Hypertension

In addition to nephrotoxicity, calcineurin inhibitor use in solid organ transplantation is associated with hypertension development within the first 12 mo in nearly 70% of patients. Several mechanisms, including endothelin-mediated systemic vasoconstriction, impaired vasodilatation secondary to reduction in nitric oxide, activation of the sympathetic and renin-angiotensin systems, abnormalities in prostaglandin metabolism, and altered cytosolic calcium translocation are implicated as mechanisms in this process *(21)*.

Combined calcium-channel blockers and angiotensin-converting enzyme inhibitors are used for treatment of this clinical problem, achieving blood pressure control in 65% of patients. Moreover, these agents may be beneficial in preventing cardiac allograft vasculopathy development, a long-term concern in cardiac transplantation *(22)*.

Osteoporosis

Glucocorticoids and calcineurin inhibitors also are associated with significant osteoporosis and related pathologic fractures. Although factors such as nutrition, gonadal status, and ambulatory status appear contributory, immunosuppressive drugs appear to be the main factor in posttransplant osteoporosis development (*see* Table 2) *(23)*.

Shane et al., from our institution, demonstrated that patients with heart failure have a 50% incidence of osteopenia and osteoporosis even prior to transplantation *(24)*. However, transplant patients may develop fractures despite even normal bone mineral density. After transplantation, the most critical period of bone loss in organ recipients appears to be within the first 6 mo, with the most dramatic bone mass reduction occurring within the first 3 mo posttransplantation and with an annualized bone loss of as much as 20%.

The trabecular bone of the spine appears to be most at risk, with vertebral fractures occurring most commonly. At 1 yr posttransplantation, documented bone mass losses include as much as 8.5% in the lumbar spine and 10.4% at the femoral neck as compared with 1.4% and 0.4%, respectively, in healthy controls *(25)*. Therefore, transplant recipients should be evaluated regularly by bone mineral densitometry and measurement of vitamin D metabolites, blood urea nitrogen, creatinine, calcium, and phosphate. Also, gonadal function should be ascertained by measurement of serum levels of testosterone in males and estradiol in females. Bone turnover markers may help assess the remodeling rate, and therapy should be directed toward bone loss prevention and

Table 2
Effects of Immunosuppressive Drugs on Bone Integrity

Agent	Effect on bone/mineral metabolism
Glucocorticoids (systemic effects)	Decrease in net calcium absorption Increase in urinary calcium excretion Increase in parathyroid hormone Decreased production of skeletal growth factors Decrease adrenal/gonadal androgen and estrogen synthesis
Direct effects on bone	Decreased bone formation by osteoblasts Increased bone resorption
Calcineurin inhibitors	Increased bone resportion Increased bone formation/serum osteocalcin Marked osteoporosis (resorption > formation) Decreased gonadal steroid synthesis
Rapamycin	Increased bone remodeling Inhibits longitudinal growth No short-term effects on bone volume
Azathioprine	Increased osteoclast number No change in bone volume
Mycophenolate mofetil	No change in bone volume

From Am J Med, with permission (23).

restoration of bone mass that is already lost. Administration of calcium, vitamin D, sex hormone replacement, and, potentially, bisphosphonates may help to attenuate these losses (26–28).

In a study of the frequency and predictors of osteporotic fractures after cardiac transplantation, investigators at Heidelberg University assessed 105 consecutive heart transplant recipients for the presence of posttransplant vertebral fractures. In yr 1 and 2 after transplantation, the proportions of patients with at least one vertebral fracture were 21 and 27%, respectively. In yr 3 and 4, one-third of patients had one or more vertebral fractures. Independent predictors of pathologic fracture, assessed by multivariate analysis, were age and lumbar bone-mineral density; interestingly, no dose-dependent effect of immunosuppressive therapy on fracture development was demonstrable (29).

Diabetes

Diabetes mellitus is a common complication after heart transplantation. Specifically, new-onset diabetes, related to continued high doses of steroids, constitutes a challenging problem. To establish the incidence of posttransplant diabetes mellitus and factors predictive of its development, a retrospective review was conducted at St. Vincent's Hospital in Sydney, Australia. Here, the cumulative incidence of posttransplantation diabetes mellitus was 15.7%, where both a family history of diabetes and insulin need beyond the first 24 h after transplantation were factors predictive of posttransplant diabetes *(30)*.

Notably, heart transplantation in patients with pre-existing diabetes mellitus, but without the stigmata of diabetic end-organ dysfunction, is performed with reasonable success. Lang et al. at our institution demonstrated equivalent 1- and 3-yr survival for patients with and without diabetes (86% and 85% vs 87% and 84%, respectively) *(31)*; these findings are in contrast with an earlier study by Czerny et al., who found significantly impaired 5-yr survival in diabetics when compared with controls (57.1% vs 67.6%) *(32)*. Insulin dependence has little effect on survival; however, concerns remain as to the integrity of wound healing and the development of nephropathy, neuropathy, peripheral arterial occlusive disease, and retinopathy in this cohort.

Gout

Immunosuppressive therapy, with pretransplantation risk factors, accounts for an elevated incidence of posttransplant gout, in which management can be challenging because of medicinal interactions between anti-gout agents and common immunosuppressants. Although it is a seemingly indolent disease in the general population, gout, and its management, can manifest significant morbidity in the posttransplant state.

To study gout's clinical impact posttransplant, an audit was conducted of all patients transplanted at the Alfred Hospital before August 1998. Two hundred twenty-five patients (81% men) were studied, with a mean posttransplant follow-up of 50.8 mo. Of these, 43 (19%) had pretransplant gout, with 19 posttransplantation recurrences; 23 patients developed gout *de novo*. Diuretic use, hypertension, and impaired renal function were more common in this subgroup. Of the 24 patients who received allopurinol, 6 developed pancytopenia and required hospitalization, 14 received a change in immunosuppression (after pancytopenia development in 5 patients, and to enable safe use of allopurinol in 9), 32 patients received colchicine, and 5 developed neuromyopathy. Nonsteroidal anti-inflammatory agents, used in 16 patients, caused serious complications in 1 (life-threatening peptic ulceration and hemorrhage, precipitating dialysis-dependent chronic renal failure). Thus, cardiac transplant recipients, when treated for gout, are at high risk of iatrogenic medication-related complications *(33)*.

Similar to patients who have not undergone cardiac transplantation, factors such as obesity, a high-purine diet, regular alcohol consumption, and diuretic therapy may be correctable in cardiac transplantation patients. However, in patients with persistent hyperuricemia, therapy must be enacted to lower the serum urate concentration to an optimal level. The continuing challenge is educating patients about correctable factors and the importance of regular medication and ensuring their compliance so that gout attacks do not recur *(34)*.

Posttransplant Lymphoproliferative Disease and Other Malignancies

Malignancies play a major role as a cause of death after cardiac transplantation, and they occur at a rate as high as 1–4% per year, a risk that is 10- to 100-fold higher than the risk in age-matched controls. Whereas malignant skin tumors and lymphomas occur most frequently, any solid organ tumor may develop (www.ctstransplant.org) *(35)*.

The risk of posttransplant lymphoproliferative disease (PTLD) was assessed in a cohort of 1563 patients who underwent cardiothoracic transplantation at Harefield Hospital from 1980 to 1994. Epstein–Barr virus (EBV) antibody titers were assessed prior to transplantation, and lymphoid neoplasms were evaluated for EBV ribonucleic acid and latent EBV gene expression. Thirty cases of PTLD occurred during follow-up, of which six were EBV-negative non-Hodgkin's lymphoma. PTLD risk was significantly elevated in the yr 1 posttransplant in those patients who were EBV-seronegative pretransplant and in young seronegative recipients of older donor organs; this risk diminished with age. In contrast, EBV-negative non-Hodgkin's lymphoma occurred entirely in men over 45 yr who were EBV-seropositive pretransplantation; this risk did not occur with greater frequency at any time posttransplant.

Thus, PTLD risk appears to coincide with EBV etiology, with greater risk incurred from primary infection than from reactivation. A second non-Hodgkin's lymphoid neoplasm, unrelated to EBV, also seems to be a consequence of transplant immunosuppression but is less likely to result from a prior infection by a ubiquitous agent *(36)*.

Investigators at our institution have demonstrated that PTLDs present along a disease spectrum pathologically as well as clinically *(37,38)*. On one hand, some patients present with a mild flu-like illness and adenopathy, which could go unnoticed to the untrained plysician. These patients may have complete resolution of their disease (labeled pathologically as atypical lymphoid hyperplasia–infectious mononucleosis-like) with small changes in their immunosuppressive regimen. On the other hand, others may present with frank carcinomatosis and extremely advanced disease, which pathologically resembles a monoclonal lymphoma; these patients generally require multimodality therapy in addition to reduction in their immunosuppression *(38)*.

We find that pathologic tumor clonality assessment assists in guiding therapy; those with polyclonal lymphoid populations are more likely to respond to less aggressive protocols, whereas those with monoclonal proliferations are less likely. For these reasons, we are aggressive in our efforts to obtain a tissue diagnosis of suspicious adenopathy and/or masses. Inevitably, first-line treatment involves a reduction in overall immunosuppressive regimen, and may or may not involve other more potent intravenous chemotherapy or radiation therapy, depending on response to intervention as well as tumor histology and grade.

LIFESTYLE AND COMPLIANCE

The success of cardiac transplantation is largely related to the recipient's understanding of the unique challenges of living with a new heart, as well as to his or her compliance with the prescribed management regimen. Investigators at Leuven examined the prevalence of appointment noncompliance and its relationship to patient profile and clinical risk. The prevalence of appointment noncompliance in 101 heart transplant recipients was 7%, with noncompliers being significantly younger, less likely to live in a stable relationship with a partner, and more likely to be depressed, perceive their health as poorer, experience symptom distress, and have more frequent drug holidays. Of the appointment noncompliers, 57% experienced one or more late acute rejection episodes, compared with 2% of appointment compliers *(39)*. These data are corroborated by Dew et al., who demonstrated a four- to sevenfold increased risk of rejection and vasculopathy in medication noncompliers. Significantly, patients who were noncompliant with a cholesterol-restricted diet had an 11-fold increased risk of mortality. Noncompliance thus represents a critical behavioral risk factor in late acute rejection episode occurrence.

Ideally, pretransplant patient profiles should allow the identification of patients at risk for appointment noncompliance. In 1995, investigators at our institution demonstrated that as many as 34% of 125 transplant recipients studied were noncompliant. In their analysis, pre-operative predictors of posttransplant noncompliance included substance abuse, suboptimal living arrangements, personality disorder, and global psychosocial risk *(40)*.

Similarly, investigators at the University of Pittsburgh evaluated 191 heart transplant recipients prospectively to examine prevalence and risk factors for posttransplant major psychiatric illness. Factors increasing the cumulative risk for posttransplant psychiatric disorders included pretransplant psychiatric history, female gender, longer hospitalization, more impaired physical functional status, and fewer social supports from caregiver and family in the perioperative period. The effect of these risk factors was additive: the presence of an increasing number of risk factors bore a dose–response relationship to the cumulative disorder risk *(41)*. Therefore, the effects of such psychiatric disorders must not be discounted. In a related study by the same investigators, posttraumatic stress disorder conferred a 13-fold increase in the risk of posttransplant mortality, and persistent depressive and anger/hostility symptoms increased the risk of arteriopathy four- to eightfold *(42)*.

Thus, noncompliance, whether in the presence or absence of psychiatric illness, is associated with a substantial increase in posttransplant morbidity and mortality. Without question, concurrent psychiatric illness further impacts negatively upon social stability and, in doing so, may further detrimentally impact therapeutic conformity and long-term survival.

TRANSPLANT VASCULOPATHY

Transplant coronary artery disease (TCAD), or transplant vasculopathy, an unusually accelerated and diffuse form of obliterative coronary arteriosclerosis, determines long-term transplanted heart function and represents the major cause of late death after cardiac transplantation. TCAD progression involves a complicated interplay between immunologic and nonimmunologic factors, ultimately resulting in repetitive vascular injury and a localized sustained inflammatory response *(43)*. Dyslipidemia, oxidant stress, immunosuppressive drugs, endothelial dysfunction and viral infection appear to be important contributors to TCAD development *(44)*.

Clearly, early identification of transplant vasculopathy is essential to improve long-term prognosis. Annual coronary angiography is performed for diagnostic and surveillance purposes; however, intravascular ultrasound represents a more sensitive diagnostic tool to detect early disease and, often, subtle lumenal stenosis. Several pharmacological agents, including the calcium-channel blocker diltiazem *(45)* and statins such as pravastatin *(46)* or simvastatin *(47)*, are effective in attenuating the disease's progression. However, because of the diffuse nature of transplant vasculopathy, neither percutaneous nor surgical revascularization procedures demonstrate efficacy. Thus, TCAD prevention represents a primary therapeutic goal to ensure long-term transplantation success *(48)*.

RETRANSPLANTATION AND ALTERNATIVES TO RETRANSPLANTATION

The incidence of transplant vasculopathy and tricuspid regurgitation (TR) require, in selected patients, consideration for elective reoperation and retransplantation. Although retransplantation results more than 6 mo after primary transplantation are comparable to results after primary transplantation, acute retransplantation is associated with such poor results at most centers as to prohibit its endorsement *(3,49)*.

For patients not expected to benefit from retransplantation, other subsequent cardiac procedures may extend patient survival and protect graft function. A review of such adjunctive procedures was performed at Vanderbilt, where 17 of 360 patients (12 adults and 5 children) underwent a subsequent procedure requiring cardiopulmonary bypass, including cardiac retransplantation (10), coronary artery bypass grafting (3), aortic root replacement (2), tricuspid valve repair (1), and myotomy and myomectomy (1). The mean interval from transplantation time to second procedure was 8.3 yr. One patient died perioperatively, two retransplant patients died late postoperatively at 22 and 84 mo. Thus, in addition to retransplantation, a variety of subsequent cardiac procedures can be performed safely in carefully selected cardiac transplant recipients for whom intermediate-term results are gratifying regarding survival and freedom from symptoms *(50)*.

A fairly frequent occurrence posttransplant is TR development, often related either to endocarditis or to iatrogenic biopsy-induced injury. Investigators at the German Heart Center Berlin evaluated 647 recipients for evidence of posttransplant TR. The overall prevalence of TR was 20.1%, with mild TR seen in 14.5%, moderate TR in 3.1%, and severe TR (with right ventricular dysfunction) in 2.5%. Tricuspid valve pathology at operation most commonly revealed biopsy-induced rupture of the chordae tendineae at various valve segments, mostly at the anterior and posterior leaflets. Eleven patients received prosthetic valve replacements (four bioprostheses and seven mechanical valves), and six patients underwent valve reconstruction. One patient died perioperatively, and five died late because of infection, arrhythmia, and trauma. Ten patients

(62.5%) were alive at a mean follow-up time of 29.9 mo (range 4–81 mo) and nine survivors are in New York Heart Association classes I and II, and one is in class III. Thus, heart transplant recipients can safely undergo valve surgery with acceptable mortality, low morbidity, and excellent intermediate-term clinical results *(51)*.

FUTURE TRENDS

Cell Transplantation and Myocyte Regrowth

The concept of regenerating the heart in heart failure via cardiomyocyte transplantation remains experimental. Several approaches, including transplantation of embryonic cardiomyocytes *(52)*, cryopreserved *(53)* or bioengineered fetal cardiomyocytes *(54)*, neonatal cardiac myocytes, skeletal myoblasts *(55)*, autologous smooth muscle cells *(56)*, and dermal fibroblasts *(57)* have been proposed. However, the further clinical application of these techniques is limited by several problems, including chronic rejection in allogeneic cells, failure to develop sufficient intercellular gap junction communications, and differential patterns in excitation–contraction coupling in skeletal and cardiac myocytes.

Alternatively, the transplantation of lineage-negative bone marrow cells *(58)* or bone marrow-derived endothelial precursor cells (with phenotypic and functional embryonic hemangioblast characteristics) is also proposed. The latter can be used directly to induce new blood vessel formation after experimental myocardial infarction, and is associated experimentally with decreased apoptosis of hypertrophied myocytes in the peri-infarct region, with long-term salvage and survival of viable myocardium, reduction in collagen deposition, and sustained improvement in cardiac function *(59)*.

Xenotransplantation

Theoretically, xenotransplantation could provide an unlimited tissue and organ supply by using other species (e.g., baboons, pigs) as donors. Unsurprisingly, however, cross-species transplant rejection prevention remains a significant barrier, as are the public and ethical dilemmas surrounding xenotranplantation's clinical application and the development of appropriate prophylaxis against so-called xenozoonoses (infections transmitted across species). A source of continuing research and generative of pertinent immunological information for allotransplantation, xenotransplantation is unlikely to offer an epidemiologically meaningful alternative to standard heart transplantation in the near future.

Mechanical Circulatory Support

Mechanical circulatory support as a bridge (or alternative) to transplantation is addressed in Chapter 12. Briefly, mechanical circulatory systems are frequently used to support patients with severe heart failure as a bridge to transplantation or recovery or as destination therapy *(60)*. Although early total artificial hearts (TAHs) and ventricular assist devices were powered mainly by external pneumatic drive units, the current generation of assist devices are electrically driven, ultracompact, and, in some cases, totally implantable. Most have small, wearable drive/control consoles, allowing patients to return to daily activities *(61)*; others in development generate power transcutaneously via magnet-based power systems.

Recent enthusiasm also surrounds the clinical application of several TAH devices. Initially proposed as an alternative for patients in whom transplantation is not an option, these devices also may hold promise for those with end-stage transplant vasculopathy, in whom the development of other comorbidities (e.g., transplant-related renal failure) has rendered them ineligible for retransplantation.

CONCLUSION

Successful long-term outcomes following heart transplantation require the transplant team's constant vigilance to identify and rectify even subtle changes in a recipient's physiology. Gradual deterioration of select organ systems (e.g., renal, bone) is anticipated and must be included in pretransplant education. However, not all immunosuppression side effects need be manifest in every patient. Whereas new immunosuppression and therapies may ultimately impact posttransplant morbidities, here, as everywhere else in transplantation, assiduous patient compliance is of paramount importance to improve long-term outcomes.

REFERENCES

1. Hunt SA. 24th Bethesda Conference: Cardiac Transplantation. J Am Coll Cardiol 1993;22,1:1–64.
2. Deng MC. Cardiac transplantation. Heart 2002;87:177–184.
3. Hosenpud JD, Bennett LE, Keck BM, et al. The Registry of the International Society for Heart and Lung Transplantation: 17th official report—2000. J Heart Lung Transplant 2000;19:909–931.
4. Laffel Gl, Barnett A, Finkelstein S, et al. The relationship between experience and outcome in heart transplantation. N. Engl J Med 1992;327:1220–1225.
5. Deng MC, Smits JMA, DeMeester J, et al. Heart transplantation is indicated only in the most severely ill patient: perspectives from the German Heart Transplant Experience. Curr Opin Cardiol 2001;16:97–104.

6. Deng MC, De Meester JMJ, Smits JMA, et al., on behalf of COCPIT Study Group. The effect of receiving a heart transplant: analysis of a national cohort entered onto a waiting list, stratified by heart failure severity. Br Med J 2000;321:540–545.

7. Aaronson KD, Schwartz JS, Chen TMC, et al. Development and prospective validation of a clinical index to predict survival in ambulatory patients referred for cardiac transplant evaluation. Circulation 1997;95:2660–2667.

8. Montoya JG, Giraldo LF, Efron B, et al. Infectious complications among 620 consecutive heart transplant patients at Stanford University Medical Center. Clin Infect Dis 2001;33:629–640.

9. Rubin RH. Prevention and treatment of cytomegalovirus disease in heart transplant patients. J Heart Lung Transplant 2000;19:731–735.

10. Knirsch CA, Jakob K, Schoonmaker D, et al. An outbreak of *Legionella micdadei* pneumonia in transplant patients: evaluation, molecular epidemiology, and control. Am J Med 2000;108:290–295.

11. Munoz P, Munoz RM, Palomo J, et al. *Pneumocystis carinii* infection in heart transplant recipients. Efficacy of a weekend prophylaxis schedule. Medicine 1997;76:415–422.

12. Aguado JM, Herrero JA, Gavalda J, et al. Clinical presentation and outcome of tuberculosis in kidney, liver, and heart transplant recipients in Spain. Spanish Transplantation Infection Study Group, GESITRA. Transplantation 1997;63:1278–1286.

13. Gallino A, Maggiorini M, Kiowski W, et al. Toxoplasmosis in heart transplant recipients. Eur J Clin Microbiol Infect Dis 1996;15:389–393.

14. Utili R, Zampino R, De Vivo F, et al. Improved outcome of pulmonary aspergillosis in heart transplant recipients with early diagnosis and itraconazole treatment. Clin Transplant 2000;14:282–286.

15. Schulman LL, Htun T, Staniloae C, et al. Pulmonary nodules and masses after lung and heart-lung transplantation. J Thorac Imaging 2000;15:173–179.

16. Grossi P, Farina C, Fiocchi R, et al. Prevalence and outcome of invasive fungal infections in 1963 thoracic organ transplant recipients: a multicenter retrospective study. Italian Study Group of Fungal Infections in Thoracic Organ Transplant Recipients. Transplantation 2000;70:112–116.

17. Hornung TS, de Goede CG, O'Brien C, et al. Renal function after pediatric cardiac transplantation: the effect of early cyclosporin dosage. Pediatrics 2001;107:1346–1350.

18. Israni A, Brozena S, Pankewycz O, et al. Conversion to tacrolimus for the treatment of cyclosporine-associated nephrotoxicity in heart transplant recipients. Am J Kidney Dis 2002;39:E16.

19. Andoh TF, Bennett WM. Chronic cyclosporine nephrotoxicity. Curr Opin Nephrol Hypertens 1998;7:265–270.

20. Olyaei AJ, de Mattos AM, Bennett WM. Immunosuppressant-induced nephropathy: pathophysiology, incidence, and management. Drug Saf 1999;21:471–488.

21. Sander M, Victor RG. Hypertension after cardiac transplantation: pathophysiology and management. Curr Opin Nephrol Hypertens 1995;4:443–451.

22. Ventura HO, Malik FS, Mehra MR, et al. Mechanisms of hypertension in cardiac transplantation and the role of cyclosporine. Curr Opin Cardiol 1997;12:375–381.

23. Rodino ME, Shane E. Osteoporosis after organ transplantation. Am J Med 1998;104:459–469.

24. Shane E, Mancini D, Aaronson K, et al. Bone mass, vitamin D deficiency, and hyperparathyroidism in congestive heart failure. Am J Med 1997;103:197–207.

25. Van Cleemput J, Daenen W, Nijs J, et al. Timing and quantification of bone loss in cardiac transplant recipients. Transplant Int 1995;8:196–200.

26. Epstein S, Shane E, Bilezikian JP. Organ transplantation and osteoporosis. Curr Opin Rheumatol 1995;7:255–261.
27. Shane E, Rivas M, McMahon DJ, et al. Bone loss and turnover after cardiac transplantation. J Clin Endocrinol Metab 1997;82:1497–1506.
28. Shane E, Rodino MA, McMahon DJ, et al. Prevention of bone loss after heart transplantation with antiresorptive therapy: a pilot study. J Heart Lung Transplant 1998;17:1089–1096.
29. Leidig-Bruckner G, Hosch S, Dodidou P, et al. Frequency and predictors of osteoporotic fractures after cardiac or liver transplantation: a follow-up study. Lancet 2001;357:342–347.
30. Depczynski B, Daly B, Campbell LV, et al. Predicting the occurrence of diabetes mellitus in recipients of heart transplants. Diabet Med 2000;17:15–19.
31. Lang CC, Beniaminovitz A, Edwards N, et al. Morbidity and mortality in diabetic patients following cardiac transplantation. J Heart Lung Transplant 2003;22: 244–249.
32. Czerny M, Sahin V, Fasching P, et al. Th impact of diabetes mellitus at the time of heart transplantation on long-term survival. Diabetologia 2002;45:1498–1508.
33. Wluka AE, Ryan PF, Miller AM, et al. Postcardiac transplantation gout: incidence of therapeutic complications. J Heart Lung Transplant 2000;19:951–956.
34. Emmerson BT. The management of gout. N Engl J Med 1996;334:445–451
35. Penn I. Tumors after renal and cardiac transplantation. Hematol Oncol Clin North Am 1993;7:431–445.
36. Swerdlow AJ, Higgins CD, Hunt BJ, et al. Risk of lymphoid neoplasia after cardiothoracic transplantation. a cohort study of the relation to Epstein–Barr virus. Transplantation 2000;69:897–904.
36. Chadburn A, Chen JM, Hsu DT, et al. The morphologic and molecular genetic categories of posttransplantation lymphoproliferative disorders (PT-LPDs) are clinical relevant. Cancer 1998;82(10):1978–1987.
37. Chen JM, Barr ML, Chadburn A, et al. Management of lymphoproliferative disorders after cardiac transplantation. Ann Thorac Surg 1993;56:527–538.
38. Garrett TP, Chadburn A, Barr ML, et al. Posttransplantation lymphoproliferative disorders treated with cyclophosphamide-doxorubicin-vincristine-prednisone chemotherapy. Cancer 1993;72:2782–2785.
39. De Geest S, Dobbels F, Martin S, et al. Clinical risk associated with appointment noncompliance in heart transplant recipients. Prog Transplant 2000;10:162–168.
40. Shapiro PA, Williams DL, Foray AT, et al. Psychosocial evaluation and prediction of compliance problems and morbidity after heart transplantation. Transplantation 1995;60:1462–1466.
41. Dew MA, Kormos RL, DiMartini AF, et al. Prevalence and risk of depression and anxiety-related disorders during the first three years after heart transplantation. Psychosomatics 2001;42:300–313.
42. Dew MA, Kormos RL, Roth LH, et al. Early posttransplant medical compliance and mental health predict physical morbidity and mortality one to three years after heart transplantation. J Heart Lung Transplant 1999;18:549–562.
43. Deng MC, Plenz G, Erren M, et al. Transplant vasculopathy: a model for coronary artery disease? Herz 2000;25:95–99.
44. Shirali GS, Ni J, Chinnock RE, et al. Association of viral genome with graft loss in children after cardiac transplantation. N Engl J Med 2001;344:1498–1503.
45. Schroeder JS, Gao SZ, Aldermann EL, et al. A preliminary study of diltiazem in the prevention of coronary artery disease in heart transplant recipients. N Engl J Med 1993;328:164–170.

46. Kobashigawa JA, Katznelson S, Laks H, et al. Effect of pravastatin on outcomes after cardiac transplantation. N Engl J Med 1995;333:621–627.
47. Wenke K, Meiser B, Thiery J, et al. Simvastatin reduces graft vessel disease and mortality after heart transplantation: a four-year ramdomized trial. Circulation 1997;96:1398–1402.
48. Behrendt D, Ganz P, Fang JC. Cardiac allograft vasculopathy. Curr Opin Cardiol 2000;15:422–429.
49. De Boer J, Cohen B, Thorogood J. Results of acute heart retransplantation. Lancet 1991;227:1158.
50. Reddy VS, Phan HH, Pierson RN III, et al. Late cardiac re-operation after cardiac transplantation. Ann Thorac Surg 2002;73:534–537.
51. Yankah AC, Musci M, Weng Y, et al. Tricuspid valve dysfunction and surgery after orthotopic cardiac transplantation. Eur J Cardiothorac Surg 2000;17:343–348.
52. Etzion S, Battler A, Barbash IM, et al. Influence of embryonic cardiomyocyte transplantation on the progression of heart failure in a rat model of extensive myocardial infarction. J Mol Cell Cardiol 2001;33:1321–1330.
53. Yokomuro H, Li RK, Mickle DA, et al. Transplantation of cryopreserved cardiomyocytes. J Thorac Cardiovasc Surg 2001;121:98–107.
54. Leor J, Aboulafia-Etzion S, Dar A, et al. Bioengineered cardiac grafts: a new approach to repair the infarcted myocardium? Circulation 2000;102(19 suppl 3): III.56–III.61.
55. El Oakley RM, Ooi OC, Bongso A, et al. Myocyte transplantation for myocardial repair: a few good cells can mend a broken heart. Ann Thorac Surg 2001;71: 1724–1733.
56. Yoo KJ, Li RK, Weisel RD, et al. Autologous smooth muscle cell transplantation improved heart function in dilated cardiomyopathy. Ann Thorac Surg 2000;70: 859–865.
57. Hutcheson KA, Atkins BZ, Hueman MT, et al. Comparison of benefits on myocardial performance of cellular cardiomyoplasty with skeletal myoblasts and fibroblasts. Cell Transplant 2000;9:359–368.
58. Orlic D, Kajstura J, Chimenti S, et al. Bone marrow cells regenerate infarcted myocardium. Nature 2001;410:701–705.
59. Kocher AA, Schuster MD, Szabolcs MJ, et al. Neovascularization of ischemic myocardium by human bone-marrow-derived angioblasts prevents cardiomyocyte apoptosis, reduces remodeling and improves cardiac function. Nat Med 2001;7: 430–436.
60. Deng MC, Loebe M, El-Banayosi A, et al. Mechanical circulatory support for advanced heart failure: effect of patient selection on outcome. Circulation 2001;103:231–237.
61. Mihaylov D, Verkerke GJ, Rakhorst G. Mechanical circulatory support systems—a review. Technol Health Care 2000;8:251–266.

10 Pediatric Heart Transplantation

Jacqueline M. Lamour, MD
and Linda J. Addonizio, MD

Contents

INTRODUCTION

A Brief History of Pediatric Cardiac Transplantation

In 1967, Kantrowitz et al. transplanted a heart from an anencephalic infant to a 3-wk-old with complex congenital heart disease *(1)*. Although the child died perioperatively, this pioneering surgery demonstrated the technical feasibility of replacing an infant heart. There was not much progress in pediatric transplantation over the following 15 yr, because, at the time, available immunosuppressive agents were inadequate to ensure long-term success. However, the introduction of cyclosporine (CyA) (Neoral, Sandoz Inc., East Hanover, NJ) in the early 1980s improved adult transplant patient survival, and, as a result, the number of centers interested in performing pediatric transplantation increased.

Through the late 1980s and early 1990s, the number of children receiving heart transplants grew significantly (Fig. 1). Concomitantly with this growth of transplantation came the expertise in complex

From: *Contemporary Cardiology: Cardiac Transplantation:*
The Columbia University Medical Center/New York-Presbyterian Hospital Manual
Edited by: N. M. Edwards, J. M. Chen, and P. A. Mazzeo © Humana Press Inc., Totowa, NJ

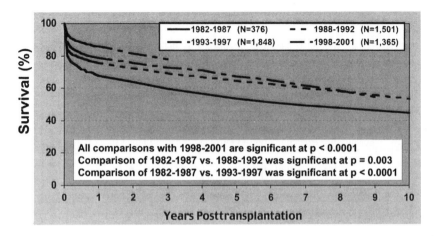

Fig. 1. Actuarial survival by era of transplantation from 1982 to 2001. Courtesy of the International Society of Heart and Lung Transplantation, with permission *(3)*.

surgical techniques needed for transplanting congenital heart malformations as well as improvement in recipient and donor selection. This rapid expansion of skill throughout the world, with increased knowledge of immunosuppression use and the introduction of new immunosuppressive therapies, has contributed to pediatric heart transplantation, which currently comprises approx 10% of all heart transplants *(2)*.

The most current data reported by the International Society of Heart and Lung Transplantation (ISHLT) registry indicate that 4,753 pediatric heart transplantations have been performed *(2)*. Actuarial survival has improved consistently since 1982 (Fig. 1). This improvement is secondary to decreased 1 yr mortality and probably reflects improved perioperative management and/or better patient selection *(3)*. For these reasons, heart transplantation is an accepted therapy for end-stage heart failure in infants and children. However, extended survival over decades remains uncertain. Late complications as a result of lifelong immunosuppression or, conversely, inadequate immunosuppression for the transplanted organ clearly limit the ultimate survival of transplant recipients. Additionally, an estimated 20% of pediatric patients continue to die waiting for a transplant *(4)*; this number increases to 30% in patients less than 6 mo of age *(5)*. Patient selection and optimal timing for listing must be weighed with respect to a finite donor pool when transplantation is considered for any child.

This chapter reviews special considerations that apply to the selection and management of the pediatric cardiac transplant recipient.

Indications for Pediatric Heart Transplantation

Cardiac transplantation is indicated in any patient with end-stage heart disease refractory to medical management in whom surgical palliation is not an option. The two major diagnostic categories in the pediatric age group are heart muscle myopathies and congenital heart disease, with the predominant diagnosis depending on the patient's age. According to the most recent ISHLT registry data, among pediatric transplant candidates, cardiomyopathy is diagnosed in less than 25% of infants below age 1 yr, 50% of children age 1–10 yr, and 62% of children age 11–17 yr. In contrast, congenital heart disease is diagnosed in greater than 75% of infants less than age 1 yr, the majority with hypoplastic left heart syndrome (HLHS), 37% of children 1–10 yr and 24% of children 11–17 yr.

Symptoms of heart failure in children vary with age. In small children, feeding difficulties or respiratory complaints may be the presenting symptom. However, in older children, abdominal complaints of nausea, vomiting, and anorexia may be the primary symptoms (6). In general, referral to a heart transplant center for evaluation should be made if heart failure signs persist despite a maximal oral cardiotonic regimen. Additionally, a patient who is frequently hospitalized for heart failure or respiratory complaints, growth failure, cardiac cachexia, anorexia and recurrent vomiting, or an unacceptably poor quality of life should be referred.

One of the major objectives of the transplant referral process is to identify a potentially treatable etiology for the heart failure, making transplant unnecessary, or, conversely, identifying an etiology that would preclude transplantation. Examples of potentially treatable causes would include carnitine or selenium deficiency, anomalies of the coronary arteries, chronic atrial or ventricular arrhythmias, and myocarditis. Dilated cardiomyopathies can also be familial or associated with more global forms of skeletal myopathies. Whereas cardiomyopathy associated with a stable skeletal myopathy is not a contraindication for transplantation, a degenerative muscular dystrophy would be. Also, other genetic, biochemical abnormalities of fatty acid, amino acid, glycogen, and mucopolysaccharide metabolism should be ruled out prior to consideration for transplant. Other contraindications are discussed later in this chapter.

Most cardiologists agree that a child with end-stage heart failure who requires inotropic support should be evaluated for transplant. However, the combination of high pulmonary vascular resistance (PVR) and inotropic dependency is associated with poor outcome and death waiting for heart transplantation *(7)*. Therefore, clinicians caring for children with heart failure should refer them for transplant evaluation prior to progression to inotropic dependency.

Optimal Timing of Referral

Once a patient is referred for heart transplantation, an extensive evaluation process begins; this includes assessments by a pediatric cardiologist, a cardiothoracic surgeon, a transplant nurse specialist, a pediatric neurologist, a pediatric psychiatrist, a social worker, and a physical therapist. There are two goals of the referral process: (a) to identify any other available treatment options that would negate the need for transplantation, and (b) if no such option exists, to decide the optimal time for listing and to delineate a therapeutic plan for the patient awaiting transplant.

The optimal timing of heart transplant referral is prior to hemodynamic compromise or irreversible end-organ damage. Often, in pediatrics, it is difficult to make this clinical prediction. To anticipate when to list a child for heart transplant, knowledge of the natural history of the particular heart disease and an understanding of donor waiting times is needed *(8)*.

Experience with pediatric retransplantation is growing as patient survival posttransplant improves. Pediatric retransplantation accounts for 10% of all pediatric transplantation *(3)*. Limited published data exist on the subject; however, a review of a multicenter experience in the early 1990s showed that the survival rate for pediatric retransplant recipients who survived beyond 6 mo was comparable to that for primary heart transplantation *(9)*. More recently, single-center experiences reported no difference in actuarial patient survival between primary transplantation and retransplantation *(10–12)*. Given the high incidence of graft vasculopathy in pediatric patients who die suddenly *(13)*, it is reasonable to consider patients for retransplantation if severe disease is found or in those who are experiencing episodes of ischemia. More investigation is needed in the pediatric age group to better define optimal retransplantation timing.

PREOPERATIVE CONCERNS

Diagnosis-Specific Considerations: Cardiomyopathy

Cardiomyopathies represent a diverse number of diseases affecting the myocardial muscle. The annual incidence of cardiomyopathy, reported by the Pediatric Cardiomyopathy Registry, is 11.8 per million patient years. When divided by functional type, 49% of the cases are dilated, 40% are hypertrophic, 3% are restrictive, and 8% are unspecified *(14)*. The most common type to require heart transplantation is dilated cardiomyopathy, and the natural history of pediatric patients with idiopathic dilated cardiomyopathy is extremely variable, with a wide range of clinical outcomes *(15–22)*. Some children with severely depressed left ventricular (LV) function can remain asymptomatic for years until a viral illness exhausts their cardiac reserves. Others become symptomatic and deteriorate quickly.

Attempts have been made to identify prognostic factors associated with outcome in dilated cardiomyopathy, but data are conflicting, not only because the disease process is variable but also because single-institution reports on children do not have sufficient numbers of patients. A favorable prognosis is associated with LV hypertrophy *(16)* and a recent viral illness *(22)*. Poor prognosis is associated with age less than 2 yr at presentation *(20)*, a family history of cardiomyopathy *(20)*, development of significant atrial or ventricular arrhythmias *(15,16,20)*, LV ejection fraction of less than 30% *(18,19,21)*, a LV end-diastolic pressure of more than 25 mmHg *(15)*, and persistent congestive heart failure *(17)*. Others dispute some of these correlations *(15–17,19,21)*. Therefore, in children, it is often difficult and overly simplistic to determine mortality risk by one or two of these factors. As heart failure research and clinical application progress, newer modalities such as β-blocker therapy in children may change existing risk stratification paradigms *(23–25)*. As more medical therapy becomes available for patients with heart failure, the need for heart transplantation may be delayed or unnecessary in some patients with dilated cardiomyopathy. Far fewer patients with hypertrophic cardiomyopathy require heart transplantation. Hypertrophic cardiomyopathies have a variable natural history and clinical expression. Although patients with this disorder have diastolic dysfunction, most have preserved LV systolic function. The unpredictable risk of sudden death resulting from ventricular tachyarrhythmia, higher in children than adults, makes this patient group particularly difficult to treat *(26)*. Because of the present availability of implantable defibrillators and newer antiarrhythmic medications, the majority of these children would not need to be considered for transplant for this reason alone. However, uncontrollable arrhythmia would justify a transplant evaluation. When present, surgical relief of severe obstruction may defer the need for cardiac transplantation for many years.

Usually, referral is indicated when a patient begins to have systolic ventricular dysfunction in addition to baseline diastolic dysfunction. In a rare patient, diastolic dysfunction alone is severe enough to warrant transplantation. An infant with severe hypertrophic cardiomyopathy should have a full genetic and metabolic work-up. The presence of a systemic metabolic derangement may affect the decision to list for transplantation.

Restrictive cardiomyopathy, the rarest myopathy form in children, carries a poor prognosis with rapid deterioration and a high mortality rate when patients experience significant heart failure *(27–31)*. In these patients, cardiac transplantation appears to be the only viable treatment option. Because there is preservation of LV systolic function, the presentation of these children can be subtle, and pulmonary vascular disease progression may precede overt heart failure symptom development and, thereby, preclude successful orthotopic transplantation. Children with idiopathic restrictive cardiomyopathy should undergo serial monitoring of their PVR indices, starting with a baseline catheterization at presentation. A rise in PVR index (PVRI) in association with even subtle symptoms should prompt a transplant evaluation and early listing.

Diagnosis-Specific Considerations: Congenital Heart Disease

Advances in surgical and medical management have greatly improved the long-term survival of patients with congenital heart disease. However, late myocardial dysfunction can occur following palliative or corrective surgery and is the most common cause of morbidity and death in these patients. Of all patients with congenital heart disease, it has been estimated that 10–20% will be potential candidates for a heart or heart–lung transplantation at some time during their lives *(32)*. These patients present multiple unique surgical and medical challenges because of their complex anatomies, palliative and corrective prior procedures, and overall debilitated health *(33,34)*. However, currently, congenital heart disease is as common an indication for transplantation as cardiomyopathy *(3)*.

The most common congenital heart lesions requiring heart transplantation are forms of complex single ventricles. In the infant population, this includes patients with hypoplastic LVs or right ventricles (RVs). Patients with HLHS comprise the largest number in this group *(35)*. Although the Norwood procedure is available and has had successful long-term results, it is a palliative operation ultimately leading to a Fontan procedure, and the outcome varies greatly among centers. However, choosing transplantation as the primary operation incurs a significant mortality risk during the wait for a donor organ and requires a commitment to lifelong immunosuppression. The decision to perform a Norwood procedure as a first operation in these patients is most often center-specific but is also driven by donor organ availability.

Other congenital lesions that are considered indications for transplantation are those for which palliative surgery carries an unacceptably high mortality risk. This includes pulmonary atresia with intact ventricular septum and coronary compromise, univentricular hearts with severe atrioventricular valve regurgitation or severe ventricular dysfunction, or complex heterotaxy syndrome.

In older children and young adults with congenital heart disease, two major diagnostic groups present for transplant. One is comprised of patients with biventricular repairs who, subsequently, develop myocardial dysfunction. The other group consists of patients with palliated single ventricles who have developed poor systemic ventricular function or have a poor hemodynamic result following palliation. The latter are most commonly patients with failed Fontan physiology. Children and young adults with failed Fontans constitute a rapidly growing group that will require future cardiac transplantation (36–38).

Overall, the majority of patients with cardiomyopathy or congenital heart disease who require transplantation have severe systemic ventricular dysfunction. However, in a patient with a single ventricle and a Fontan repair, there is no pulmonary ventricle; therefore, the cardiac output from the ventricle is dependent on passive pulmonary blood flow. In these patients, even a mild decrease in LV function or a decrease in diastolic compliance, particularly in combination with an abnormality in lung function or perfusion, could be responsible for low cardiac output (a failure of forward flow) and makes transplantation the only survival option. Sometimes, other conditions, such as pulmonary disease or bronchopulmonary collaterals, may compete with the passive pulmonary flow; treatment of these conditions or embolization may obviate or delay the need for a transplant.

Additional transplant referral criteria for patients with congenital heart disease and relatively normal ventricular function would include growth failure, severe protein-losing enteropathy, cardiac cachexia, and severe cyanosis secondary to arteriovenous malformations (39). The complexity of these lesions dictates that all children and young adults with congenital heart disease who require a transplant be evaluated at an established congenital heart surgical center to ensure that other operative and medical alternatives are exhausted and that all necessary preoperative questions are answered.

Contraindications in Children

Improvements in surgical techniques and perioperative and postoperative care have allowed successful transplantation in high-risk patients. Consequently, many historical absolute contraindications to transplantation have become relative. Orthotopic cardiac transplantation is feasible for most complex congenital heart lesions if the pulmonary arteries (PAs) and veins are of reasonable size and PVR is not excessive *(40,41)*.

A high, fixed PVR is an absolute contraindication for orthotopic cardiac transplantation. However, elevated PVR should be considered a continuum of risk, and the absolute upper limit resistance is not well defined. Generally, patients with a PVRI less than 6 indexed Woods units are at low risk for developing right heart failure (RHF) *(42)*. If the PVRI is greater than 6 indexed Woods units, pharmacological testing with pulmonary vasodilators in the catheterization lab is warranted to assess reactivity of the PA bed *(42–44)*. At the same time, the medical regimen should be optimized by adding intravenous inotropes and vasodilator therapy, when the cardiac index is extremely low, or altering the patient's oral regimen, if he or she is stable. If acute testing is initially unsuccessful in dropping the PVRI, a course of tailored inotropes and vasodilators, including various combinations of dobutamine, milrinone, nitroprusside, nitric oxide (NO), and prostacyclin, may achieve a decrease in PVRI *(42–44)*.

Transplantation with a PVRI greater than 6 Woods units, even after drug testing, is possible, although RHF risk is reported to be as high as 40% with a mortality of 15% *(42)*. Patients with a fixed PVRI greater than 10 indexed Woods units despite all treatment should be evaluated for a heart–double lung, heart–single lung, or heterotopic transplantation, unless a longer-term vasodilator and inotrope trial are deemed useful.

Active malignancy is a contraindication to heart transplantation. However, growing experience with transplantation in survivors of childhood cancers shows excellent survival in children who have developed adriamycin cardiomyopathy *(45,46)*. An optimal disease-free interval is hard to estimate and may be based on the nature of the primary tumor and disease progression at diagnosis time. Some investigators recommend a 1-yr disease-free interval after completion of adequate cancer therapy prior to transplantation *(45)*.

Other medical exclusion criteria include irreversible multi-organ failure, degenerative neurological disorders, or other systemic diseases that are life-limiting despite treatment.

Additionally, psychosocial stability in the child and family has a major effect on the successful organ transplantation outcome. An intact family support structure or a legal guardian is necessary before transplantation is considered. Lack of an adequate caretaker, active drug or alcohol abuse, or an untreated major psychiatric disorder are absolute exclusion criteria for transplantation. Similarly, a documented history of significant medical noncompliance in the patient or family is a risk factor associated with a poor outcome and should be considered a relative contraindication to transplant *(47–49)*.

Pretransplant Management Unique to Children

When the evaluation is complete, data are reviewed by the Pediatric Cardiac Transplant Team, which is responsible, with the family, for the decision to list a patient for transplantation. If a child's immunizations are not current, or if the child is nonimmunized but clinically stable, he or she can receive an age-appropriate set at listing time, with the exception of live viral vaccines. Patients on the active waiting list who are not hospitalized need close outpatient follow-up and repeat hemodynamic monitoring every 6–12 mo, depending on their diagnoses, to recheck PVR and determine the necessity and suitability of remaining on the list.

The majority of children waiting for heart transplantation are in the hospital. Many require permanent central venous access for inotropic support, monitoring hemodynamics, nutrition, anticoagulation, and blood draws. Swan–Ganz catheters are appropriate management in the hospital setting, though they are contraindicated in some children with congenital lesions and are not possible in others. Anticoagulation therapy is strongly recommended in pediatric patients with poor ventricular function, as these patients are at risk for both acute pulmonary emboli and cerebrovascular accidents *(50)*.

Many infants with congenital heart disease waiting for transplantation have ductal-dependent lesions and must remain in the hospital on continuous prostglandin E1 infusions to maintain ductal patency after birth. Patients with HLHS comprise the largest part of this group. Stenting of the ductus arteriosus to avoid long-term prostaglandin has been reported *(51)*.

After birth, PVR gradually falls. As a result, those patients with mixing lesions have an increase in pulmonary blood flow at the expense of systemic blood flow. The challenge in managing these children to a successful transplant is balancing the flow to both the pulmonary and systemic circulation, ideally as a 1:1 shunt. Some strategies to limit pulmonary blood flow in the face of falling PVR include decreasing the prostaglandin E1 dose to the minimal necessary to maintain ductal patency and maintaining the patient on room air. In the event that the patient requires mechanical ventilation, mild hypoventilation to keep pC_{O2} greater than 40 mmHg may also improve pulmonary-to-systemic circulation balance.

Also, maintaining adequate nutrition and avoiding infection is important while these infants wait for transplant. Infants and small children are at particular risk for anemia while waiting for transplantation because of frequent blood draws and poor nutritional states. In this population, daily erythropoietin injections decrease the need for blood transfusions and, therefore, may decrease the risk of preformed antibody development *(52)*.

As end-stage heart failure worsens, so does end-organ perfusion and function. Intervention with mechanical support prior to severe low output and cardiac arrest may reverse end-organ dysfunction and allow the patient to remain a potential transplant recipient. Extracorporeal membrane oxygenation (ECMO) with decompression of the LV has been used successfully as a bridge to transplant *(53–55)*. Although ECMO is the most widely used support system in pediatrics because of patient size restrictions, its complications are considerable, including bleeding, infection, and thromboembolism. It is a circuit based on nonpulsatile flow so that, although end-organ function may be recovered initially, its optimal use is usually limited to 2 or 3 wk. In adolescents, who have larger body surface area, implantable LV assist devices can successfully bridge patients to transplant *(56)*.

Experience with paracorporeal pneumatic ventricular assist devices (VADs) is growing in Europe *(57,58)*. These devices have been used in children weighing 3.2–52 kg. The smallest child in this series was a patient with pulmonary atresia and an intact ventricular septum who underwent a Blalock–Taussing shunt and had a myocardial infarct postsurgery. This patient did not survive, and the authors suggest that these devices are not appropriate for patients with intracardiac shunts *(57)*. However, successful bridging to transplant was achieved in both series, with the longest device used for 98 d.

DONOR AND OPERATIVE CONCERNS

Donor Heart Procurement

Children with congenital heart disease account for almost 50% of heart transplants in the pediatric age group *(3)*. Over the past 20 yr, experience transplanting numerous congenital heart variants has contributed to an expertise level such that few anatomic combinations are considered a contraindication to heart transplantation *(59–68)*. Often, heart transplantation for congenital heart defects is performed after multiple palliative operations and presents special surgical challenges. Success depends on recognition of the recipient anatomic needs by the harvesting surgical team at procurement time. These recipients' complex hearts may have abnormalities in their situs, systemic venous return, pulmonary venous return, and great vessels. Orientation of the heart relative to the systemic and pulmonary venous return is important to avoid obstruction at the anastomosis sites. Previous palliative operations may result in discontinuous, shunted, or banded PAs. Creative use of donor tissue is necessary when recreating normal anatomy in complex hearts. Therefore, in such a situation, the donor heart should be procured with additional length of superior vena cava (SVC), aorta, and PA, as needed.

There is a limited supply of adequate donor hearts. In choosing a donor for a pediatric patient, donor–recipient size mismatch is common. Experience shows that the acceptable weight range for a particular donor can be broad and sometimes triples that of the recipient weight *(69)*. This is particularly true in recipients who have significant cardiomegaly, because there is greater pericardial space to accommodate a larger organ. In the operating room (OR), special attention to tailoring the mismatch in great vessel size is necessary. In recipients whose native hearts are not enlarged, such as in restrictive cardiomyopathy and some congenital lesions, donor size must match more closely to prevent postoperative restriction and tamponade caused by the smaller pericardial space.

In January 1999, the United Network for Organ Sharing (UNOS) in the United States changed its algorithm for donor heart allocation *(70)*. In the past, both blood group O and pediatric candidates were at a disadvantage when compared with other groups. Children, mostly in the adolescent age group, were competing with adults for donor organs. Often, advanced-age donor hearts were given to adolescents, and adult recipients received adolescent donor hearts, based solely on length of time on the waiting list.

However, data show that receiving a heart from an advanced-age donor adversely affects survival in pediatric heart transplant recipients. One-yr survival is reported as low as 20% using donor hearts greater than 40 yr of age *(71)*. The new UNOS allocation system mandates that an adolescent donor heart be offered to a pediatric patient in the most urgent status before being given to an adult. Because pediatric patients represent a small percentage of the heart transplant waiting list, this change could make a tremendous difference on a child's life span without greatly affecting donor acquisition in the adult population.

Transplanting ABO-incompatible hearts is a potentially unique procedure in infants requiring heart transplantation. This practice is contraindicated in adults, because of hyperacute rejection risk caused by preformed recipient antibodies to the donor blood group antigens. However, infants do not produce antibody to blood group antigens until approx 1 yr. Additionally, the newborn's complement system remains immature for some time. These factors spare the infant from hyperacute rejection. Pioneering clinical work on transplantation across ABO blood groups was performed at the Hospital for Sick Children and University of Toronto because of an almost 50% recipient demise on the infant wait list. The investigators reported transplantation of ABO-incompatible hearts in infants with favorable results *(72)*. Isolated centers around the world have followed suit to improve donor availability for infants.

Operative Management

Heart transplantations in children with complex congenital heart lesions are now easily performed using technically creative surgical solutions devised to repair systemic and venous anomalies, heterotaxy syndromes, HLHS, dextrocardia, and transposition of the great arteries. These specific strategies are discussed in Chapter 5.

Orthotopic heart transplantation has been performed successfully to a "physiologic" single lung. This term is used in any patient in whom, because of unilateral pulmonary hypertension or an anatomical reason, there is only cardiac blood flow to a single lung. Such cases arise when there is PA discontinuity caused by a classic Glenn anastomosis (SVC to right pulmonary artery [RPA]) or an isolated left pulmonary artery (LPA). In these cases, RPA anatomy and pressures are normal; however, the LPA is hypertensive or absent as a result of aortopulmonary shunts, collaterals, or unilateral pulmonary vein stenosis. Previously, such patients required a heart–lung transplant because of donor RHF risk. Patients have been successfully transplanted with an orthotopic heart to a single lung with excellent results *(73)*. PA reconstruction can be accomplished successfully at transplantation time and even connected to the "hypertensive" lung; however, blood flows only to the normotensive lung.

Perioperative management

The intraoperative and immediate postoperative management of transplant patients is directed at optimizing allograft function in the face of three variables: acute denervation, prolonged ischemia, and acclimation to the recipient's hemodynamic environment. The newly transplanted heart has a relatively fixed stroke volume, and, therefore, an increased heart rate is necessary to augment cardiac output. Typically, a heart rate of 100 beats per minute (bpm) in an adolescent or 120 bpm in a smaller child is desirable early after transplant. In infants, faster heart rates are often necessary. Augmented heart rates can be achieved with inotropes or atrial pacing. In addition, agents such as isoproterenol are helpful in that they offer inotropy, chonotropy, and pulmonary vasodilatation.

Often, despite the ischemic insult the donor organ receives, systolic function recovers rapidly. Diastolic dysfunction may persist for several weeks. The newly transplanted heart benefits from the addition of low-dose inotropes in the early postoperative period, although they are frequently not necessary for long in a patient with a short ischemic time and low PVR.

Similarly to other pediatric patients who undergo open heart procedures, early extubation is desirable and achievable in patients with good graft function and low PVR. In children who receive a large donor heart, maximizing pulmonary toilet is warranted to alleviate potential left lower lung compression caused by the oversized heart. A period of nasal continuous positive airway pressure after extubation may be helpful.

Immediate postoperative care in children with high PVR varies significantly. Efforts begin preoperatively to decrease resistance with a tailored regimen based on trials in the catheterization laboratory. Beginning in the OR when coming off bypass, these patients are restarted on vasodilators, such as nitric oxide, milrinone, dobutamine, or prostacyclin, and are continued on them as needed for an extended time. Initially, deep sedation and an effort to maintain a mildly alkalotic state with PO_2 30–40 mmHg with adequate oxygenation, maintaining PCO_2 greater than 100 mmHg and no metabolic acidosis, are necessary to minimize the PVR. A more prolonged intubation may be required. Usually, the RV responds to its new hemodynamic environment within the first 2 or 3 d. The right heart may seem unaffected in the first 24 h; however, failure can occur following this honeymoon period. For persistent elevated PVR after transplant and RV failure, the right heart may need to be rested and then trained for a short period on a VAD *(74)*. In these circumstances, the RV usually shows recovery signs within 3–6 d and is then able to support the circulation *(75)*.

POSTOPERATIVE MANAGEMENT
Immunosuppression

In the absence of data available from pediatric clinical trials, most management is patient-tailored *(76–79)*. Approximately 40% of patients receive induction therapy in the form of a polyclonal anti-T-cell preparation. The remaining patients receive either OKT3 or interleukin-2 receptor antibody *(3)*.

Between October 1999 and December 2001, at the time of discharge from the hospital, CyA and tacrolimus (Prograf, Fujisawa Healthcar, Deerfield, IL) were used to nearly the same extent. However, more recipients reported taking CyA at 1-yr follow-up. Mycophenolate mofetil (MMF) was used in 50% of patients at the time of discharge and in 30% at 1-yr follow-up. Prednisone was used in 67% of patients at the time of discharge and in less than 50% at 1-yr follow-up. Rapamycin (Rapamune, Wyeth-Ayerst Laboratories, Madison, NJ) is now used in a small percentage of patients at hospital discharge *(3)* (Fig. 2).

In contrast, from April 1994 through December 1999, CyA was used in 80% of patients at discharge and in 75% at 1-yr follow-up; aziothioprine was used in 75% of patients at discharge; and MMF was used in less than 20% of patients at discharge. The practice of weaning patients from steroids shortly after transplant has remained consistent, with 50% of patients on prednisone at 1-yr follow-up *(80)*.

The greater diversity of immunosuppressive agents currently available allows the clinician to tailor management to each patient. However, several principles guide the choice of immunosuppression at each center. First, combination therapy minimizes the side effects of any single drug while targeting multiple steps in the T-cell activation cascade. Calcineurin inhibitors are the primary immunosuppressants.

The nephrotoxic effects of the calcineurin inhibitors in children are similar to those in adults; however children are anticipated to be on these drugs for several additional years. Some specific side effects of each drug may be minimized if lower doses can be used with additional drugs. For instance, gingival hyperplasia and the hypertrichosis associated with CyA are usually less severe if lower doses are allowed by multiple immunosuppressive drug use. Common adjunct therapy consists of azathioprine and MMF.

Corticosteroids are used in the majority of initial immunosuppressive regimens. The side effects of steroids (most notably the growth retardation associated with them) have encouraged many to attempt steroid withdrawal as soon as possible, a strategy that yields mixed success *(76,79)*.

In general, children metabolize drugs more quickly than adults, thus blood trough levels are needed to monitor and correctly dose CyA, tacrolimus, and MMF. In some circumstances, it is necessary to greatly increase the amount and/or frequency of the dose to achieve therapeutic levels. Because metabolism in children changes with time, particularly during growth, it is necessary to monitor drug levels more frequently than in adults. It is common to find an unexpected rejection late after transplant in a patient who has not been monitored closely or who has "outgrown" his or her drugs.

Another, more common, problem in childhood transplantation is the frequent use of antibiotics and their interaction with immunosuppressants. Young children have an increased incidence of infections as they grow and gain natural immunity. Many newer antibiotics that are prescribed by pediatricians can dramatically change CyA or tacrolimus

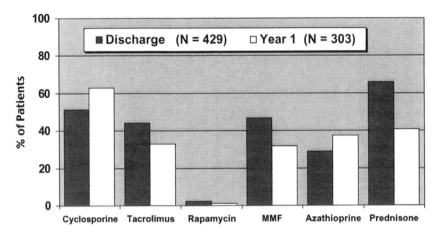

Fig. 2. Maintenance immunosuppression in pediatric heart transplant recipients from 1999 to 2001. Courtesy of the International Society of Heart and Lung Transplantation, with permission *(3)*.

metabolism and, thereby, their associated blood levels. Families and physicians should be counseled to review antibiotics choices with the transplant team to prevent toxicity or inadequate immunosuppression.

Noncompliance with medications occurs in at least 25% of pediatric patients and is a risk factor for acute rejection, late rejection, graft vasculopathy, and death *(47,81–85)*. The transplant team's assessment of stress, resources, and coping of the recipient and family is as integral and essential to the patient's longevity as the proper immunosuppressive regimen. The evaluation must focus not only on the child at various ages and developmental levels but also on the parents, including their parenting skills and ability to understand and follow directions. Heightened vigilance and education, particularly as the patient reaches adolescence (even if he or she was compliant during childhood), is important for preventing the sequela of noncompliance *(85,86)*.

Acute Rejection

Most pediatric heart transplant recipients experience at least one rejection episode during their lifetimes, and the majority of these are in the first 3 mo after transplantation *(87–89)*. The ideal method for diagnosing acute rejection remains controversial in the pediatric population. The "gold standard" of rejection surveillance is endomyocardial biopsy, which, at present, remains the only direct method for early rejection detection, as well as an important means for determining adequacy of rejection episode treatment. However, those centers that have a large neonatal and infant population rely primarily on physical examination and echocardiography *(87,90)*.

In the newborn and young child, rejection may have more manifest symptoms in a less aggressive stage. Symptoms including irritability, poor feeding, nausea, abdominal pain, or changes in sleep pattern and signs including fever, tachycardia, hepatosplenomegaly, new murmur, gallop, or arrhythmia are described as consistent with rejection *(87)*. Because endomyocardial biopsies are not typically performed frequently on infants and children, it remains unclear whether histologic findings precede symptoms and for how long.

In older children, clinical parameters are usually insensitive rejection indicators, often until myocardial performance is compromised. Rejection with hemodynamic compromise, an unambiguous clinical finding, is associated with a poor outcome *(91)*.

Graft Vasculopathy

The prevalence of graft vasculopathy is reported to be between 7% and 19% and remains the most significant obstacle to longevity in pediatric patients *(47,84,92–94)*. However, this may be an underestimation given the screening tools available to detect disease. Graft vasculopathy is associated with late rejection episodes, increased numbers of rejections, and noncompliance *(47,93,94)*.

When coronary artery disease has been detected, modification of immunosuppression to halt or slow disease progression has been attempted. Coronary artery stents and coronary artery bypass, used with limited success in the adult population, generally are not feasible in the pediatric population but have been attempted in select patients *(95–97)*. Graft vasculopathy increases the risk of a poor outcome and sudden death in the pediatric population, especially in the face of noncompliance *(47)*. Currently, there are no treatment options proven to prevent or halt disease progression, and retransplantation is the only option when disease is severe. Unfortunately, numerous of patients are found to have coronary artery disease after they have died suddenly, a phenomenon resulting from both the inadequacy of angiography to detect small vessel disease and the rapidity of the immune-based pathologic process *(13,92)*.

Posttransplant Lymphoproliferative Disease

The incidence of posttransplant lymphoproliferative disease (PTLD) in pediatric heart transplant recipients is reported between 13% and 26% *(84,98–100)*. The majority of cases are related to a primary Epstein–Barr virus (EBV) infection and seroconversion of EBV titers *(98,99,101)*. The incidence is higher in children because most children are EBV-negative prior to transplant; many convert during normal childhood illness or contract the virus from their grafts. Clinical manifestations can be as vague as fever and malaise or fulminant, as with gastrointestinal bleeding. In cases where involvement is localized to the tonsils and adenoids, a history of recurrent sinusitis and snoring is common *(98)*.

Treatment for the disease includes reduction or temporary cessation of immunosuppression. This approach is effective in the majority of cases, especially when the disease is polyclonal. The addition of antiviral medication, immunoglobulin, and anti-monoclonal antibodies, such as rituximab (Rituxan, Genentech Inc., South San Francisco, CA), may provide benefit in treating polyclonal disease, although limited data are available *(98–101)*. It is important to monitor closely for allograft rejection when reducing immunosuppression, as it frequently occurs and may be the cause of death following successful cure of PTLD *(99,100)*. Polymorphic disease is more common and tends to respond to treatment better than the rare monomorphic disease forms that do not respond to this therapy. In these cases, chemotherapy is required *(98,100,101)*.

Infection

Although most infectious concerns in heart transplantation are similar for adults and the older child, the young child warrants special mention. Age at transplantation is an important risk factor for infection. The young infant has an increased risk of mortality from infection compared to the older heart transplant recipient *(102)*. Age is also relevant when considering the chance of prior exposure to certain infectious agents. Younger children are less likely to have been exposed to cytomegalovirus and EBV. They are less likely to have had varicella and more likely to be exposed after transplantation.

Age also determines the number of immunizations the patient has received. Children who are not fully immunized prior to transplantation require vaccination after transplantation. Immunizations should be delayed following transplant until immunosuppression is weaned to maintenance levels. Prior to this, the child's ability to mount an immune response may be deficient. Live viral vaccines are not recommended *(103)*.

Growth After Transplantation

A pediatric cardiac allograft must increase in size over the course of a lifetime. Even when markedly oversized donors are used, ventricular volumes, indexed to recipient body size, tend to normalize early after transplant. During follow-up, ventricular volumes remain approximate for recipient body size. Great vessel growth is also appropriate *(104–106)*. Somatic growth is variable. In general, infant heart transplant recipients grow normally, although patients' height percentiles tend to be below age normal means in the lowest quartile *(106–108)*. This appears true despite the different immunosuppressive protocols used by pediatric centers with variable steroid use *(106,108)*. In children and adolescents, growth is normal despite a lack of catch-up growth initially after transplant, which ultimately may impinge on final adult height. Weight usually increases dramatically in patients in yr 1 after transplant, particularly in those pediatric patients with a predilection to be overweight, but tends to slow over time when immunosuppression medications are weaned. Pubertal development in adolescence is normal *(108)*.

CONCLUSION

Enormous progress has been made in pediatric heart transplantation over the last 20 yr. The use of VADs and the continued development of these devices for the smallest patients will allow more infants and children to be bridged to transplant successfully. Late complications and the long-term effects of immunosuppression are ongoing challenges for clinicians caring for these patients. Newer immunosuppressive drugs and therapeutic modalities have enhanced ability to treat acute and chronic rejection and PTLD. However, with the inflexible medication regimen currently required for success, noncompliance risk continues to jeopardize long-term survival, particularly in the adolescent age group. Continued therapy refinement and the discovery of ways to induce tolerance promise to improving longevity and quality of life in the pediatric transplant recipient.

Although it is not a cure for end-stage heart disease, as a palliative therapy, cardiac transplantation potentially allows the recipient to enjoy a full and active life inhibited only by daily medications and chronic medical surveillance.

REFERENCES

1. Kantrowitz A, Haller JD, Joos H, et al. Transplantation of the heart in an infant and an adult. Am J Cardiol 1968;22:783–790.
2. Hosenpud JD, Bennett LE, Keck BM, et al. The registry of the International Society for Heart and Lung Transplantation: 18th official report—2001. J Heart Lung Transplant 2001;20:805–815.
3. Boucek MM, Edwards LB, Keck BM, et al. The registry of the International Society for Heart and Lung Transplantation: fifth official report—2001 to 2002. J Heart Lung Transplant 2002;21:827–840.
4. McGiffin DC, Naftel DC, Kirklin JK, et al. Predicting outcome after listing for heart transplantation in children: comparison of Kaplan–Meier and parametric competing risk analysis. J Heart Lung Transplant 1997;16:713–722.

5. Morrow WR, Naftel D, Chinnock R, et al. Outcome of listing for heart transplantation in infants younger than six months: predictors of death and interval to transplantation. J Heart Lung Transplant 1997;16:1255–1266.
6. Rosenthal DN, Addonizio L, Chin C, et al. Heart failure symptoms vary with age in pediatric patients. J Heart Lung Transplant 2002;21:128.
7. Addonizio LJ, Hsu DT, Fuzesi L, et al. Optimal timing of pediatric heart transplantation. Circulation 1989;80(suppl III):III.84–III.89.
8. Fricker FJ, Addonizio LJ, Bernstein D, et al. Heart transplantation in children indications. Pediatr Transplant 1999;3:333–342.
9. Michler RE, Edwards NM, Hsu DT, et al. Pediatric retransplantation. J Heart Lung Transplant 1993;12:S319–S327.
10. Kanter KR, Vincent RN, Berg AM, et al. Twelve-year experience with pediatric cardiac retransplantation. J Heart Lung Transplant 2001;20:231.
11. Sehra R, Checchia P, Johnston J, et al. Outcomes following repeat cardiac transplantation. Suppl Circulation 2001;104:II–677.
12. Addonizio LJ, Kichuk MR, Hsu DT, et al. Improved surgery following pediatric cardiac retransplantation using total lymphoid irradition. J Heart Lung Transplant 1997;16:76.
13. Lamour JM, Addonizio LJ, Korsin RL, et al. Sudden cardiac death following heart transplantation in children. Suppl Circulation 2001;104:II–677.
14. Lipshultz SE, Sleeper LA, Towbin JA, et al. The incidence of pediatric cardiomyopathy: the prospective pediatric cardiomyopathy registry. JACC 2001;37:465A.
15. Lewis AB, Chabot M. Outcome of infants and children with dilated cardiomyopathy. Am J Cardiol 1991;68:365–369.
16. Wiles HB, McArthur PD, Taylor AB, et al. Prognostic features of children with idiopathic dilated cardiomyopathy. Am J Cardiol 1991;68:1372–1376.
17. Friedman RA, Moak JP, Garson A. Clinical course of idiopathic dilated cardiomyopathy in children. JACC 1991;18:152–156.
18. Akagi T, Benson LN, Lightfoot NE, et al. Natural history of dilated cardiomyopathy in children. Am Heart J 1991;121:1502–1506.
19. Chen S, Nouri S, Balfour I, et al. Clinical profile of congestive cardiomyopathy in children. J Am Coll Cardiol 1990;15:189–193.
20. Griffin ML, Hernandez A, Martin TC, et al. Dilated cardiomyopathy in infants and children. J Am Coll Cardiol 1988;11:139–144.
21. Ino T, Benson LN, Freedom RM, et al. Natural history and prognostic risk factors in endocardial fibroelastosis. Am J Cardiol 1988;62:431–434.
22. Taliercio CP, Seward JB, Driscoll DJ, et al. Idiopathic dilated cardiomyopathy in the young: clinical profile and natural history. J Am Coll Cardiol 1985;6:1126–1131.
23. Williams RV, Tani LY, Shaddy RE. Intermediate effects of treatment with metoprolol or carvedilol in children with left ventricular systolic dysfunction. J Heart Lung Transplant 2002;21:906–909.
24. Bruns LA, Christant MK, LamourJM, et al. Carvedilol as therapy in pediatric heart failure: an initial multicenter experience. J Pediatr 2001;138:457–458.
25. Azeka E, Franchini Ramires JA, Valler C, et al. Delisting of infants and children from the heart transplantation waiting list after carvedilol treatment. J Am Coll Cardiol 2002;40:2034–2038.
26. McKenna W, Deanfield J, Faruqui A, et al. Prognosis in hypertrophic cardiomyopathy: role of age and clinical, electrocardiographic and hemodynamic features. Am J Cardiol 1981;47:532–538.

27. Lewis, AB. Clinical profile and outcome of restrictive cardiomyopathy in children. Am Heart J 1992;123(6):1589–1593.
28. Cetta F, O'Leary PW, Seward JB, et al. Idiopathic restrictive cardiomyopathy in childhood: diagnostic features and clinical course. Mayo Clin Proc 1995;70:634–640.
29. Denfield SW, Rosenthal G, Gajarski RJ, et al. Restrictive cardiomyopathies in childhood. Etiologies and natural history. Texas Heart Institute J 1997;24(1):38–44.
30. Chen SC, Balfour IC, Jureidini S. Clinical spectrum of restrictive cardiomyopathy in children. J Heart Lung Transplant 2001;20(1):90.
31. Weller RJ, Weintraub R, Addonizio LJ, et al. Outcome of idiopathic restrictive cardiomyopathy in children. Am J Cardiol 2002;90:501–506.
32. Penoske P, Freedom R, Rowe R, et al. The future of heart and heart–lung transplantation in children. Heart Transplant 1984;3:233–238.
33. Hsu DT, Quaegebeur JM, Michler RE, et al. Heart transplantation in children with congenital heart disease. J Am Coll Cardiol 1995;26:743–749.
34. Lamour JM, Addonizio LJ, Galantowicz ME, et al. Outcome after orthotopic cardiac transplantation in adults with congenital heart disease. Circulation 1999; 100[suppl II]:II.200–II.205.
35. Chiavarelli M, Boucek MM, Nehlsen-Cannarella SL, et al. Neonatal cardiac transplantation intermediate-term results and incidence of rejection. Arch Surg 1992;127:1072–1076.
36. Carey JA, Hamilton L, Hilton CJ, et al. Orthotopic cardiac transplantation for the failing Fontan circulation. Eur J Cardiothorac Surg 1998;14:7–14.
37. Addonizio LJ, Hsu DT, Michler RE, et al. Cardiac transplantation in children after failed Fontan operations. J Heart Lung Transplant 1993;12:S93.
38. Bernstein D, Naftel DC, Hsu DT, et al. Outcome of listing for failed Fontan: a multi-institutional study. J Heart Lung Transplant 1999;18:69.
39. Lamour JM, Hsu DT, Kichuk MR, et al. Regression of pulmonary venous malformations following heart transplantation. Pediatr Transplant 2000;4:280–284.
40. Benson L, Freedom RM, Gersony WM, et al. Session II: cardiac replacement in infants and children: indications and limitations. J Heart Lung Transplant 1991;10:791–801.
41. Bailey LL. Heart transplantation techniques in complex congenital heart disease. J Heart Lung Transplant 1993;12:S168–S175.
42. Addonizio LJ, Gersony WM, Robbins RC, et al. Elevated pulmonary vascular resistance and cardiac transplantation. Circulation 1987;76(suppl V):V.52–V.55.
43. Zales VR, Pahl E, Backer CL, et al. Pharmacologic reduction of pretransplantation pulmonary vascular resistance predicts outcome after pediatric heart transplantation. J Heart Lung Transplant 1993;12:965–973.
44. Gajarski RJ, Towbin JA, Bricker T, et al. Intermediate follow-up of pediatric heart transplant recipients with elevated pulmonary vascular resistance index. J Am Coll Cardiol 1994;23:1682–1687.
45. Goldstein DJ, Seldomridge JA, Addonizio LJ, et al. Orthotopic heart transplantation in patients with treated malignancies. Am J Cardiol 1995;75:968–971.
46. Armitage JM, Kormos RL, Griffith B, et al. Heart transplantation in patients with malignant disease. J Heart Transplant 1990;9:627–630.
47. Addonizio LJ, Hsu DT, Smith CR, et al. Late complications in pediatric cardiac transplant recipients. Circulation 1990;82(suppl IV):IV.295–IV.301.
48. Douglas JF, Hsu DT, Addonizio LJ. Noncompliance in pediatric heart transplant patients. J Heart Lung Transplant 193;12:S92.
49. Douglas JF, Slater J, Hsu DT, et al. Can we treat noncompliance and decrease graft loss and death? J Heart Lung Transplant 2000;19:60.

50. Hsu DT, Addonizio LJ, Hordof AJ, et al. Acute pulmonary embolism in pediatric patients awaiting heart transplantation. J Am Coll Cardiol 1991;17:1621–1625.

51. Ruiz CE, Gamra H, Zhang HP, et al. Stenting of the ductus arterious as a bridge to cardiac transplantation in infants with the hypoplastic left heart syndrome. N Engl J Med 1993;328:1605–1608.

52. Shaddy RE, Bullock EA, Tani LY, et al. Epoetin alfa therapy in infants awaiting heart transplantation. Arch Pediatr Adolesc Med 1995;149:322–325.

53. Galantowicz ME, Stolar CJH. Extracorporeal membrane oxygenation for perioperative support in peditric heart transplantation. J Thorac Cardiovasc Surg 1991;102:148–152.

54. DelNido PJ, Armitage JM, Fricker FJ, et al. Extracorporeal membrane oxygenation support as a bridge to pediatric heart transplantation. Circulation 1994;90: II.66–II.69.

55. Ishino K, Weng Y, Alexi-Meskishvili V, et al. Extracorporeal membrane oxygenation as a bridge to cardiac transplantation in children. Artif Organs 1996;20: 728–732.

56. Helman DN, Addonizio LJ, Morales DL, et al. Implantable left ventricular assist devices can successfully bridge adolescent patients to transplant. J Heart Lung Transplant 2000;19:121–126.

57. Ishino K, Loebe M, Uhlemann F, et al. Circulatory support with paracorporeal pneumatic ventricular assist device in infants and children. Eur J Cardio Thorac Surg 1997;11:965–972.

58. Weyand M, Kececioglu D, Hekl HG, et al. Neonatal mechanical bridging to total orthotopic heart transplantation. Ann Thorac Surg 1998;66:519–522.

59. Doty DB, Renlund DG, Caputo GR, et al. Cardiac transplantation in situs inversus. J Thorac Cardiovasc Surg 1990;99:493–499.

60. Mayer JE, Perry S, O'Brien P, et al. Orthptopic heart transplantation for complex congential heart disease. J Thorac Cardiovas Surg 1990;99:484–492.

61. Yacoub M, Mankad P, Ledingham S. Donor procurement and surgical techniques for cardiac transplantation. Seminars Thorac and Cardiovasc Surg 1990;l2: 153–161.

62. Chartrand C, Guerin R, Kangah M, et al. Pediatric heart transplantation: surgical considerations for congenital heart diseases. J Heart Transplant 1990;9:608–617.

63. Cooper MM, Fuzesi L, Addonizio LJ, et al. Pediatric heart transplantation after operations involving the pulmonary arteries. J Thorac Cardiovasc Surg 1991; 102:386–395.

64. Allard M, Assaad A, Bailey L, et al. Session IV: surgical techniques in pediatric heart transplantation. J Heart Lung Transplant 1991;10:808–827.

65. Menkis AH, McKenzie FN, Novick RJ, et al. Expanding applicability of transplantation after multiple prior palliative procedures. Ann Thorac Surg 1991; 52:722–726.

66. Hasan A, Au J, Hamilton RJL, et al. Orthotopic heart transplantation for congenital heart disease. Eur J Cardio Thorac Surg 1993;7:65–70.

67. Vouhe PR, Tamisier D, Le Bidios J, et al. Pediatric cardiac transplantation for congenital heart defects: surgical considerations and results. Ann Thorac Surg 1993;56:1239–1247.

68. Razzouk AJ, Gundry SR, Chinnock RE, et al. Orthotopic transplantation for total anamolous pulmonary venous connection associated with complex congenital heart disease. J Heart Lung Transplant 1995;14:713–717.

69. Mitchell MB, Campbell DN, Clarke DR, et al. Infant heart transplantation: improved intermediate results. J Thorac Cardiovasc Surg 1998;116:242–252.

70. Renlund DG, Taylor DO, Kfoury AG, et al. New UNOS rules: historical background and implications for transplantation management. J Heart Lung Transplant 1999;18:1065–1070.
71. Chin C, Miller J, Robbins R, et al. The use of advanced-age donor hearts adversely affects survival in pediatric heart transplantation. Pediatr Transplant 1999;3:309.
72. West LJ, Phil D, Pollock-Barziv SM, et al. ABO-incompatible heart transplantation in infants. New Engl J Med 2001;344:793–800.
73. Addonizio LJ, Hsu DT, Lamour JM, et al. Successful orthotopic heart transplantation to a single lung in patients with congenital heart disease. Circulation 1998;98:I–688.
74. Chen JM, Levin HR, Rose EA, et al. Experience with right ventricular assist devices for peri-operative right-sided circulatory failure. Ann Thorac Surg 1996;61: 305–310.
75. Addonizio LJ, Hsu DT, Douglas JF, et al. Cardiac transplantation in children with markedly elevated pulmonary vascular resistance. J Heart Lung Transplant 1993;12:S93.
76. Bailey L, Gundry S, Razzouk A, et al. Bless the babies: one hundred fifteen late survivors of heart transplantation during the first year of life. J Thorac Cardiovasc Surg 1993;105:805–815.
77. Armitage JM, Fricker FJ, del Nido P, et al. A decade (1882 to 1992) of pediatric cardiac transplantation and the impact of FK 506 immunosuppression. J Thorac Cardiovasc Surg 1993;105:464–473.
78. Parisi F, Abbattista AD, Vinciguerra G, et al. Twelve years of cyclosporine in pediatric heart transplantation: what is the future? Transplant Proc 1998;30: 1967–1968.
79. Nohria A, Ehtisham J, Ramahi TM. Optimum maintanence trough levels of cyclosporine in heart transplant recipients given cortiosteriod-free regimen. J Heart Lung Transplant 1998;17:849–853.
80. Boucek MM, Faro A, Novick RJ, et al. The registry of the International Society for Heart and Lung Transplantation: fourth official pediatric report—2000. J Heart Lung Transplant 2001;20:39–52.
81. Chartrand C, Servando ES, Chartrand S. Risk factors for acute rejection after heart transplantation. Transplant Proc 2001;33:1732–1734.
82. Griffin KJ, Elkin TD. Nonadherence in pediatric transplantation: a review of the existing literature. Pediatr Transplant 2001;5:246–249.
83. Ringewald JM, Gidiing SS, Crawford SE, et al. Nonadherence is associated with late rejection in pediatric heart transplant recipients. J Pediatr 2001;139:75–78.
84. Sigusson G, Fricker FJ, Berstein D, et al. Long-term survivors of pediatric heart transplantation: a multicenter report of sixty-eight children who have survived longer than five years. J Pediatr 1997;130:862–871.
85. Uzark KC, Sauer SN, Lawrence KS, et al. The psychosocial impact of pediatric heart transplantation. J Heart Lung Transplant 1992;11:1160–1167.
86. Slater, JA. Psychiatric aspects of organ transplantation in children and adolescents. Child and Adolescent Psychiatric Clinic of North America 1994;3:557–598.
87. Chinnock RE, Baum MF, Larsen R, et al. Rejection management and long-term surveillance of the pediatric heart transplant recipient: the Loma Linda experience. J Heart Lung Transplant 1993;12:S255–S264.
88. Rotundo K, Naftel D, Boucek R, et al. Allograft rejection following cardiac transplantation in infants and children: a multi-institiutional study. J Heart Lung Transplant 1996;15:S80.

89. Balzer DT, Moorhead S, Saffitz JE, et al. Utility of surveillance biopsies in infant heart transplant recipients. J Heart Lung Transplant 1995;14:1095–1101.

90. Tanengco MV, Dodd D, Frist WH, et al. Echocardiographic abnormalities with acute cardiac allograft rejection in children: correlation with endomyocardial biopsy. J Heart Lung Transplant 1993;12:S203–S210.

91. Pahl E, Naftel DC, Canter CE, et al. Death after rejection with severe hemodynamic compromise in pediatric heart transplant recipients: a multi-institutional study. J Heart Lung Transplant 2001;20:279–287.

92. Pahl E, Zales VR, Fricker FJ, et al. Posttransplant coronary artery disease in children. Circulation 1994;90(pt 2):II.56–II.60.

93. Mulla NF, Johnston JK, Dussen V, et al. Late rejection is a predictor of transplant coronary artery disease in children. J Am Coll Cardiol 2001;37:243–250.

94. Addonizio LJ, Hsu DT, Douglas JF, et al. Decreasing incidence of coronary disease in pediatric cardiac transplant recipients using increased immunosuppression. Circulation 1993;88(pt 2):224–229.

95. Aranda JM, Pauly DF, Kerensky RA, et al. Percutaneous coronary intervention versus medical therapy for coronary allograft vasculopathy. One center's experience. J Heart Lung Transplant 2002;21:860–866.

96. Musci M, Pasic M, Meyer R, et al. Coronary artery bypass grafting after orthotopic heart transplantation. Eur J Cardiothorac Surg 1999;16:163–168.

97. Shaddy RE, Revenaugh JA, Orsmond GS, et al. Coronary intervention procedures in pediatric heart transplant recipients with cardiac allograft vasculopathy. Am J Cardiol 2000;85:1370–1372.

98. Zangwill SD, Hsu DT, Kichuk MR, et al. Incidence and outcome of primary Epstein–Barr virus infection and lymphoproliferative disease in pediatric heart transplant Recipients. J Heart Lung Transplant 1998;17:1161–1166.

99. Boyle GJ, Michaels GJ, Webber SA, et al. Posttransplantation lymphoproliferative disorders in pediatric thoracic organ recipients. J Pediatr 1997;131:309–313.

100. Berstein D, Baum D, Berry G, et al. Neoplastic disorders after pediatric heart transplantation. Circulation 1993;88(pt 2):230–237.

101. Green M, Michaels MG, Webber SA, et al. The management of Epstein–Barr virus associated posttransplant lymphoproliferative disorders in pediatric solid organ transplant recipients. Pediatr Transplant 1999;3:271–281.

102. Schowengerdt KO, Naftel DC, Seib PM, et al. Infection after pediatric heart transplantation: results of a multi-institional study. J Heart Lung Transplant 1997;16:1207–1216.

103. Bork J, Chinnock R, Ogata K, et al. Infectious complications in infant heart transplantation. J Heart Lung Transplant 1993;12:S199–S202.

104. Zales VR, Wright KL, Muster AJ, et al. Ventricular volume growth after cardiac transplantation in infants and children. Circulation 1992;86(suppl II):II.272–II.275.

105. Bernstein D, Kolla S, Miner M, et al. Cardiac growth after heart transplantation. Circulation 1992;85:1433–1439.

106. Hirsch R, Huddleston CB, Mendeloff EN, et al. Infant and donor organ growth after heart transplantation in neonates with hypoplastic left heart syndrome. J Heart Lung Transplant 1996;15:1093–1100.

107. Baum M, Chinnock R, Ashwal S, et al. Growth and neurodevelopmental outcome of infants undergoing heart transplantation. J Heart Lung Transplant 1993; S211–S217.

108. De Broux E, Huot CH, Chartrand S, et al. Growth and pubertal development following pediatric heart transplantation: a 15-year experience at Ste. Justine hospital. J Heart Lung Transplant 2000;19:825–833.

11 Surgical Alternatives to Transplantation

Deon W. Vigilance, MD
and Michael Argenziano, MD

CONTENTS

INTRODUCTION
REVASCULARIZATION FOR ISCHEMIC CARDIOMYOPATHY
REPARATIVE SURGERY: CORRECTING MITRAL VALVE
    REGURGITATION
LV GEOMETRY RESTORATION
CONCLUSION
REFERENCES

INTRODUCTION

Congestive heart failure (CHF) is a leading cause of hospital admissions in the United States (1). Heart failure affects over 400,000 people in the United States each year and accounts for a 1-yr mortality rate of 60% in this population (2,3). When maximal medical therapy is insufficient in stabilizing myocardial function and surgical options fail or do not exist, heart transplantation is the final recourse. Because a limited donor organ pool exists, with only 2500 heart transplants in the United States each year (4), priority is given to patients with limited life expectancy and no medical or surgical alternatives.

Currently, optimal medical management of patients awaiting cardiac transplantation is confined to inotropic support, afterload-reducing agents, diuretics, and internal cardioverter-defibrillators (3). However, despite aggressive nonsurgical management, the mortality rates for

From: *Contemporary Cardiology: Cardiac Transplantation:*
The Columbia University Medical Center/New York-Presbyterian Hospital Manual
Edited by: N. M. Edwards, J. M. Chen, and P. A. Mazzeo © Humana Press Inc., Totowa, NJ

patients on the heart transplant waiting list remains high *(1,5)*. To address this problem, many alternative surgical procedures have been conceived and used in heart failure treatment . These procedures have been used with varying indications, degrees of efficacy, and associated risks. For the purposes of this chapter, the major surgical approaches to heart failure management are categorized according to their principal mode of therapeutic benefit: (a) revascularization of ischemic myocardium, (b) repair of structural defects causing pressure overload, and (c) anatomic remodeling of the ventricle. Mechanical ventricular assistance and replacement will be described in Chapter 12.

REVASCULARIZATION FOR ISCHEMIC CARDIOMYOPATHY

Myocardial ischemia is the most common cause of heart failure and the most frequently documented indication for heart transplantation in the United States *(6)*. Coronary artery disease (CAD) resulting in myocardial ischemia is responsible for approx 60% of heart failure cases *(6,7)*. The majority of patients with CAD and severe left ventricle (LV) dysfunction receive medical management, which often results in poor long-term survival. Because heart transplantation is available only to approx 2500 patients per year because of a limited donor organ supply, the only recourse for most patients who are unresponsive to medical therapy is surgical revascularization.

Because it is difficult to predict which patients will show improvements in ventricular function postoperatively, and because of the high mortality in patients who do not benefit from revascularization, many patients are not offered coronary artery bypass grafting (CABG) surgery. Nonetheless, several studies document the feasibility of surgical revascularization in patients with severe ventricular dysfunction. In one multi-institutional study, 83 patients (mean ejection fraction = 24%) underwent CABG, and 39 patients (mean ejection fraction = 18%) were surgically revascularized *(8)*. In both series, patients experienced improvements in ventricular function with a low perioperative mortality and a 3-yr survival greater than 80%. In another study, 42 patients (ejection fraction < 20%) underwent CABG and showed improved postoperative ventricular function, operative mortality of 4.8%, and 1-yr survival of 88% *(9)*. Finally, in a retrospective review of patients undergoing either medical therapy or surgical revascularization while awaiting heart transplantation, those undergoing CABG had a 5-yr survival of 80% compared to only 28% in the medically managed group *(10)*. The operative mortality in this series was 20%, illustrating the potentially high risk of surgery in this patient population.

As a result of the unpredictability of functional improvement after high-risk surgical revascularization, a number of studies have attempted to identify preoperative factors associated with improved outcome. Currently, resurrection of ischemic but viable (hibernating) myocardium is thought to be the main mechanism by which ventricular function may improve after surgical revascularization; this concept is supported by the historical observation that patients with heart failure and angina fare better after revascularization than those without angina.

In a study of 57 patients (mean ejection fraction = 28%), the only clinical variable predictive of a favorable outcome was the presence of significant hibernating myocardium areas, manifested as a large reversible defect on preoperative thallium-201 scanning *(11)*. Because the presence of revascularizable ischemic myocardium is highly correlated with the presence of angina or previous myocardial infarction *(12)*, these factors are considered positive predictors of outcome after high-risk CABG.

Finally, the current ability to identify viable myocardium areas by thallium-201 scintigraphy, single-photon emission computed tomography, and positron emission tomography allows more precise identification of patients who are likely to benefit from surgical revascularization.

Despite the positive prognostic significance of hibernating myocardium, various other preoperative variables influence surgical results in patients with ischemic cardiomyopathy. In a retrospective study of patients undergoing CABG (ejection fraction < 20%), poor outcome predictors included advanced age, female gender, increased CAD severity, and the presence of ventricular arrhythmias *(13)*. In another study, peripheral vascular disease, hypertension, and increased LV filling pressures were associated with decreased postoperative survival *(14)*. Thus, although the presence of ischemic but viable myocardium should weigh heavily in the decision to proceed with surgical revascularization in patients with ventricular dysfunction, numerous other factors that may predict a significantly increased risk of failure must be considered.

In summary, patients with end-stage heart failure resulting from ischemic heart disease present a significant therapeutic challenge. Despite the recent development of pharmacologic agents that may prolong life expectancy in these patients, surgical revascularization represents a potentially life-saving option while awaiting heart transplantation. Advanced diagnostic techniques may aid in the identification of patients with hibernating myocardium who generally benefit from revascularization. Thus, proper patient selection for revascularization optimizes benefits while limiting associated procedural risks. However, significant comorbid conditions, heart failure severity, and the quality of the distal coronary vasculature are important determinants of functional recovery and survival that should not be ignored. A representative diagnostic and management algorithm for ischemic cardiomyopathy management has been provided in Fig. 1.

REPARATIVE SURGERY: CORRECTING MITRAL VALVE REGURGITATION

The major etiology of mitral regurgitation (MR) in the United States is degenerative valvular damage *(15)*. The pathophysiologic basis of myocardial dysfunction in MR resulting from degenerative valve disease is chronic volume overload leading to ventricular dilatation. Ventricular dilatation potentiates MR, and MR potentiates dilatation, resulting in perpetuation of a positive-feedback cycle *(16)*.

In ischemic mitral insufficiency, myocardial ischemia or infarction may be the dominant causative mechanism. In this case, papillary muscle dysfunction results in mitral valve prolapse and clinically significant MR. Although loss of papillary contractile function because of ischemia or infarction is necessary for ischemic MR development, ventricular dilatation or mitral annulus widening are also considered critical in this process *(17)*. In early ischemic MR stages, myocardial revascularization may be sufficient to reverse the pathologic process, but if permanent ventricular damage was sustained or irreversible ventricular or annular dilatation ensued, concomitant mitral valve repair (MVP) or replacement may (MVR) be necessary as well.

Although surgical intervention is recommended and highly successful in patients with MR and preserved systolic function, a more challenging cohort of potential surgical candidates are patients with signs of clinical heart failure or evidence of depressed systolic function. In these patients, MVR can further depress myocardial performance, and is associated with high perioperative mortality and poor long-term survival *(18)*. For these reasons, alternatives to MVR have been developed to avoid or minimize the pathologic processes responsible for postoperative deterioration in systolic performance.

An important pathogenetic determinant of ventricular dysfunction after conventional MVR is elimination of valvular–ventricular interactions induced by subvalvular apparatus disruption *(19)*. The specific mechanisms by which papillary–ventricular attachments enhance sys-

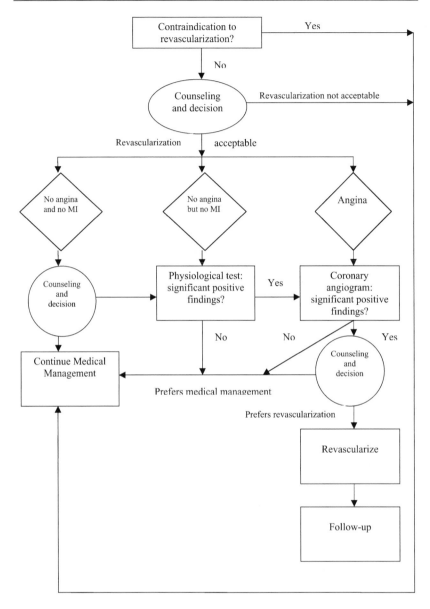

Fig. 1. Algorithm of high risk coronary artery revascularization.

tolic function include preload enhancement of midwall LV fibers (via LV sphericalization inhibition) *(20)* and reduction of regional midwall afterload *(21)*. Thus, techniques of MVR with chordal preservation have been developed (Fig. 2). Several experimental and clinical studies com-

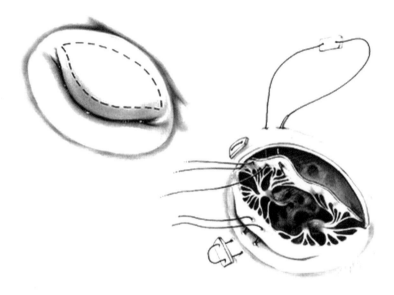

Fig. 2. Mitral valve replacement with preservation of subvalvular apparatus. From ref. *52* with permission.

pare the effects of conventional MVR and chord-preserving procedures on ventricular function. In a recent comparison of conventional MVR to chord-preserving procedures, chordal sparing was associated with superior preservation of ventricular geometry *(22)*. These and other studies confirm the clinical importance of subvalvular apparatus preservation when feasible. Clinical reports demonstrate a significant reduction in operative mortality and improvement in long-term survival in patients undergoing chord-sparing procedures *(23–25)*. The decreased morbidity and mortality noted after MVR procedures are likely because of improved ventricular function preservation as well as decreased operative time and technical complexity. Recognizing the importance of maintaining an intact subvalvular apparatus, Bolling et al. placed great emphasis on repairing the mitral valve rather than replacing it in patients with cardiomyopathy and severe MR *(26)*. Bowling et al. demonstrated effective correction of MR by means of annuloplasty during intermediate-term follow-up *(26)*.

Therefore, the modern MR surgical management is based on a continually evolving understanding of pathologic determinants of valvular and ventricular dysfunction.

LV GEOMETRY RESTORATION

LV Aneurysmorrhaphy (Dor Procedure)

Left ventricular aneurysms (LVAs) are characterized: (a) anatomically, by thinning of the ventricular wall in a scarred area resulting from a transmural myocardial infarction *(27)*, and (b) functionally, by paradoxic motion of the aneurysmal segment with ventricular geometry distortion. Although the majority of ventricular aneurysms are chronic, developing over time after the initial myocardial injury, LVA may develop immediately after acute myocardial infarction (AMI). Usually, acute LVA are not managed surgically but are allowed to mature while hemodynamic stability is established by pharmacologic agents, mechanical support, or myocardial revascularization.

Because of recent improvements in the medical management of AMI, CHF, and ventricular arrhythmias, the number of patients requiring surgery to repair chronic ventricular aneurysm treatment has decreased. However, the primary indications for surgical intervention have not changed; they include medically refractory heart failure, angina pectoris, ventricular tachyarrhythmias, and thromboembolism.

Whereas patients manifesting these symptoms are known to have a poor long-term survival without surgical intervention, asymptomatic patients have reported a 5-yr survival of 90% with medical therapy alone *(28)*. Although this suggests that surgical intervention should be reserved for symptomatic patients only, it is observed that asymptomatic patients are at risk for rapidly progressing to heart failure resulting from decompensation of a chronically volume-overloaded and dilated LV, leading to global ventricular dysfunction. Therefore, surgical management is offered to asymptomatic patients with chronic LVA who manifest evidence of progressive ventricular dilation or dysfunction, increasing MR, or aneurysmal enlargement *(27)*.

The pathophysiologic effects of an LVA on ventricular function are mediated by two major mechanisms. First, paradoxic motion of the aneurysmal freewall and septum results in volume overloading and dilitation of the remaining functional myocardium. Pathologically, this paradoxic motion is caused not only by stretching the aneurysmal scar but also by stretching the border zones of viable myocardium surrounding the aneurysm *(29)*. The second mechanism responsible for progressive ventricular function deterioration involves normal ventricular geometry distortion. As the base of an enlarging ventricular aneurysm dilates, it carries the adjacent normal freewall away from the septum, disturbing the normal parallel relationship between the septum and lateral freewall. This and other ventricular geometry distortions may significantly decrease contractile efficiency, even in the face of normal local myocardial contractility *(30,31)*.

Early attempts at surgical LVA treatment were based on the assumption that simple resection was the optimal way to relieve volume overload of the remaining ventricular myocardium. Consequently, open aneurysm resection with linear closure of the ventriculotomy, introduced by Cooley in 1958 *(32)*, remained the standard technique for greater than 25 yr. However, frequent inability to document improvement in ventricular performance and continued high mortality led to modifications of this approach based on an improved understanding of the underlying pathologic basis of ventricular dysfunction. Simply resecting dysfunctional myocardium and closing the aneurysmal segment only addresses the regurgitant volume, but does not eliminate the septum's paradoxic motion or restore normal ventricular geometry.

The Dor procedure *(33)* of ventricular aneurysmorrhaphy was conceived to correct the constellation of pathophysiologic defects. This procedure's main objective is to improve ventricular function by eliminating paradoxic motion of the freewall and septum and restoring global ventricular geometry. In the Dor endoventricular circular patch ventriculoplasty (Fig. 3), the aneurysmal freewall is resected, and the defect is bridged with an endocardial patch. In this operation, the aneurysmal septum is not imbricated but is excluded from the ventricular cavity by fixation of the endocardial patch to the junction of the septal endocardial scar and normal septal myocardium. After placing a pursestring suture around the base of the defect, the endocardial patch is sewn circumferentially to the edges of remaining myocardium. While restoring ventricular geometry, this maneuver also prevents paradoxic motion of the diseased septum and border zone by excluding these areas from ventricular contraction forces.

The theoretic advantages of the Dor procedure of ventricular aneurysmorrhaphy over traditional simple closure are supported by encouraging clinical results. In Dor's experience, surgical mortality is less than 7%, and postoperative evaluation confirms improvement in ejection fraction and control of ventricular arrhythmias in the majority of patients *(34)*. Nonetheless, attempts to compare this procedure's results with new modifications of the linear closure technique *(35)* have been inconclusive because of a lack of randomization and failure to control for variables such as infarct size and the effect of concomitant revascularization on ventricular function.

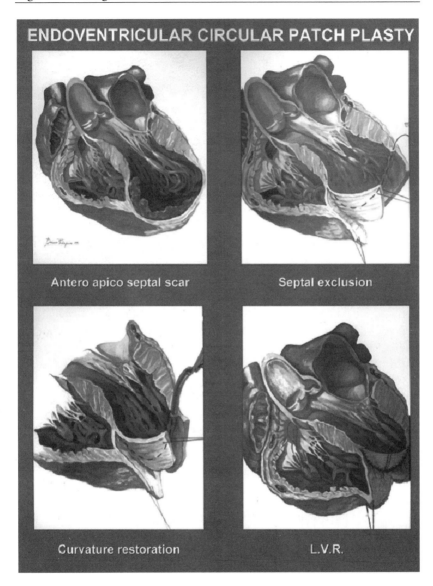

Fig. 3. Left ventricular aneurysmorrhaphy (Dor Procedure). From ref. *53* with permission.

Therefore, as in the case of chord-preserving mitral valve operations, surgical ventricular aneurysm management has undergone significant evolution as an improved understanding of underlying pathogenetic processes has been achieved. In this respect, the Dor procedure represents an example of surgical interventions designed to specifically address complex and multifactorial pathologic processes that were previously unappreciated or ignored.

Surgical Anterior Ventricular Endocardial Restoration

Anterior wall myocardial infarction may result in ventricular shape and size alterations *(36,37)*. Dramatic systolic functional LV recovery is not commonly achieved following revascularization *(38)*. Loss of contractile function of the anterior wall and septum causes remote ventricular myocardium to dilate as an adaptive mechanism to maintain stroke volume. This remodeling process results in ventricular dysfunction, and, ultimately, CHF *(39)*. Surgical anterior ventricular endocardial restoration (SAVER) excludes akinetic LV segments following anterior wall myocardial infarction that resulted in LV dilatation. This intervention, using Dor procedure principles with some technical modifications (Fig. 4), was performed in 439 patients for postinfarction dilated cardmyopathy.

After CABG or MVR is performed, the infarcted anterior wall segment is incised parallel to the left anterior descending artery. The transition point between viable and scarred myocardium is identified. Placing an encircling suture at the transitional zone excludes the scar from the ventricular cavity, creating an approx 2 × 3 cm purse orifice. The opening is closed with a Dacron patch. To enhance hemostasis, the patch is covered by the excluded scar tissue *(39)*.

Like the Dor procedure, SAVER also improved ejection fraction in studies. LV end systolic volume index also improved during the SAVER experience. The multicenter SAVER experience supported Dor's experience with dilated cardiomyopathy after anterior myocardial infarction.

Dynamic Cardiomyoplasty

Dynamic cardiomyoplasty (DCM) is a surgical treatment of dilated cardiomyopathy. In DCM, the latissimus dorsi muscle is mobilized and wrapped circumferentially around the heart and then stimulated synchronously with the cardiac cycle (Fig. 5). Effectively, the muscle wrap acts as an autologous external compression device, providing synchronized systolic pressure augmentation. At medium-term follow-up, the

---

Fig. 4. SAVER (*opposite and next page*)
(**A**) After opening the anterior ventricular scar, the region is palpated to better delineate myocardial scar from viable tissue. (**B**) Placement of an encircling suture between the viable and nonviable myocardial tissue. (**C**) Sewing the dacron patch into place. (**D**) Noncontracting scar is sewn over the dacron patch. From ref. *39* with permission.

A

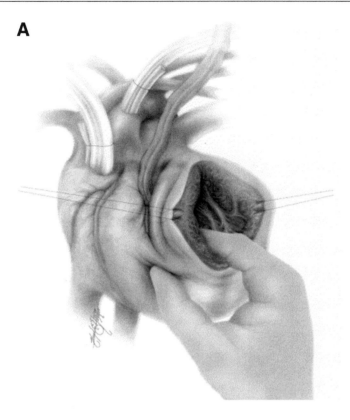

B

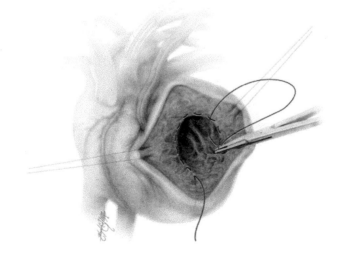

C

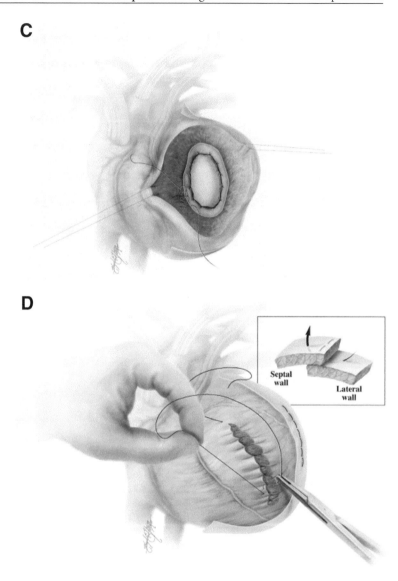

D

majority of patients undergoing DCM enjoy substantial improvements in functional status, although objective hemodynamic improvements are often not demonstrable *(40)*.

Although, originally, DCM was thought to improve cardiac function simply by providing systolic "squeeze" to the failing ventricle, subsequent experimental and clinical studies suggest that the mechanisms by which DCM influences myocardial function may be considerably more

A   **B**

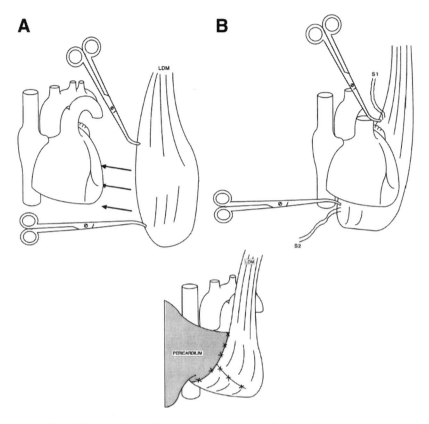

Fig. 5. Dynamic cardiomyoplasty. From ref. *54* with permission.

complex and may include ventricular volume stabilization by the girdling effect of the muscle wrap *(41)*.

In recent well-controlled experimental *(42)* and clinical *(43)* studies, DCM increased ejection fraction and peak ejection rate while decreasing end-diastolic volume, end-systolic volume, and end-diastolic pressure. Although reduction of ventricular volume and pressure had no effect on cardiac index, it enhanced effective contractility and reduced myocardial wall stress. The latter finding supports previous studies that reported beneficial effects of DCM on myocardial stress–strain relationships *(44,45)*. An additional effect noted in these studies was a reduction in wall motion asynchrony, a common characteristic of failing ventricles. Finally, it is postulated that, by contracting at the appropriate point in mid- to late-systole, the muscle wrap could improve ejection dynamics by acting as a "time-varying afterload reducer," lowering ventricular volumes and pressures near the end of the systolic contraction phase *(43,46)*.

Significant evidence points to the existence of at least two dominant mechanisms by which DCM ameliorates clinical heart failure severity . First, the passive constraint (or girdling effect) of the muscle wrap, whether stimulated or not, restrains the ventricle from further dilation and prevents continuing increases in myocardial tension by stabilizing cavitary radius *(47)*. Second, the reduction in wall stress affected by dynamic systolic compression may reduce the stimulation of pathologic myocyte hypertrophy and remodeling. Thus, by limiting ventricular dilatation and decreasing wall stress, DCM may halt, or even reverse, pathologic ventricular remodeling *(47)*.

Acorn Cardiac Support Device

The Acorn cardiac support device (CSD; Acorn Cardiovascular, Inc, St. Paul, MN) is a mesh-like wrapping device that is circumferentially placed around the heart (Fig. 6) to provide end-diastolic ventricular support *(48)*. This surgical approach to dilated cardiomyopathy is aimed at preventing the spheroidal reshaping that the heart undergoes in end-stage heart failure. Passive ventricular restraint devices halt or reverse cardiac remodeling by reducing wall stress and myocyte overstretch.

Typically, the Acorn device is placed via a sternotomy and is sutured in place near the atrioventricular groove. Prior to placement, the device is tailored to fit snugly around the ventricle. Device placement can be accomplished as a lone procedure or during concomitant CABG and/or valve surgery. Preclinical studies demonstrate significant promise in LV end-diastolic volume reduction *(49)*. Early clinical results (6–12-mo follow-up) from a safety study reveal CSD support to be effective in limiting cardiac dilatation progression and increasing LV ejection fraction *(50,51)*.

CONCLUSION

In the United States, data clearly demonstrate that cardiac transplantation has plateaued at approx 2500 cases annually, illustrating the limitation of donor organ availability. As average life expectancy increases, the demand for interventions to tackle the varying degrees of heart failure is also expected to increase.

Although aggressive medical management demonstrates some success in treating end-stage heart failure patients, many patients require surgical intervention. These surgical interventions range from straightforward and efficacious mitral valve repair for early mitral regurgitation to the complex Dor procedure for end-stage dilated cardiomyopathy with associated ventricular aneurysm. Although some procedures aim to

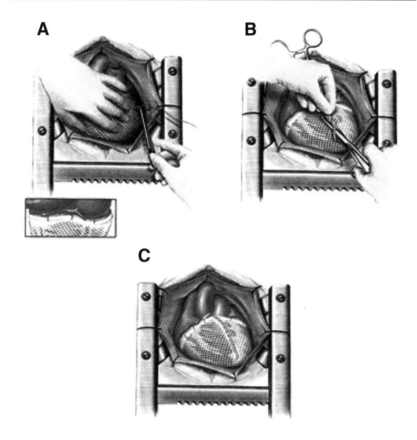

Fig. 6. Placement of Acorn textile support. From ref. *48.*

correct specific abnormalities responsible for ventricular function deterioration, others more ambitiously attempt to reverse this deterioration by physically reconstructing the ventricle or providing direct mechanical assistance.

REFERENCES

1. Bolling SF, Smolens IA, Pagani FD. Surgical alternatives for heart failure. J Heart Lung Transplant 2001;20:729–733.
2. Chen FY, Cohn LH. The surgical treatment of heart failure. A new frontier: nontransplant surgical alternatives in heart failure. Cardiol Rev 2002;10(6): 326–333.
3. Novitzky D. Alternatives to organ transplantation. Trans Proceed 1997;29: 3766–3769.
4. Starling RC, Young JB. Surgical therapy for dilated cardiomyopathy. Cardiol Clin 1998;16:727–737.

5. Tavazzi L. Epidemiology of dilated cardiomyopathy: a still undetermined entity. Eur Heart J 1997;18:4–6.
6. Kherani AR, Garrido MJ, Cheema FH, et al. Nontransplant surgical options for congestive heart failure. Congest Heart Fail 2003;9(1):17–24.
7. Teerlink J, Goldhaber S, Pfeffer M. An overview of contemporary etiologies of congestive heart failure. Am Heart J 1991;121:1852–1853.
8. Elefteriades JA, KronIL. CABG in advance left ventricular dysfunction. Cardiol Clin 1995;1:35–42.
9. Lansman SL, Cohen M, Galla JD, et al. Coronary bypass with ejection fraction of 0.20 or less using centigrade cardioplegia: long-term follow-up. Ann Thorac Surg 1993;56:480–485.
10. Luciani GB, Faggian G, Razzolini R. Severe left ventricular failure: coronary operation of heart transplantation. Ann Thorac Surg 1993;55:719–723.
11. Chan RKM, Raman J, Lee KG, et al. Prediction of outcome after revascularization in patients with poor left ventricular function. Ann Thorac Surg 1996;61;1428–1434.
12. Konstam M, Dracup K, Baker D, et al. Heart failure: evaluation and care of patients with left ventricular systolic dysfunction. Clinical practice No. 11 AHCPR Publication No. 94-0612. Rockville, MD. Agency for Health Care Policy and Research, Public Health Service, U.S. Department of Health and Human Services. June 1994, 67–77.
13. Kern JA, Kron IL. High-risk myocardial revascularization. In: Rose EA, Stevenson LW, eds. Management of end-stage heart disease. Lippincott-Raven, Philadelphia, PA: 1998, pp. 149–153.
14. Milano CA, White WD, Smith LR, et al. Coronary artery bypass in patients with severely depressed ventricular function. Ann Thorac Surg 1993;56:487–493.
15. Enriquez-Sarano M, Tajik A, Schaff H, et al. Echocardiographic prediction of survival after surgical correction of organic mitral regurgitation. Circulation 1994;90:830–837.
16. Chen FY, Adams DH, Aranki SF, et al. Mitral valve repair in cardiomyopathy. Circulation 1998;98:124–127.
17. Spence PA, Peniston CM, David TE, et al. Toward a better understanding of the etiology of left ventricular dysfunction after mitral valve replacement: an experimental study with possible clinical implications. Ann Thorac Surg 1986;17:363–371.
18. Sarris GE, Miller DC. Role of the mitral subvalvular apparatus in left ventricular systolic mechanics. Semin Thorac Cardiovasc Surg 1989;1:133–142.
19. Phillips HR, Levine FH, Carter JE, et al. Mitral valve replacement for isolated mitral regurgitation: analysis of clinical course and late postoperative left ventricular ejection fraction. Am J Cardiol 1981;48:647–654.
20. March RJ, Waters KA, Talbot T, et al. Influence of native mitral apparatus on three-dimensional left ventricular geometry following mitral valve replacement. Surg Forum 1986;17:306–308.
21. McBride LR, Carpentier A. Surgical anatomy of cardiac valves and techniques of valve reconstruction. In: Baue AE, et al., eds. Glenn's Thoracic and Cardiovascular Surgery, vol. II, 6th ed. Appleton & Lange, Norwalk, CT: pp. 1967–1971.
22. Galloway AC, Colvin SB, Baumann FG, et al. A comparison of mitral valve reconstruction with mitral valve replacement: intermediate-term results. Ann Thorac Surg 1989;47:655–662.
23. Sand ME, Naftel DC, Blackstone EH, et al. A comparison of repair and replacement for mitral valve incompetence. J Thorac Cardiovasc Surg 1987;94:208–219.
24. Perier P, Deloche A, Chauvaud S, et al. Comparative evaluation of mitral valve repair and replacement with Starr, Bjork, and porcine valve prostheses. Circulation 1984;70(suppl I):I.187–I.192.

25. Rankin JS, Livesey SA, Smith R, et al. Trends in the surgical treatment of ischemic mitral regurgitation: effects of mitral valve repair on hospital mortality. Semin Thorac Cardiovasc Surg 1989;1:149–163.
26. Bolling SF, Pagani FD, Deeb GM, et al. Intermediate-term outcome of mitral reconstruction in cardiomyopathy. J Thorac Cardiovasc Surg 1998;115:381–388.
27. Cox JL. Left ventricular aneurysm: pathophysiologic observations and standard resection. Semin Thorac Cardiovasc Surg 1997;9:113–122.
28. Grondin P, Kretz JG, Bical O, et al. Natural history of succular aneurysms of the left ventricle. J Thorac Cardiovasc Surg 1979;77:57–62.
29. Moulton MJ, Downing SW, Creswell LI, et al. Mechanical dysfunction in the border zone of an ovine model of left ventricular aneurysm. Ann Thor Surg 1995;60:986–988.
30. Cox JL. Surgical management of left ventricular aneurysms: a clarification of the similarities and differences between the Jatene and Dor techniques. Semin Thorac Cardiovasc Surg 1997;9:131–138.
31. Jatene AD. Surgical treatment of left ventricular aneurysm. In: Baue AE, et al., eds. Glenn's Thoracic and Cardiovascular Surgery, vol. II, 5th ed. Appleton & Lange Publishers, Norwalk, CT: p. 1829.
32. Cooley DA, Collins HA, Morris GC, et al. Ventricular aneurysm after myocardial infarction. Surgical excision with use of temporary cardiopulmonary bypass. JAMA 1958;167:557.
33. Dor V, Saab M, Coste P, et al. Left ventricular aneurysm. A new surgical approach. Thorac Cardiovasc Surg 1989;37:11–19.
34. Dor V, Sabatier M, Di Donato M, et al. Late hemodynamic results after left ventricular patch repair associated with coronary grafting in patients with postinfarction akinetic or dyskinetic aneurysm of the left ventricle. J Thorac Cardiovasc Surg 1995;110:1291–1301.
35. Mickleborough LL. Ventricular aneurysmectomy and surgical ablative approaches for malignant arrhythmias. In: Rose EA, Stevenson LW, eds. Management of End-stage Heart Disease. Lippincott-Raven Publishers, Philadelphia, PA: 1998, pp. 155–164.
36. Zardini P, Marino P, Golia G, et al. Ventricular remodeling and infarct expansion. Am J Cardiol 1993;72:98G–106G.
37. Baur LH, Schipperheyn JJ, van der Wall EE, et al. Regional myocardial shape alteration in patients with anterior myocardial infarction. Int J Card Imag 1996;12:89–96.
38. Harrison JK, Califf RM, Woodlief LH, et al. Systolic left ventricular function after reperfusion therapy for acute myocardial infarction. Analysis of determinants of improvement. The TAMI Study Group. Circulation 1993;87:1531–1541.
39. Athanasuleas CL, Stanley AWH Jr., Buckberg GD, et al. Surgical anterior ventricular endocardial restoration in the dilated remodeled ventricle after anterior myocardial infarction. J Am Coll Cardiol 2001;37:1199–1209
40. Furnary AP, Jessup M, Moreira LFP. Multicenter trial of dynamic cardiomyoplasty for chronic heart failure. The American Cardiomyoplasty Group. J Am Coll Cardiol 1995;28:1175–1180.
41. Hagege AA, Desnos M, Fernandez F, et al. Clinical study of the effects of latissimus dorsi muscle flap stimulation after cardiomyoplasty. Circulation 1995; 92(suppl):II.210–II.215.
42. Patel HJ, Lankford EB, Polidori DJ, et al. Dynamic cardiomyoplasty: its chronic and acute effects on the failing heart. J Thorac Cardiovasc Surg 1997;114:169–178.
43. Schreuder JJ, van der Veen FH, van der Velde ET, et al. Left ventricular pressure–volume relationships before and after cardiomyoplasty in patients with heart failure. Circulation 1997;96:2978–2986.

44. Lee KL, Dignan RJ, Dyke CM, et al. Effects of dynamic cardiomyoplasty on left ventricular performance and myocardial mechanics in dilated cardiomyopathy. J Thorac Cardiovasc Surg 1991;102:124–131.
45. Bellotti G, Moraes A, Bocchi E, et al. Late effects of cardiomyoplasty on left ventricular mechanics and diastolic filling. Circulation 1993;88:304–308.
46. Brutsaert DL, Sys SU. Relaxation and diastole of the heart. Physiol Rev 1989; 69:1228–1315.
47. Capouya ER, Gerber RS, Drinkwater DC Jr., et al. Girdling effect of nonstimulated cardiomyoplasty on left ventricular function. Ann Thorac Surg 1993;56:867–871.
48. Mott BD, Oh JH, Misawa Y, et al. Mechanisms of cardiomyoplasty: comparative effects of adynamic versus dynamic cardiomyoplasty. Ann Thorac Surg 1998; 65:1039–1045.
49. Konertz WF, Shapland JE, Hotz H, et al. Passive containment and reverse remodeling by a novel textile cardiac support device. Circulation 2001;104(suppl I): I.270–I.275.
50. Sabbah H, Chaudhry P, Kleber F, et al. Passive mechanical containment of progressive left ventricular dilation: a surgical approach to the treatment of heart failure. J Heart Failure 2000;6(1):115.
51. Konertz W, Kebler FX, Dushe S, et al. Efficacy trends with the acorn cardiac support device in patients with heart failure: a one year follow-up. J Heart Lung Transplantation 2001;20(2):217.
52. Sintek CF, Pfeffer TA, Kochamba GS, et al. Mitral valve replacement: technique to preserve the subvalular apparatus. Ann Thorac Surg 1995;59:1027–1029.
53. Dor V. The endoventricular circular patch plasty (Dor procedure) in ischemic akinetic dilated ventricles.Heart Fail Rev 2001;6(3):187–193.
54. Chachques JC, Marino JP, Lajos P, et al. Dynamic cardiomyoplasty: clinical follow-up at 12 years. Eur J Cardiothorac Surg 1997;12(4):560–568.

12 Mechanical Circulatory Assistance As a Bridge to Transplantation

Takushi Kohmoto, MD, PhD and Yoshifumi Naka, MD, PhD

CONTENTS

INTRODUCTION
SYSTEMS
PREOPERATIVE CONCERNS
SURGICAL IMPLANTATION TECHNIQUES
POSTOPERATIVE MANAGEMENT
COMPLICATIONS
NEAR FUTURE
CONCLUSION
REFERENCES

INTRODUCTION

Mechanical circulatory assistance has become the standard of care for potential heart transplant patients with life-threatening heart failure refractory to medical and other surgical therapies *(1–5)*. Significant advances in technology and clinical experience have occurred during the past 10 yr. Indications for ventricular assist device (VAD) placement have broadened to include patients who were thought to be unsuitable for device insertion. Improving long-term success with device support has even led to the possibility of permanent support *(6)*. Currently, there is a wide array of devices available and in development.

From: *Contemporary Cardiology: Cardiac Transplantation:*
The Columbia University Medical Center/New York-Presbyterian Hospital Manual
Edited by: N. M. Edwards, J. M. Chen, and P. A. Mazzeo © Humana Press Inc., Totowa, NJ

This chapter describes the use of mechanical assist devices as a bridge to transplantation. Currently available devices, patient and device selection, surgical technique, postoperative management, and complications are discussed. Finally, the new devices that are under development or evaluation are mentioned.

SYSTEMS

Short-Term Support: Abiomed BVS (5000i)

The Abiomed BVS 5000i (Abiomed Cardiovascular Inc., Danvers, MA) is a short-term uni- or biventricular support system comprised of external pumps driven by a computer-controlled drive console. In 1992, the Food and Drug Administration (FDA) approved the product for postcardiotomy support *(7)*. Since then, the indications for use have expanded to include acute myocardial infarction (AMI), myocarditis, right ventricle (RV) support in conjunction with a long-term left ventricle (LV) support device, bridge to recovery and bridge to transplant. As a result, the device is one of the most commonly used means of short-term mechanical cardiac support *(8,9)*.

Advantages that make the BVS system popular are the ease of insertion and simplicity in operation, obviating the need for a full-time perfusionist. The system functions reliably for several days, with average support duration between 5 and 9 d. This is particularly helpful in hospitals where it may be necessary to transfer the patient to a transplant center for further treatment *(10,11)*. The system has proven its efficacy in the treatment of acute myocarditis and postcardiotomy cardiogenic shock (PCCS) *(8,12–14)*. In addition, the cost may be closer to that of centrifugal pumps than was expected *(15)*. For these reasons, the BVS system is the standard for short-term bridging.

Disadvantages of this device include the requirement for continuous anticoagulation, limited mobility compared to implantable devices, and the requirement to remain in an intensive care unit (ICU). Flow rates are also limited compared to those of other devices. The maximum flow rate of 6 L/min may not be enough for septic or larger patients. Although patients have been supported as long as 90 d, the device is best suited for short-term use (less than 10 d).

Short-Term Systems: Extracorporeal Membrane Oxygenation

Extracorporeal membrane oxygenation (ECMO) provides mechanical cardiac support (uni- or biventricular) as well as pulmonary support. Although neonatal use has been successful, the adult experience has been mixed.

The main indications for ECMO are the need for mechanical assistance in the face of combined pulmonary failure and pure respiratory failure. When initially used for PCCS, survival was low (25%) *(16)*. With experience and improved circuits, survival increased to 40% *(17)*. ECMO benefits include potential peripheral cannulation and the versatility of small consoles. This allows potential implementation in areas outside the operating room for both cardiac and pulmonary support.

Major limitations include the requirement for sedation, with possible paralysis and heparinization. Also, a full-time perfusionist is necessary to run the equipment. Although it may last for several days, the duration of support is usually only 2–3 d. Complications are common, including leg ischemia, renal failure, bleeding, and oxygenator failure, especially with veno-arterial ECMO support. Overall, successful ECMO use in adults has been limited to select centers *(18)*.

Implantable Pulsatile Devices: HeartMate Left Ventricular Assist Device

The HeartMate left ventricular assist device (LVAD) (Thoratec Corporation, Pleasanton, CA) was designed in 1975 *(19)*. The system was originally an implantable pneumatic (IP) vented system requiring a large, cumbersome console that did not allow patients much mobility outside the hospital. Since 1986, this system has been effective as a long-term support device with an end goal of heart transplantation. The system underwent years of development, and, in 1991, a clinical trial of the vented electric (VE) model began *(20)*. The electric system allowed a great amount of mobility, with portable battery units worn in a holster. Since then, both models have shown a 60–70% rate of survival to transplantation *(21–23)*. The worldwide average implant duration is 80–100 d, and maximum duration of support has exceeded 2 yr *(23)*. The probability of device failure is 35% at 2 yr *(6)*, which is much higher than that of the Novacor left ventricular assist system (LVAS).

The HeartMate is made out of a titanium alloy external housing, with inflow and outflow tracts that use porcine xenograft valves (25mm). The unique characteristic of the device is its internal blood-contacting surface, which is made of textured titanium on one side and textured polyurethane on the other. This textured surface results in the deposition of a fibrin-cellular matrix that forms a pseudoneointima. The formation of this surface decreases the need for anticoagulation, because thrombus formation is greatly reduced *(23)*. Patients with these devices take aspirin (for anti-inflammation, but not primarily for anticoagulation) and have a remarkably low rate of thromboembolic complications *(2,23)*.

The device has a pumping capacity in excess of 10 L/min and a stroke volume of 83 mL. Pulsatile flow is created using a pusher-plate system *(23)*. The device is operated in a fixed-rate or automatic mode. In automatic mode, the pump senses when the chamber is full and activates the pusher plate.

The pump is inserted into the left upper quadrant of the abdomen either pre- or intraperitoneally. The driveline, consisting of an air vent and power cables, is tunneled and brought out of the skin in the right upper quadrant. Small battery units, worn in a harness, are connected to the cables. Battery life is between 4 and 6 h, depending on the patient's activity level *(23)*. In case of an emergency, a portable hand pump can activate the device.

The patient's body size is an important factor in allowing device placement, because of the device's size and flow limitation. Because the device requires flow greater than 3.0 L/min to avoid thromboembolic complications caused by blood stagnation, patients should have a body surface area (BSA) greater than 1.5 m^2 (cardiac index greater than 2.0 L/min/m^2).

Although the HeartMate LVAD and the Novacor LVAS are the first generation of relatively reliable mechanical cardiac assist devices, they have achieved significant clinical success. As a result, the Randomized Evaluation of Mechanical Assistance for the Treatment of Congestive Heart Failure (REMATCH) study used the HeartMate LVAD as a destination therapy, rather than as a bridge to transplantation *(6)*. Based on these data supporting mechanical therapy over medical therapy, the FDA approved the HeartMate LVAD for use as a destination therapy.

Implantable Pulsatile Pumps: Novacor

The Novacor (World Heart Corp., Ottawa, ON, Canada) LVAS was first used in 1984 in a successful bridge-to-transplant application *(1)*. Initially, it was designed as a console-based controller system, but, since 1993, it has been available with a wearable controller. This system is reliable, with about 55–65% of patients surviving to transplantation *(1,24,25)*. The worldwide mean time of LVAS support using this system is 85 d, with the device lasting as long as 962 d *(24)*. The company currently claims a 3-yr pump reliability greater than 90% *(26)*, which is much higher than that of the HeartMate LVAD.

The pump works using dual pusher plates that compress a polyurethane sac. Twenty-one mm bioprosthetic valves are used in both the in- and outflow tracts. Stroke volume reaches 70 mL. Similarly to the HeartMate device, the pump is placed in the left upper abdominal quadrant. The inflow tract is connected to the LV apex and the outflow tract to the ascending aorta. The percutaneous driveline is brought out in the right upper quadrant of the abdomen and connected to a controller worn on a belt system. Unlike the HeartMate system, patients require anticoagulation with warfarin to avoid embolic events. Currently, the Investigation of Nontransplant-Eligible Patients who are Inotrope Dependent trial is evaluating this device as a long-term alternative to transplantation. Recently, a new inflow cannula made with Gore-Tex® was introduced, and the thromboembolic rate is reported to be reduced (1,5).

Paracorporeal Pulsatile Devices: Thoratec

The Thoratec paracorporeal VAD (Thoratec Laboratories Corp., Pleasanton, CA) is another reliable and often-used system for ventricular support. Unlike the Novacor and HeartMate systems, this is a paracorporeal system that can be applied for uni- or biventricular support. Because the actual pump chamber is outside of the body, this device can be used on patients with body sizes too small to house the HeartMate or Novacor devices. However, a paracorporeal system also limits mobility and presents an obstacle for patients in a long-term setting. In 1984, the first Thoratec system was used as a successful bridge to transplantation. The system received FDA approval for bridging to transplantation in 1995 and for postcardiotomy support in 1998 (27).

The pump consists of a prosthetic ventricle with a maximum stroke volume of 65 mL and cannulae for ventricular or atrial inflow and arterial outflow. Currently, a large pneumatic drive console is available, and a smaller briefcase-sized power driver unit is in trial (27). Pneumatic drivers provide alternating air pressure to fill and empty the blood pump. The pump flow rate ranges from 1.3 to 7.2 L/min (27). Inflow cannula placement can occur in an atrial or ventricular position. Ventricular cannula placement is better for left-sided support, as it allows for greater flow rates than does atrial cannulation. Anticoagulation with warfarin is necessary, as it is in patients with mechanical valves (27).

This device has been used in over 1000 patients for uni- and biventricular support for both bridge-to-transplantation and post-cardiotomy recovery. Survival to transplantation is in the 60–80% range, depending on which ventricle was supported (27,28). The great benefit of this system is its versatility. It is easy to place with less surgical dissection, can be used for patients of various sizes, can be attached to the atrium or ventricle, and can be used for right and left heart support. However, its paracorporeal location limits the patient's activity and its use as a long-term device.

Total Artificial Heart: CardioWest

The CardioWest total artificial heart (TAH) (CardioWest Technologies, Inc., Tucson, AZ) is a pneumatic, biventricular, orthotopically implanted TAH with an externalized driveline to its console. It consists of two spherical polyurethane chambers with polyurethane diaphragms. In- and outflow conduits are constructed of Dacron™ and contain Medtronic-Hall™ (Medtronic, Inc., Minneapolis, MN) valves. It began as the Jarvik-7 TAH used in the early 1980s (29,30). Despite early obstacles, in 1993, a new investigational device exemption study began. The trial showed support durations of 12–186 d with a 93% survival to transplant (31). European experience with the CardioWest TAH has been slightly worse, although encouraging (32,33).

The TAH benefits from the ability to provide excellent, early support avoiding irreversible end-organ damage in rapidly decompensating, critically ill patients (31). Unlike the other devices, it obviates the presence of the native heart. This is particularly useful in situations where leaving the native heart in place would be detrimental or impossible (e.g., infection or cardiac tumors).

To accommodate the TAH, adequate intrathoracic space is required. Fitting criteria includes BSA greater than 1.7 m², cardiothoracic ratio greater than 0.5, LV diastolic dimension greater than 66 mm, anteroposterior distance greater than 10 cm, and combined ventricular volume greater than 1500 mL. Careful intraoperative fitting is critical. In addition to size requirements, strict anticoagulation with warfarin, aspirin, and pentoxifylline is needed (34). Rehabilitation is limited as well because of the large console. A portable console is in development.

PREOPERATIVE CONCERNS

Indications for LVAD Implantation

The traditional indication for VAD support has been refractory cardiac failure in patients eligible for heart transplantation. Recently, the patient population has expanded from patients with chronic heart failure to include a large proportion of patients with acute heart failure. Although some reports show better outcomes in stable patients awaiting heart transplant (34,35), acceptable results have been obtained in this emerging acute patient population (10,12,13,36–38).

Currently, there are several clinical scenarios in which VADs are implanted. These include PCCS, AMI, acute decompensation of chronic heart failure, myocarditis, chronic heart failure in transplantation candidates, ventricular arrhythmia, and high-risk cardiac operations.

PCCS patients have shown significant survival benefits if identified early and appropriately treated *(10)*. Because most centers have the capability for short-term VAD support but not for long-term VAD support or transplant, the authors created a so-called "Bridge-to-Transplant Network" *(10)*. This system rapidly identifies and transfers appropriate patients in the authors' region. Initial evaluation optimizes patients with short-term VAD support and transfers patients within 72 h of decompensation. Long-term LVAD implantation, if necessary, is then performed within 5 d after evaluation.

AMI patients suffer from cardiogenic shock at an approximate rate of 6% and, with cardiogenic shock, have a mortality rate of almost 80% *(39,40)*. Even with early revascularization, 1-yr survival remains less than 50% in those patients *(41)*. Many of these patients suffer unrecoverable myocardial damage or lack suitable coronary anatomy for revascularization. Advanced mechanical support may be the only therapy available for these patients. Mechanical support can successfully bridge these patients to recovery or transplant *(42,43)*.

Patients with long-standing heart failure may decompensate acutely or over longer time periods. These patients may not have been listed for transplant at the time of failure, although often they are followed at transplant centers. Acute decompensation can be triggered by several etiologies, including new ischemic injuries, arrhythmias, and infections. Patients already listed for heart transplant are the traditional group that comprises VAD populations. These patients tend to do well with VAD placement, as rehabilitation can be optimized before transplant *(22)*.

LVAD implantation for acute myocarditis, particularly in young patients, is used most often as a bridge to recovery rather than to transplantation. Unfortunately, it is difficult to determine which patients will benefit from short-term support and which patients will require long-term devices with subsequent transplantation *(44)*. Because recovery is more likely in this population, short-term VADs are placed more often with subsequent transition to long-term VADs if necessary *(12)*.

Patients with ventricular arrhythmias are unique in that, aside from the arrhythmia, their native cardiac function may not be compromised significantly. If pharmacologic therapy and defibrillators fail, VAD support may be warranted. VAD support has been implemented successfully in these cases *(45–47)*.

Patients undergoing high-risk cardiac surgery may need mechanical ventricular support if the surgical procedure is not successful. Patients need to be screened for transplant candidacy preoperatively. Cardiac surgery is then scheduled with LVAD back-up, in the event that LVAD support and subsequent heart transplant are needed.

Patient Selection

The selection process for VAD implantation must reach a balance between an extremely liberal listing of highest-risk patients with unacceptably high mortality rates, and an exceedingly conservative approach that passes over patients who would otherwise have benefited from VAD support. Judicious use is also important, as VAD implantation incurs significant social and financial investment.

According to the FDA, approval for transplant is required for VAD implantation (except for specific exemptions as part of destination therapy trials), although this requirement may be difficult to meet in the setting of acute cardiac failure. Generally, the accepted hemodynamic criteria include systolic blood pressure less than 80 mmHg (or mean arterial blood pressure less than 65 mmHg), pulmonary capillary wedge pressure greater than 20 mmHg, systemic vascular resistance more than 2100 dynes*s/cm^5, urine output less than 20 cc/h (in adults) despite diuretics, and a cardiac index of less than 2 L/min/m^2 despite maximal inotropic or intra-aortic balloon pump support *(48)*. In addition, several other factors must be taken into account.

In 1995, Columbia University, in conjunction with the Cleveland Clinic Foundation, devised a scoring system to predict which patients would have successful outcomes after LVAD implantation *(49)*. However, as the technology evolved, use of these devices widened and extended, and, in 2001, the old score was revised to better reflect the current LVAD-eligible population *(50)*. The old score was based on a system proposed by Norman et al. and included a cardiac index of less than 2 L/min/m^2 and a pulmonary capillary wedge pressure greater than 20 mmHg *(51)*. It utilized 10 factors significant for mortality, using univariate analysis with a score of less than 5 corresponding to a 33% postimplantation death risk *(49)*. The revised score was based on 130 patients receiving VE HeartMate devices from 1996 to 2001.

Interestingly, unlike in the old system, preoperative renal insufficiency did not impact survival in the new scoring system. This is likely because of aggressive renal insufficiency treatment with ultrafiltration and hemodialysis. After multivariate analysis, the five factors in the new scoring system were: ventilatory support (score of 4), redo surgery (score of 2), previous LVAD insertion (score of 2), central venous pressure (CVP) greater than 16 mmHg (score of 1) and prothrombic time greater than 16 s (score of 1). After adding the scores of these risk factors, a sum greater than 5 corresponds to a 47% mortality, as opposed to a 9% mortality for a score less than 5 *(50)*.

Device placement urgency has plays a part in survival. In a study by Deng et al., patients receiving emergent LVADs because of acute heart failure, such as AMI, acute myocarditis, and postcardiotomy low output syndrome, had a lower survival to transplantation when compared with those receiving devices for chronic failure or those who did not need devices while on the heart transplant list *(35)*.

Device Selection

Invariably, device selection is influenced both by availability and physicians' experiences. Although much is published on individual devices, few studies compare assist devices at a single institution *(4,15)*. Currently, there are five FDA-approved assist devices, in addition to the intra-aortic balloon pump, for these indications. These devices include:

- Abiomed BVS 5000
- Thoratec paracorporeal device
- Novacor LVAS
- Thoratec HeartMate IP LVAD
- Thoratec HeartMate VE LVAD

In addition to the FDA-approved devices, there are several other VADs in development and in clinical use. Characteristics of each device were discussed previously in this chapter.

Important clinical issues to consider when choosing a device include the expected duration of support, need for biventricular support, cost, device-related risks (such as the need for anticoagulation and device failure rates), patient characteristics (especially the patient's size), and United Network for Organ Sharing (UNOS) classification rules. Institutional standards of care, ranging from community practice to tertiary heart failure/transplant centers, also influence device selection.

First, the implantable HeartMate VE LVAD and the Novacor LVAS require a patient BSA greater than 1.5 m^2. Patients smaller than 1.5 m^2 require support with the Abiomed BVS, a centrifugal pump, or the Thoratec paracorporeal device, depending on the estimated support period *(52–54)*.

Patients requireing mechanical circulatory support can be divided into the three main categories listed below. These clinical scenarios and patient needs dictate the best type of device to use.

- Profound shock: those in acute, profound shock (e.g., PCCS), potentially with end-organ failure and right heart failure (RHF)
- Decompensating congestive heart failure (CHF): chronically ill patients who are transplant candidates
- Nontransplant candidates: these patients may become transplant-eligible when supported with assist devices and if other organ function recovers

Patients in profound shock with end-organ dysfunction and RHF need early, efficacious support to avoid permanent end-organ damage and increase their survival chances. The preferred devices are the Abiomed BVS 5000, the Thoratec paracorporeal device, and the TAH, if available. These devices provide full biventricular support, re-establishing nearly normal hemodynamics and, potentially, allowing myocardial recovery *(7)*. Early implementation of biventricular support is critical in patients with severe biventricular failure *(12–14)*.

The potential for myocardial recovery and neurological status need to be determined while a patient is on ventricular support. If a prolonged support period is expected, a longer-term device can be implanted as a LVAD with concomitant use of a short-term device as a right ventricular assist device (RVAD). Despite severe cardiac failure, these patients can be salvaged successfully with survival rates approaching those of the general cardiac transplantation population *(55,56)*. Patients at non-transplant centers, who may benefit from a longer-term device and transplant evaluation, can be transferred safely to transplant centers when stabilized on short-term devices *(11)*. The preferred device for use in this setting is the Abiomed BVS 5000.

Patients with chronic CHF who are transplant candidates may decompensate before receiving a transplant. In these patients, long-term support must be considered. Hospital discharge and rehabilitation become important factors in choosing a device *(21,57)*. Longer-term support with end-organ recovery and better rehabilitation is associated with better long-term survival *(58)*. Therefore, the current recommended devices are the implantable HeartMate VE LVAD and Novacor LVAS. If RHF is present and the patient is a transplant candidate, treatment is mandatory and can be accomplished medically or with a short-term VAD such as the Abiomed BVS.

SURGICAL IMPLANTATION TECHNIQUES

HeartMate LVAD Implantation

The techniques for assist device implantation vary. HeartMate LVAD placement is briefly described here. These systems, similarly to the Novacor LVAS, have several hemodynamic benefits. The short inflow cannula, which is connected to the LV apex, allows lower left atrial pressure (LAP) for filling the pump. Also, the LV apical cannulation, unlike cannulation of the left atrium, prevents blood stasis and thrombus formation in a hypokinetic LV.

The patient is placed on supine and prepped. Median skin incision is extended to the abdomen, usually up to the umbilicus. A preperitoneal (or intraperitoneal) LVAD pocket is created in the abdominal left upper quadrant. A driveline is tunneled to the right upper quadrant of the abdomen prior to heparinization. The device is primed and brought into the field. Pericardium is opened and the heart is cannulated for bypass. The aortic cannulation site needs to be chosen carefully to leave room for outflow graft anastomosis. If a patent foramen ovale (PFO) is identified by transesophageal echocardiogram (TEE), bicaval venous cannulation is chosen. If not, single right atrial cannulation is used.

On cardiopulmonary bypass (CPB), the outflow graft length is measured, the aortic crossclamp is applied, and an ellipticolongitudinal aortotomy is created. The graft is sewn into place using 4–0 Prolene suture. To ensure hemostasis, BioGlue (CryoLife Inc., Kennesaw, GA) is applied over the anastomosis. Hemostasis is confirmed immediately after clamp release. A circular core bored out of the apex of the LV allows for inflow cannula placement. Pledgetted sutures (2–0 Tevdek) are placed circumferentially around the cored opening and passed through the inflow cuff. When all the sutures are placed, the cuff is brought down to the ventricle, and the sutures are tied. The inflow cannula is secured to the LVAD body. The pump is primed manually and vented through the outflow tract as the patient is weaned from bypass. Drains are placed in the mediastinum, the pericardium, and the LVAD pocket. After hemostasis is achieved, the chest and upper abdomen are closed in the standard fashion. The authors use #2 Vicryl interrupted figure-of-eight sutures to close abdominal fascia; if the patient is small, and the abdominal fascia cannot be reapproximated safely without tension, they insert a Gore-Tex® patch to prevent herniation.

Technical Considerations

We outline several important technical points to consider when implanting devices. First, pericardium dissection and choice of aortic cannulation site must be performed carefully to help outflow cannula placement and to help subsequent reoperation for heart transplantation. Perfect hemostasis must be confirmed carefully prior to chest closure, because surgical bleeding can cause hemodynamic instability and, moreover, necessitates multiple blood transfusions. These may subsequently lead patients to volume overload and RHF, as described later in this chapter. Finally, appropriate wound closure technique is also important, because these patients are prone to infection and wound dehiscence (59).

INTRAOPERATIVE TEE USE TO ASSESS VALVULAR PATHOLOGY AND PFO

Intraoperative TEE is necessary when implantation is planned, especially to evaluate presence of aortic insufficiency (AI) and PFO, because
both can cause significant problems immediately or chronically.

If AI is present, blood ejected from the LVAD into the ascending aorta
can enter the LV cavity, resulting in circuitous blood flow through the
LVAD and limiting forward (or actual) cardiac output despite high
LVAD flows *(60)*. If the patient has more than moderate AI, the aortic
leaflets can be sutured closed, or, if the leaflets are defective, the leaflets
can be excised and the orifice closed with a Dacron or bovine pericardial
patch. This can be done through the aortotomy for the outflow graft
anastomosis. These methods apply only if recovery of cardiac function
is not anticipated. Prior to LVAD insertion, the aortic valve normally
closes only in diastole and is exposed only to diastolic pressure. However,
the aortic valve leaflets frequently remain closed in systole after LVAD
implantation, and they are exposed to the high systolic pressure generated
by LVAD ejection. Therefore, AI can become evident in a chronic phase
and, if it is significant, reoperation may be required to close the aortic
valve *(60)*. Also, if the aortic valve remains closed, commissural fusion
of the native aortic valve leaflets has been reported after 26–689 d of
LVAD support *(61)*.

If a temporary device, such as Abiomed BVS, is used and the inflow
cannula is inserted from the LV apex, care must be taken not to advance
the inflow cannula too deeply; if it is inserted deeply enough that the tip
passes across the aortic valve, it can also cause circuitous blood flow
through the LVAD and can decrease the forward flow.

If a PFO is present, it must be closed. If left open, significant right-to-
left shunting can continue after LVAD implantation; the LAP decreases
through the emptying of the LV and decreasing of the left ventricular
end-diastolic pressure (LVEDP), and the right atrial pressure (RAP)
increases with continuing RHF and fluid load. This right-to-left shunting
can result in significant deoxygenation despite increased LVAD flow.
Although a PFO is not identified intra-operatively, it can become evident
later if the RAP remains high for a longer period.

Other valvular pathologies that should be assessed before or during
LVAD implantation include:

- Mitral stenosis, which can prevent filling of the LVAD and subsequently cause pulmonary edema. If present, mitral commissurotomy
  should be performed through the apical ventriculotomy for the inflow
  cannula.
- Mitral regurgitation (MR), which usually does not affect LVAD flow *(62)*.

- Tricuspid insufficiency. The authors used to perform repairs (annuloplasty); however, the repair did little to improve RV performance, and their recent strategy is to perform tricuspid repair only if severe tricuspid regurgitation and ascites is present *(60)*. Use of inhaled nitric oxide (NO) also helps RV performance.

PROSTHETIC VALVES

Assist device use in patients with prosthetic valves was once considered absolutely contraindicated *(63)*. However, recently, such patients have been considered candidates for assist devices; if the duration of support is expected to be short and myocardial recovery is expected, short-term assist devices are used with appropriate anticoagulation *(64,65)*. In patients requiring long-term LVAD support as a bridge to transplantation, the authors' preferred strategy is as follows *(60)*:

- If a patient has an aortic mechanical valve, it is oversewn with a Dacron patch from the aortic side to prevent thrombus at the mechanical valve with resultant embolism if the mechanical valve occasionally opens with LV ejection, or in the event of device failure *(60,66)*. If the patient has a tissue valve and the LVAD empties the LV cavity sufficiently, most often the valve does not open. However, if the valve is damaged or insufficient, its orifice must be sewn closed, either primarily or with a pericardial patch.
- If a patient has a mechanical mitral valve, appropriate anticoagulation is mandatory to prevent valve thrombosis. The authors also recommend anticoagulation for tissue mitral valves after experiencing a case with thrombus formation under the cusps of a tissue mitral valve *(62)*.

CORONARY ARTERY LESIONS

Pre-existing coronary artery disease (CAD) is common in LVAD candidates. Adequate CAD evaluation is important to maximize the benefits of VAD implantation. Coronary artery bypass to the right coronary system may be necessary when implanting a LVAD to support RV function. This is especially important for early postoperative RV protection, including arrhythmia prevention. Refractory, malignant arrhythmias can be an indication for VAD implantation *(46,47)*. However, the authors usually do not perform left-sided bypass for angina, as post-LVAD angina is uncommon. If a coronary bypass is performed, proximal anastomosis placement should take into account the LVAD outflow anastomosis site. Therefore, we recommend proximal bypass anastomosis from the lesser aortic curvature, providing ample room on the anterolateral aspect of the aorta to accommodate the LVAD outflow graft.

AIR EMBOLISM PREVENTION

Air can be entrained from the LV inflow cannula, and this can cause fatal air embolism *(2)*. This catastrophic event can occur at the time of device implantation or explantation *(2,67)*. During implant, care must be taken to discontinue CPB or reduce CPB flow prior to starting the device to prevent suctioning of air from the LV inflow cannula. Intraoperative TEE is useful in detecting air in the ascending aorta. Also, if a temporary device such as the Abiomed BVS5000 is used, the inflow cannula is usually inserted from the LV apex with pursestring sutures, thus, the mobilization and dislocation of the cannula needs to be prevented.

Conversely, during explant, the LV inflow cannula should not be manipulated before achieving full CPB. The device must be turned off prior to starting CPB. In the Thoratec paracorporeal device, the vacuum (or suction) pressure needs to be adjusted to less than 20 mmHg if chest is open to prevent suctioning air from the inflow cannulation site. The vacuum pressure can be increased up to 40 mmHg when the chest is closed (Thoratec Manual).

POSTOPERATIVE MANAGEMENT

Early Postoperative Period

There are several factors that are important in the postoperative management of patients with mechanical support. Antibiotic prophylaxis starts preoperatively and continues for at least 3 d postimplant. RHF is treated immediately or prophylactically with milrinone and inhaled NO *(68)*. In addition, vasodilatory hypotension is treated with intravenous arginine vasopressin (Parke-Davis, Morris Plains, NJ) *(69)*. Aprotinin is continued in the postoperative period until hemorrhage stops *(70)*. Ventricular arrhythmias are managed with appropriate pharmacologic agents and cardioversion, if necessary. Anticoagulation with aspirin is used for patients with all devices. Additional anticoagulation with heparin and, subsequently, warfarin is used for patients receiving the Thoratec paracorporeal, Novacor, and axial flow devices. Physical therapy and nutrition are addressed early.

Late Postoperative Period

Late postoperative care focuses on rehabilitation and monitoring of the immunologic changes *(71)* induced by the LVAD during the wait for heart transplantation. Patients with the VE Thoratec LVAD and the Novacor LVAS are eligible for discharge to home while awaiting transplant *(1,21,72,73)*. General criteria for discharge include physical rehabilitation, echocardiographic evidence of marginal heart function (to keep the patient alive until manual pumping can be instituted in the event of device failure), and a training course in device use and care. Support from the family is important. When these criteria are met, patients undergo a gradual program with longer trips outside the hospital and, finally, discharge with weekly returns *(21,74)*. Panel-reactive antibody levels are measured in LVAD patients biweekly. This topic is discussed in detail in other chapters.

LVAD Explant vs Transplant

Except for destination-therapy patients, LVAD patients in the United States are listed as heart transplant candidates. However, the profound ventricular unloading provided by LVAD support can lead to reverse remodeling evident at genetic, biochemical, and histological levels *(75,76)*.

Long-term LVAD explantation is considered only if there is significant myocardial recovery evidenced by an exercise testing protocol. LVAD flow is reduced to 2 L/min while the patient exercises on a treadmill. Right heart catheterization and echocardiography are performed to determine the adequacy of ventricular function *(77)*. Although functional recovery allowing LVAD explantation is reported *(78)*, our experience shows that only a small number of patients can be weaned successfully from their devices *(79,80)*, whereas others report better recovery rates *(81–83)*. The question of which patients are suitable for bridge-to-recovery and device explantation requires further clinical evaluation.

COMPLICATIONS

Bleeding

Bleeding is a major complication after LVAD implantation. It can occur both in the immediate perioperative period and later postoperatively.

Immediate postoperative bleeding occurs in 20–40% of patients who receive assist devices *(1–5)*. Preoperative heart failure leading to hepatic dysfunction, preoperative anticoagulation, coagulopathy caused by blood–device surface interaction, extensive surgical dissection, and prolonged cardiopulmonary bypass time contribute to a higher bleeding rate after these procedures. In the immediate postoperative period, coagulation parameters as well as complete blood counts must be monitored closely, and products can be replaced as necessary. Because excessive blood product transfusions can cause volume overload and, subsequently, exacerbate RHF, unnecessary transfusions must be avoided. Although meticulous surgical technique is the mainstay of hemostasis, several medications can prevent postoperative bleeding.

It is well established that aprotinin reduces blood loss and blood use in patients receiving assist devices *(70)*. Desmopressin can be used as an adjunct for uremic patients or those on aspirin *(84,85)*. Re-exploration for bleeding should be performed in a timely fashion, if needed. However, if excessive bleeding is noted at the time of chest closure, the chest can be left open and packed, and the patient can be taken to the ICU. The chest is closed when coagulation is normalized.

Bleeding can also occur late postoperatively. The Novacor LVAS and Thoratec paracorporeal device require heparin, and, subsequently, warfarin is started to achieve an INR of 2.5–3.5. Aspirin is added to this regimen with both devices. Aspirin is also used for patients with Thoratec HeartMate LVAD. Adequate anticoagulation levels must be maintained carefully. LVADs can activate coagulation and fibrinolytic pathways, and there is potential to exacerbate bleeding or clotting complications *(86)*. Therefore, clinical signs of late bleeding need to be monitored carefully in those patients. In one report, there was a peak of occurrence of cerebral bleeding 3 mo after implantation *(5)*.

Anticoagulative management for patients who have heparin-induced thrombocytopenia type II and who require LVAD implantation is not common, but, nonetheless, careful assessment and continued vigilance are mandatory *(87)*.

Infection

Infection is one of the most serious complications common after LVAD implantation, affecting short- and long-term survival for patients on mechanical circulatory support. Although the definition of device-related infection varies among publications, LVAD infection, in general, can manifest as driveline, pocket, or bloodstream infections or, ultimately, as device endocarditis. In addition to device-related infections, these patients are susceptible to the common infections seen in critically ill patients such as pneumonia, line sepsis (in multiple catheters and intravenous lines), and urinary tract infections. Therefore, it is sometimes difficult to identify the infection source of when a patient on LVAD support has positive blood cultures.

The reported infection rates in these patients are from 12 to 55% *(88,89)*. Pocket infection rates are reported to be 11–24% for the HeartMate and Novacor systems, and the driveline infection rate is even higher, in the range of 18–30% for the two devices *(88,90)*. Again, there is much variability in these data because definitions for these infections are not standardized. Sepsis accounts for 21–25% of LVAD deaths and occurs at a rate of 11–26% *(1,6,88,90)*.

Various microorganisms are responsible for these infections. Gram-positive cocci are seen most commonly *(91,92)*, but Gram-negative bacilli and fungi can be identified. If organisms are identified, timely and appropriate systemic and topical infection management is necessary. Infection is not a contraindication to transplantation in this population, and transplantations have been accomplished successfully in infected patients *(91–94)*. Topical driveline infection treatments include exit site immobilization, local sterilization, drainage, and, ultimately, surgical debridement *(95)*.

Appropriate cavity drainage is needed for a LVAD pocket infection. Device endocarditis can be treated with systemic antibiotics as well as emergent heart transplantation, device explantation, or device replacement *(96)*.

The interaction between device and human that occurs after VAD implantation is a topic of much interest. LVAD implantation is accompanied by progressive defects in cellular immunity caused by an aberrant state of T-cell activation and apoptosis. These defects predispose LVAD patients to become infected *(97)*. More research is needed in this area to further understand this phenomenon.

Thromboembolic Events

Thromboembolism is a major concern in any patient with mechanical circulatory support, because of the blood–device interface. The prevalence of embolism varies from 2 to 47%, with the majority occurring in cerebral distribution in the 25% range, although embolism's definition varies among publications *(1–5,88,90,98)*. The HeartMate LVAD has the lowest thromboembolic rate of the devices, although these patients receive only aspirin. This likely results from the device's unique textured blood–interface surface that promotes formation of a neointimal surface that resists thrombus formation *(99)*. Other devices require heparin in the immediate postoperative period and, subsequently, warfarin as well as antiplatelet agents such as aspirin. The Novacor LVAS is known to have a higher thromboembolic event rate *(1,4,5)*. However, this was significantly reduced after the inflow cannula was changed to a gelatin-coated Vascutek conduit *(1,5)*. A new Gore-Tex® inflow cannula was introduced later, which further decreased the rate. Whether the rate of thromboembolic events with the Novacor LVAS decreases to as low as that of the HeartMate LVAD needs further evaluation.

Device Failure

Device failure is a major concern, because the number of heart transplantations is declining *(100)* and, according to a new UNOS rule, the status of patients awaiting heart transplant on mechanical assist devices changes from 1A to 1B 30 d after implantation *(101)*.

Device failure involves various events, although the definition and, therefore, the reported event rate also vary among publications. Major failures, such as disconnection of the outflow assembly from the pump body or pump diaphragm rupture, require emergent device replacement to prevent the patient's death *(102)*. Minor failures, such as controller or battery malfunction, usually do not require emergency surgery but require appropriate treatment such as controller replacement *(102,103)*.

The HeartMate IP and VE devices reported a failure rate of approx 10%, including major and minor failures *(2,4,5,102)*. Of note, although no system failed within 12 mo of implantation, the probability of device failure was 35% at 24 mo in the REMATCH trial, in which those devices were used as destination therapy *(6)*. However, recent system modifications have reduced this incidence significantly *(5,102)*. In the event of electronic failure, the HeartMate device can be operated by a pneumatic console, and the reported survival rate to heart transplantation with the HeartMate is comparable (72%) to that of other devices even when backup components are used *(102)*.

According to recent publications, the Novacor LVAS has better durability, with a failure rate between 0% and 2% *(1,4,5)* and with devices replaced after 3–4 yr of support. The main failure mode is bearing wear, and this can be monitored periodically in vivo. If signs of wear are detected, the patient can be upgraded to UNOS status 1A or device replacement can be scheduled on a nonemergency basis *(104)*. The Thoratec paracorporeal device is reported to have a lower incidence (3.5%) of major failures *(3,103,105)*. In any event, pump design modifications and improvements must be continued, and these will result in more reliable and durable systems.

Right Heart Failure

RHF is reported in 10–30% of patients who received an implantable HeartMate LVAD or Novacor LVAS, and an RVAD was used in 1–11% of all cases *(2,4,68,102,106)*. In those patients who had implantable LVADs with additional RVAD, the survival to transplant was low (5–32%) *(70,102,106)*. In patients with Thoratec paracorporeal devices, RVAD use was as high as 38–42% *(3,103)*. This may be related to differences in device selection criteria and device availability among institutions.

In patients with end-stage heart failure, pulmonary vascular resistance (PVR) is usually elevated because of long-standing left heart failure and is further increased in the early postoperative period by the effects of CPB and blood products *(107)*. These factors, individually or in combination, can lead to impaired RV contractility, increased RV afterload, and subsequent RV dysfunction *(68)*. In most cases, unloading and supporting the LV helps decrease PVR and improve RV performance. Interestingly, two independent analyses elucidated low preoperative RV stroke work index and low preoperative mean pulmonary arterial pressure (PAP) as risk factors for either postoperative development of RHF or postoperative RVAD use*(68,106)*. This indicates that, in these cases, the RV is weakened and unable to generate high PAP against elevated PVR preoperatively.

Because perioperative blood transfusions can cause patients to develop RHF, intraoperative use of aprotinin is strongly recommended *(70)*. If there is any sign of RHF perioperatively, such as increased CVP or decreased LVAD flow with appropriate LV decompression and without tamponade, RHF treatment must be initiated immediately with pulmonary vasodilators (inhaled NO and type III phosphodiesterase inhibitors) and inotropic agents for RV contractility *(68)*. If the RV function does not improve, RVAD insertion may be required. Although the reported survival to transplant is low if an RVAD is used, the decision to insert an RVAD should not be delayed.

Multisystem Organ Failure

Multisystem organ failure (MSOF) is another frequent complication in this patient population. Because of the significant amount of preoperative end-organ dysfunction and numerous comorbid conditions, some of these patients do not fully recover after device implantation. In many situations, MSOF is the end result of a long cascade of complications including sepsis, bleeding, and other events. At other times, MSOF may be the result of significant preoperative multiorgan dysfunction that worsens after the insult of surgery. In these scenarios, MSOF accounts for 11–29% of deaths with the device *(90)* and careful evaluation of preoperative end-organ function is important.

Sensitization

LVAD implantation is associated with an increased risk of developing circulating anti-human lymphocyte antigen class I and II antibodies (sensitization) *(108–110)*. As many as 66% of patients with a LVAD are sensitized before transplantation *(108,111)*. This increased antibody level is a significant risk for early graft failure and poorer patient survival as a result of complement-mediated humoral rejection *(112,113)*. To avoid sensitization, aprotinin should be used intraoperatively to reduce the number of necessary blood product (especially platelet) transfusions *(83,114)*. If the patient is sensitized, donor-specific cross-matching is mandatory, and this results in increased waiting time *(108)*. Recent studies demonstrate that pretransplantation immunomodulatory therapy with intravenously administered cyclophosphamide with intravenous immunoglobulin successfully reduced serum alloreactivity and reduced waiting list times and acute rejection risk *(108–112)*. Details are described in other chapters.

NEAR FUTURE

Axial Flow Pumps

Axial flow pumps represent one of the newest generations of assist devices. They provide full cardiac support in a much smaller pump with fewer moving parts and a smaller blood-contacting surface than pusher-plate devices. In addition to their small size, their design is notable for continuous flow. Several studies demonstrate metabolic and neurohumoral changes in organ perfusion with nonpulsatile flows *(115–127)*. However, both clinical and long-term animal studies failed to show significant differences in morbidity and mortality with axial flow pumps *(128–136)*. Currently, the most promising devices are the HeartMate II (Thoratec Laboratories Corp., Pleasanton, CA), the DeBakey VAD (MicroMed Technology, Inc., Houston, TX), and the Jarvik 2000 (Jarvik Heart, Inc., New York, NY). These devices weigh between 53 and 176 g and can generate flows in excess of 10 L/min.

As mentioned above, these axial flow pumps have similar features. Their small size allows implantation into smaller patients than most pulsatile pumps. This also eases placement and explantation. With fewer moving parts, there are fewer friction points; therefore, expected durability is increased. Although there is controversy over the risks and benefits of long-term continuous flow, most patients maintain some native cardiac function and, therefore, continue to have pulsatile patterns of blood flow.

Unfortunately, if there is a device failure, there are few options or backup mechanisms in place other than replacement. Additionally, because these pumps lack valves, if device malfunction does occur, the patient can develop hemodynamics equivalent to those seen with wide-open AI.

The DeBakey pump has been implanted successfully in a small number of patients in Europe *(137,138)*. In addition, the Heartmate II and the Jarvik 2000 have been implanted successfully in humans *(139)*.

Centrifugal Pumps

Years after the invention of centrifugal pumps, researchers are looking into these pumps as the "third" generation of implantable circulatory assist devices. The HeartQuest System (MedQuest Products Inc., Salt Lake City, UT) is a pump built on the Maglev (Magnetic Levitation) concept, which allows for frictionless pumping, no thrombogenicity, minimal noise and vibration, and durability because of lack of metal-to-metal contact. These pumps have been tested in animals with promising results *(140)*. The VentrAssist (Micromedical Industries, Ltd., Chatswood, New South Wales, Australia) is another promising centrifugal pump currently undergoing animal testing. The centrifugal pump is hydrodynamically suspended, resulting in no wear, no hemolysis, and no need for anticoagulation *(141)*. Another centrifugal pump in development is the HeartMate III from the Thoratec Corporation. It is about one-third the size of the HeartMate I pump and has about three times the volume of the HeartMate II *(142,143)*. These centrifugal pumps share the advantages of ease of operation and dependability, with few moving parts. However, careful experimental and clinical evaluation needs to be performed in terms of safety and durability of these new devices.

Total Artificial Heart

The new TAHs in development will allow for full implantability and hospital discharge. The AbioCor TAH (Abiomed Cardiovascular Inc. Danvers, MA) consists of an internal thoracic pump, an internal rechargeable battery, internal electronics, and an external battery pack. External power is delivered via a transcutaneous energy transmission coil located under the skin of the chest wall. The pump consists of two ventricles with corresponding artificial valves. Its stroke volume is between 60 and 65 cc with an output between 4 and 10 L/min. A centrifugal pump moves hydraulic fluid between the ventricles, providing alternate LV and RV pulsatile flow. There is an atrial balance chamber that adjusts for left and RAPs. As with previous TAHs, fitting is critical. Anticoagulation is maintained with warfarin and clopidogrel (Plavix). The first human implantation was performed in July 2001 at Jewish Hospital in Louisville, KY *(144)*. This device is currently under evaluation by the FDA.

CONCLUSION

Mechanical circulatory assistance, especially LVAD support, is currently the standard of care for potential heart transplant patients with life-threatening heart failure refractory to medical therapy. Technological advances, increased clinical experience, and broadened indications for insertion allow more patients to benefit from VAD support. For some patients, with a decreasing donor supply and with the FDA approval of the HeartMate LVAD as destination therapy, mechanical circulatory assistance may become an alternative to transplant. In turn, such a strategy may result in the listing of more appropriate transplant candidates, increased survival, and better quality of life for patients with end-stage heart disease.

ACKNOWLEDGMENT

Dr. Naka is the Herbert Irving Assistant Professor of Surgery at Columbia University.

REFERENCES

1. Deng MC, Loebe M, El-Banayosy A, et al. Mechanical circulatory support for advanced heart failure—effect of patient selection on outcome. Circulation 2001;103:231–237.
2. McCarthy PM, Smedira NO, Vargo RL, et al. One hundred patients with the HeartMate left ventricular assist device: evolving concepts and technology. J Thorac Cardiovasc Surg 1998;115:904–912.
3. McBride LR, Naunheim KS, Fiore AC, et al. Clinical experience with 111 Thoratec ventricular assist devices. Ann Thorac Surg 1999;67:1233–1238, discussion 1238–1239.
4. El-Banayosy A, Arusoglu L, Kizner L, et al. Novacor left ventricular assist system versus HeartMate vented electric left ventricular assist system as a long-term mechanical circulatory support device in bridging patients: a prospective study. J Thorac Cardiovasc Surg 2000;119:581–587.
5. Navia JL, McCarthy PM, Hoercher KJ, et al. Do left ventricular assist device (LVAD) bridge-to-transplantation outcomes predict the results of permanent LVAD implantation? Ann Thorac Surg 2002;74:2051–2063.
6. Rose EA, Gelijns AC, Moskowitz AJ, et al. Randomized Evaluation of Mechanical Assistance for the Treatment of Congestive Heart Failure (REMATCH) Study Group. Long-term mechanical left ventricular assistance for end-stage heart failure. N Engl J Med 2001;345:1435–1443.
7. Guyton RA, Schonberger JP, Everts PA, et al. Postcardiotomy shock: clinical evaluation of the BVS 5000 Biventricular Support System. Ann Thorac Surg 1993;56:346–356.
8. Jett GK. ABIOMED BVS 5000: experience and potential advantages. Ann Thorac Surg 1996;61:301–304.
9. Wassenberg PA. The Abiomed BVS 5000 biventricular support system. Perfusion 2000;15:369–371.
10. Helman DN, Morales DL, Edwards NM, et al. Left ventricular assist device bridge-to-transplant network improves survival after failed cardiotomy. Ann Thorac Surg 1999;68:1187–1194.
11. McBride LR, Lowdermilk GA, Fiore AC, et al. Transfer of patients receiving advanced mechanical circulatory support. J Thorac Cardiovasc Surg 2000; 119:1015–1020.

12. Chen JM, Spanier TB, Gonzalez JJ, et al. Improved survival in patients with acute myocarditis using external pulsatile mechanical ventricular assistance. J Heart Lung Transplant 1999;18:351–357.

13. Marelli D, Laks H, Amsel B, et al. Temporary mechanical support with the BVS 5000 assist device during treatment of acute myocarditis. J Card Surg 1997; 12:55–59.

14. Samuels LE, Kaufman MS, Thomas MP, et al. Pharmacological criteria for ventricular assist device insertion following postcardiotomy shock: experience with the Abiomed BVS system. J Card Surg 1999;14:288–293.

15. Couper GS, Dekkers RJ, Adams DH. The logistics and cost-effectiveness of circulatory support: advantages of the ABIOMED BVS 5000. Ann Thorac Surg 1999;68:646–649.

16. Pennock JL, Pierce WS, Wisman CB, et al. Survival and complications following ventricular assist pumping for cardiogenic shock. Ann Surg 1983;198:469–478.

17. Stolar CJ, Delosh T, Bartlett RH. Extracorporeal life support organization 1993. ASAIO J 1993;39:976–979.

18. Levi D, Marelli D, Plunkett M, et al. Use of assist devices and ECMO to bridge pediatric patients with cardiomyopathy to transplantation. J Heart Lung Transplant 2002;21:760–770.

19. Poirier VL. Heartmate VE LVAS improvements. Oral presentation. International Society for Heart and Lung Transplantation. 3rd Fall education meeting. Mechanical Cardiac Support and Replacement II, Nov. 9–10, 2001.

20. Frazier OH. First use of an untethered, vented electric left ventricular assist device for long-term support. Circulation 1994;89:2908–2914.

21. DeRose JJ Jr., Umana JP, Argenziano M, et al. Implantable left ventricular assist devices provide an excellent outpatient bridge to transplantation and recovery. J Am Coll Cardiol 1997;30:1773–1777.

22. Sun BC, Catanese KA, Spanier TB, et al. 100 long-term implantable left ventricular assist devices: the Columbia–Presbyterian interim experience. Ann Thorac Surg 1999;68:688–694.

23. Poirier VL. Worldwide experience with the TCI HeartMate system: issues and future perspective. Thorac Cardiovasc Surg 1999;49(suppl):316–320.

24. Murali S. Mechanical circulatory support with Novacor LVAS: worldwide clinical results. Thorac Cardiovasc Surg 1999;47(suppl):321–325.

25. Robbins RC, Kown MH, Portner PM, et al. The totally implantable novacor left ventricular assist system. Ann Thorac Surg 2001;71(suppl):S162–S165.

26. Portner P. Oral presentation. International Society for Heart and Lung Transplantation. 3rd Fall education meeting. Mechanical Cardiac Support and Replacement II, Nov. 9–10, 2001.

27. Farrar DJ. The Thoratec ventricular assist device: a paracorporeal pump for treating acute and chronic heart failure. Semin Thorac Cardiovasc Surg 2000;12:243–250.

28. El-Banayosy A, Korfer R, Arusoglu L, et al. Bridging to cardiac transplantation with the Thoratec Ventricular Assist Device. Thorac Cardiovasc Surg 1999; 47(suppl 2):307–310.

29. Anderson FL, DeVries WC, Anderson JL, et al. Evaluation of total artificial heart performance in man. Am J Cardiol 1984;54:394–398.

30. DeVries WC, Anderson JL, Joyce LD, et al. Clinical use of the total artificial heart. N Engl J Med 1984;310:273–278.

31. Copeland JG, Arabia FA, Banchy ME, et al. The CardioWest total artificial heart bridge to transplantation: 1993 to 1996 national trial. Ann Thorac Surg 1998;66: 1662–1669.

32. Arabia FA, Copeland JG, Smith RG, et al. International experience with the CardioWest total artificial heart as a bridge to heart transplantation. Eur J Cardiothorac Surg 1997;11(suppl):S5–S10.

33. Copeland JG, Pavie A, Duveau D, et al. Bridge to transplantation with the CardioWest total artificial heart: the international experience 1993 to 1995. J Heart Lung Transplant 1996;15:94–99.

34. Schmid C, Deng M, Hammel D, et al. Emergency versus elective/urgent left ventricular assist device implantation. J Heart Lung Transplant 1998;17:1024–1028.

35. Deng MC, Weyand M, Hammel D, et al. Selection and outcome of ventricular assist device patients: the Muenster experience. J Heart Lung Transplant 1998;17: 817–825.

36. Minami K, El Banayosy A, Posival H, et al. Improvement of survival rate in patients with cardiogenic shock by using nonpulsatile and pulsatile ventricular assist device. Int J Artif Organs 1992;15:715–721.

37. Copeland JG, Smith RG, Arabia FA, et al. The CardioWest total artificial heart as a bridge to transplantation. Semin Thorac Cardiovasc Surg 2000;12:238–242.

38. Hendry PJ, Masters RG, Mussivand TV, et al. Circulatory support for cardiogenic shock due to acute myocardial infarction: a Canadian experience. Can J Cardiol 1999;15:1090–1094.

39. Goldberg RJ, Gore JM, Thompson CA, et al. Recent magnitude of and temporal trends (1994–1997) in the incidence and hospital death rates of cardiogenic shock complicating acute myocardial infarction: the second National Registry of Myocardial Infarction. Am Heart J 2001;141:65–72.

40. Goldberg RJ, Gore JM, Alpert JS, et al. Cardiogenic shock after acute myocardial infarction. Incidence and mortality from a community-wide perspective, 1975 to 1988. N Engl J Med 1991;325:1117–1122.

41. Hochman JS, Sleeper LA, White HD, et al. One-year survival following early revascularization for cardiogenic shock. JAMA 2001;285:190–192.

42. Mueller HS. Role of intra-aortic counterpulsation in cardiogenic shock and acute myocardial infarction. Cardiology 1994;84:168–174.

43. Champsaur G, Ninet J, Vigneron M, et al. Use of the Abiomed BVS System 5000 as a bridge to cardiac transplantation. J Thorac Cardiovasc Surg 1990;100:122–128.

44. Houel R, Vermes E, Tixier DB, et al. Myocardial recovery after mechanical support for acute myocarditis: is sustained recovery predictable? Ann Thorac Surg 1999;68:2177–2180.

45. Farrar DJ, Hill JD, Gray LA, et al. Successful biventricular circulatory support as a bridge to cardiac transplantation during prolonged ventricular fibrillation and asystole. Circulation 1989;80:III.147–III.151.

46. Holman WL, Roye GD, Bourge RC, et al. Circulatory support for myocardial infarction with ventricular arrhythmias. Ann Thorac Surg 1995;59:1230–1231.

47. Swartz MT, Lowdermilk GA, McBride LR. Refractory ventricular tachycardia as an indication for ventricular assist device support. J Thorac Cardiovasc Surg 1999;118:1119–1120.

48. Oz MC, Rose EA, Levin HR. Selection criteria for placement of left ventricular assist devices. Am Heart J 1995;129:173–177.

49. Oz MC, Goldstein DJ, Pepino P, et al. Screening scale predicts patients successfully receiving long-term implantable left ventricular assist devices. Circulation 1995;92(suppl):II.169–II.173.

50. Rao V, Oz MC, Flannery MA, et al. Revised screening scale to predict survival following left ventricular assist device insertion. J Thorac Cardiovasc Surg 2003;125:855–862.

51. Norman JC, Cooley DA, Igo SR, et al. Prognostic indices for survival during postcardiotomy intra-aortic balloon pumping: methods of scoring and classification, with implications for LVAD utilization. J Thorac Cardiovasc Surg 1977; 74:709–720.

52. Copeland JG, Arabia FA, Smith RG. Bridge to transplantation with a Thoratec left ventricular assist device in a 17-kg child. Ann Thorac Surg 2001;71:1003–1004.

53. Sadeghi AM, Marelli D, Talamo M, et al. Short-term bridge to transplant using the BVS 5000 in a 22-kg child. Ann Thorac Surg 2000;70:2151–2153.

54. Reinhartz O, Keith FM, El-Banayosy A, et al. Multicenter experience with the Thoratec ventricular assist device in children and adolescents. J Heart Lung Transplant 2001;20:439–448.

55. Farrar DJ, Hill JD. Univentricular and biventricular Thoratec VAD support as a bridge to transplantation. Ann Thorac Surg 1993;55:276–282.

56. Farrar DJ, Hill JD, Pennington DG, et al. Preoperative and postoperative comparison of patients with univentricular and biventricular support with the thoratec ventricular assist device as a bridge to cardiac transplantation. J Thorac Cardiovasc Surg 1997;113:202–209.

57. Kormos RL, Murali S, Dew MA, et al. Chronic mechanical circulatory support: rehabilitation, low morbidity, and superior survival. Ann Thorac Surg 1994;57:51–57.

58. Ashton RC, Goldstein DJ, Rose EA, et al. Duration of left ventricular assist device support affects transplant survival. J Heart Lung Transplant 1996;15:1151–1157.

59. Hutchinson OZ, Oz MC, Ascherman JA. The use of muscle flaps to treat left ventricular assist device infections. Plast Reconstr Surg 2001;107:364–373.

60. Rao V, Slater JP, Edwards NM, et al. Surgical management of valvular disease in patients requiring left ventricular assist device support. Ann Thorac Surg 2001;71:1448–1453.

61. Rose AG, Park SJ, Bank AJ, et al. Partial aortic valve fusion induced by left ventricular assist device. Ann Thorac Surg 2000;70:1270–1274.

62. Barbone A, Rao V, Oz MC, et al. LVAD support in patients with bioprosthetic valves. Ann Thorac Surg 2002;74:232–234.

63. Frazier OH, Rose EA, Macmanus Q, et al. Multicenter clinical evaluation of the HeartMate 1000 IP left ventricular assist device. Ann Thorac Surg 1992;53: 1080–1090.

64. Swartz MT, Lowdermilk GA, Moroney DA, et al. Ventricular assist device support in patients with mechanical heartvalves. Ann Thorac Surg 1999;68:2248–2251.

65. Tisol WB, Mueller DK, Hoy FB, et al. Ventricular assist device use with mechanical heart valves: an outcome series and literature review. Ann Thorac Surg 2001; 72:2051–2054,discussion 2055.

66. Stringham JC, Bull DA, Karwande SV. Patch closure of the aortic anulus in a recipient of a ventricular assist device. J Thorac Cardiovasc Surg 2000;119: 1293–1294.

67. Helman DN, Addonizio LJ, Morales DL, et al. Implantable left ventricular assist devices can successfully bridge adolescent patients to transplant. J Heart Lung Transplant 2000;19:121–126.

68. Kavarana MN, Pessin-Minsley MS, Urtecho J, et al. Right ventricular dysfunction and organ failure in left ventricular assist device recipients: a continuing problem. Ann Thorac Surg 2002;73:745–750.

69. Argenziano M, Choudhri AF, Oz MC, et al. A prospective randomized trial of arginine vasopressin in the treatment of vasodilatory shock after left ventricular assist device placement. Circulation 1997;96:II.286–II.290.

70. Goldstein DJ, Seldomridge JA, Chen JM, et al. Use of aprotinin in LVAD recipients reduces blood loss, blood use, and perioperative mortality. Ann Thorac Surg 1995;59:1063–1067.
71. Ankersmit H-J, Itescu S. Immunobiology of left ventricular assist devices. In: Goldstein DJ, Oz MC, eds. Cardiac Assist Devices. Futura Publishing Company, Inc., Armonk, NY: 2000, pp. 193–211.
72. Morales DL, Catanese KA, Helman DN, et al. Six-year experience of caring for forty-four patients with a left ventricular assist device at home: safe, economical, necessary. J Thorac Cardiovasc Surg 2000;119:251–259.
73. Catanese KA, Goldstein DJ, Williams DL, et al. Outpatient left ventricular assist device support: a destination rather than a bridge. Ann Thorac Surg 1996;62: 646–652.
74. El-Banayosy A, Fey O, Sarnowski P, et al. Midterm follow-up of patients discharged from hospital under left ventricular assistance. J Heart Lung Transplant 2001;20:53–58.
75. Levin HR, Oz MC, Chen JM, et al. Reversal of chronic ventricular dilation in patients with end-stage cardiomyopathy by prolonged mechanical unloading. Circulation 1995;91:2717–2720.
76. Frazier OH, Benedict CR, Radovancevic B, et al. Improved left ventricular function after chronic left ventricular unloading. Ann Thorac Surg 1996;62:675–681.
77. Foray A, Williams D, Reemtsma K, et al. Assessment of submaximal exercise capacity in patients with left ventricular assist devices. Circulation 1996;94: II.222–II.226.
78. Mueller J, Wallukat G, Weng Y, et al. Predictive factors for weaning from a cardiac assist device. An analysis of clinical, gene expression, and protein data. J Heart Lung Transplant 2001;20:202.
79. Mancini DM, Beniaminovitz A, Levin H, et al. Low incidence of myocardial recovery after left ventricular assist device implantation in patients with chronic heart failure. Circulation 1998;98:2383–2389.
80. Helman DN, Maybaum SW, Morales DL, et al. Recurrent remodeling after ventricular assistance: is long-term myocardial recovery attainable? Ann Thorac Surg 2000;70:1255–1258.
81. Hetzer R, Muller JH, Weng YG, et al. Midterm follow-up of patients who underwent removal of a left ventricular assist device after cardiac recovery from end-stage dilated cardiomyopathy. J Thorac Cardiovasc Surg 2000;120:843–853.
82. Hetzer R, Muller JH, Weng Y, et al. Bridging-to-recovery. Ann Thorac Surg 2001;71:S109–S113.
83. Yacoub MH. A novel strategy to maximize the efficacy of left ventricular assist devices as a bridge to recovery. Eur Heart J 2001;22:534–540.
84. Ansell J, Klassen V, Lew R, et al. Does desmopressin acetate prophylaxis reduce blood loss after valvular heart operations? A randomized, double-blind study. J Thorac Cardiovasc Surg 1992;104:117–123.
85. Czer LS, Bateman TM, Gray RJ, et al. Treatment of severe platelet dysfunction and hemorrhage after cardiopulmonary bypass: reduction in blood product usage with desmopressin. J Am Coll Cardiol 1987;9:1139–1147.
86. Spanier T, Oz M, Levin H, et al. Activation of coagulation and fibrinolytic pathways in patients with left ventricular assist devices. J Thorac Cardiovasc Surg 1996;112:1090–1097.
87. Christiansen S, Jahn UR, Meyer J, et al. Anticoagulative management of patients requiring left ventricular assist device implantation and suffering from heparin-induced thrombocytopenia type II. Ann Thorac Surg;2000;69:774–777.

88. El-Banayosy A, Korfer R, Arusoglu L, et al. Device and patient management in a bridge-to-transplant setting. Ann Thorac Surg 2001;71:S98–S102.
89. El-Banayosy A, Minami K, Arusoglu L, et al. Long-term mechanical circulatory support. Thorac Cardiovasc Surg 1997;45:127–130.
90. Minami K, El-Banayosy A, Sezai A, et al. Morbidity and outcome after mechanical ventricular support using Thoratec, Novacor, and HeartMate for bridging to heart transplantation. Artif Organs 2000;24:421–426.
91. Holman WL, Skinner JL, Waites KB, et al. Infection during circulatory support with ventricular assist devices. Ann Thorac Surg 1999;68:711–716.
92. Gordon SM, Schmitt SK, Jacobs M, et al. Nosocomial bloodstream infections in patients with implantable left ventricular assist devices. Ann Thorac Surg 2001;72:725–730.
93. Oz MC, Argenziano M, Catanese KA, et al. Bridge experience with long-term implantable left ventricular assist devices. Are they an alternative to transplantation? Circulation 1997;95:1844–1852.
94. Vilchez RA, McEllistrem MC, Harrison LH, et al. Relapsing bacteremia in patients with ventricular assist device: an emergent complication of extended circulatory support. Ann Thorac Surg 2001;72:96–101.
95. Pasque MK, Hanselman T, Shelton K, et al. Surgical management of Novacor drive-line exit site infections. Ann Thorac Surg 2002;74:1267–1268.
96. Nurozler F, Argenziano M, Oz MC, et al. Fungal left ventricular assist device endocarditis. Ann Thorac Surg 2001;71:614–618.
97. Ankersmit HJ, Tugulea S, Spanier T, et al. Activation-induced T-cell death and immune dysfunction after implantation of left-ventricular assist device. Lancet 1999;354:550–555.
98. Thomas CE, Jichici D, Petrucci R, et al. Neurologic complications of the Novacor left ventricular assist device. Ann Thorac Surg 2001;72:1311–1315.
99. Rafii S, Oz MC, Seldomridge JA, et al. Characterization of hematopoietic cells arising on the textured surface of left ventricular assist devices. Ann Thorac Surg 1995;60:1627–1632.
100. Hertz MI, Taylor DO, Trulock EP, et al. The registry of the International Society for Heart and Lung Transplantation: 19th official report—2002. J Heart Lung Transplant 2002;21:950–956.
101. Renlund DG, Taylor DO, Kfoury AG, et al. New UNOS rules: historical background and implications for transplantation management. United Network for Organ Sharing. J Heart Lung Transplant 1999;18:1065–1070.
102. Frazier OH, Rose EA, Oz MC, et al. HeartMate LVAS investigators. Left ventricular assist system, multicenter clinical evaluation of the HeartMate vented electric left ventricular assist system in patients awaiting heart transplantation. J Thorac Cardiovasc Surg 2001;122:1186–1195.
103. Korfer R, El-Banayosy A, Arusoglu L, et al. Single-center experience with the thoratec ventricular assist device. J Thorac Cardiovasc Surg 2000;119:596–600.
104. Wheeldon DR, LaForge DH, Lee J, et al. Novacor left ventricular assist system long-term performance: comparison of clinical experience with demonstrated in vitro reliability. ASAIO J 2002;48:546–551.
105. McBride LR, Naunheim KS, Fiore AC, et al. Risk analysis in patients bridged to transplantation. Ann Thorac Surg 2001;71:1839–1844.
106. Fukamachi K, McCarthy PM, Smedira NG, et al. Pre-operative risk factors for right ventricular failure after implantable left ventricular assist device insertion. Ann Thorac Surg 1999;68:2181–2184.

107. Cave AC, Manche A, Derias NW, et al. Thromboxane A2 mediates pulmonary hypertension after cardiopulmonary bypass in the rabbit. J Thorac Cardiovasc Surg 1993;106:959–967.

108. John R, Liez K, Schuster M, et al. Immunologic sensitization in recipients of left ventricular assist devices. J Thorac Cardiovasc Surg 2003;125:578–591.

109. Itescu S, Tung TC, Burke EM, et al. Preformed IgG antibodies against major histocompatibility complex class II antigens are major risk factors for high-grade cellular rejection in recipients of heart transplantation. Circulation 1998;98: 786–793.

110. Massad MG, Cook DJ, Schmitt SK, et al. Factors influencing HLA sensitization in implantable LVAD recipients. Ann Thorac Surg 1997;64:1120–1125.

111. Pagani FD, Dyke DB, Wright S, et al. Development of anti-major histocompatibility complex class I or II antibodies following left ventricular assist device implantation: effects on subsequent allograft rejection and survival. J Heart Lung Transplant 2001;20:646–653.

112. John R, Lietz K, Burke E, et al. Intravenous immunoglobulin reduces anti-HLA alloreactivity and shortens waiting time to cardiac transplantation in highly sensitized left ventricular assist device recipients. Circulation 1999;100(suppl): II.229–II.235.

113. Smith JD, Danskine AJ, Laylor RM, et al. The effect of panel reactive antibodies and the donor specific crossmatch on graft survival after heart and heart–lung transplantation. Transplant Immunol 1993;1:60–65.

114. Moazami N, Itescu S, Williams MR, et al. Platelet transfusions are associated with the development of anti-major histocompatibility complex class I antibodies in patients with left ventricular assist support. J Heart Lung Transplant 1998;17: 876–880.

115. Angell James JE, Daly M. Effects of graded pulsatile pressure on the reflex vasomotor responses elicited by changes of mean pressure in the perfused carotid sinus-aortic arch regions of the dog. J Physiol 1971;214:51–64.

116. Gaer JA, Shaw AD, Wild R, et al. Effect of cardiopulmonary bypass on gastrointestinal perfusion and function. Ann Thorac Surg 1994;57:371–375.

117. Hickey PR, Buckley MJ, Philbin DM. Pulsatile and nonpulsatile cardiopulmonary bypass: review of a counterproductive controversy. Ann Thorac Surg 1983;36:720–737.

118. Hornick P, Taylor K. Pulsatile and nonpulsatile perfusion: the continuing controversy. J Cardiothorac Vasc Anesth 1997;11:310–315.

119. Levine FH, Philbin DM, Kono K, et al. Plasma vasopressin levels and urinary sodium excretion during cardiopulmonary bypass with and without pulsatile flow. Ann Thorac Surg 1981;32:63–67.

120. Moores WY, Gago O, Morris JD, et al. Serum and urinary amylase levels following pulsatile and continuous cardiopulmonary bypass. J Thorac Cardiovasc Surg 1977;74:73–76.

121. Noris M, Morigi M, Donadelli R, et al. Nitric oxide synthesis by cultured endothelial cells is modulated by flow conditions. Circ Res 1995;76:536–543.

122. Taylor KM, Wright GS, Bain WH, et al. Comparative studies of pulsatile and nonpulsatile flow during cardiopulmonary bypass. III. Response of anterior pituitary gland to thyrotropin-releasing hormone. J Thorac Cardiovasc Surg 1978;75:579–584.

123. Taylor KM, Wright GS, Reid JM, et al. Comparative studies of pulsatile and nonpulsatile flow during cardiopulmonary bypass. II. The effects on adrenal secretion of cortisol. J Thorac Cardiovasc Surg 1978;75:574–578.

124. Watkins WD, Peterson MB, Kong DL, et al. Thromboxane and prostacyclin changes during cardiopulmonary bypass with and without pulsatile flow. J Thorac Cardiovasc Surg 1982;84:250–256.
125. Sezai A, Shiono M, Orime Y, et al. Major organ function under mechanical support: comparative studies of pulsatile and nonpulsatile circulation. Artif Organs 1999;23:280–285.
126. Sezai A, Shiono M, Orime Y, et al. Comparison studies of major organ microcirculations under pulsatile- and nonpulsatile-assisted circulations. Artif Organs 1996;20:139–142.
127. Sezai A, Shiono M, Orime Y, et al. Renal circulation and cellular metabolism during left ventricular assisted circulation: comparison study of pulsatile and nonpulsatile assists. Artif Organs 1997;21:830–835.
128. Wakisaka Y, Taenaka Y, Chikanari K, et al. Long-term evaluation of a nonpulsatile mechanical circulatory support system. Artif Organs 1997;21:639–644.
129. Taenaka Y, Tatsumi E, Sakaki M, et al. Peripheral circulation during nonpulsatile systemic perfusion in chronic awake animals. ASAIO Trans 1991;37:M365–M366.
130. Sakaki M, Taenaka Y, Tatsumi E, et al. Influences of nonpulsatile pulmonary flow on pulmonary function. Evaluation in a chronic animal model. J Thorac Cardiovasc Surg 1994;108:495–502.
131. Reddy RC, Goldstein AH, Pacella JJ, et al. End organ function with prolonged nonpulsatile circulatory support. ASAIO J 1995;41:M547–M551.
132. Macha M, Litwak P, Yamazaki K, et al. Survival for up to six months in calves supported with an implantable axial flow ventricular assist device. ASAIO J 1997;43:311–315.
133. Kawahito K, Damm G, Benkowski R, et al. Ex vivo phase 1 evaluation of the DeBakey/NASA axial flow ventricular assist device. Artif Organs 1996;20:47–52.
134. Hindman BJ, Dexter F, Smith T, et al. Pulsatile versus nonpulsatile flow. No difference in cerebral blood flow or metabolism during normothermic cardiopulmonary bypass in rabbits. Anesthesiology 1995;82:241–250.
135. Hindman BJ, Dexter F, Ryu KH, et al. Pulsatile versus nonpulsatile cardiopulmonary bypass. No difference in brain blood flow or metabolism at 27 degrees C. Anesthesiology 1994;80:1137–1147.
136. Dapper F, Neppl H, Wozniak G, et al. Effects of pulsatile and nonpulsatile perfusion mode during extracorporeal circulation—a comparative clinical study. Thorac Cardiovasc Surg 1992;40:345–351.
137. Wieselthaler GM, Schima H, Hiesmayr M, et al. First clinical experience with the DeBakey VAD continuous-axial-flow pump for bridge to transplantation. Circulation 2000;101:356–359.
138. Potapov EV, Loebe M, Nasseri BA, et al. Pulsatile flow in patients with a novel nonpulsatile implantable ventricular assist device. Circulation 2000;102: III.183–III.187.
139. Westaby S, Banning AP, Jarvik R, et al. First permanent implant of the Jarvik 2000 Heart. Lancet 2000;356:900–903.
140. Khanwilkar P. Oral presentation. International Society for Heart and Lung Transplantation. 3rd Fall education meeting. Mechanical Cardiac Support and Replacement II, Nov. 9–10, 2001.
141. Woodard J. Oral presentation. International Society for Heart and Lung Transplantation. 3rd Fall education meeting. Mechanical Cardiac Support and Replacement II, Nov. 9–10, 2001.
142. Maher TR, Butler KC, Poirier VL, et al. HeartMate left ventricular assist devices: a multigeneration of implanted blood pumps. Artif Organs 2001;25:422–426.

143. Loree HM, Bourque K, Gernes DB, et al. The Heartmate III: design and in vivo studies of a maglev centrifugal left ventricular assist device. Artif Organs 2001;25:386–391.

144. SoRelle R. Cardiovascular news. Totally contained AbioCor artificial heart implanted July 3, 2001. Circulation 2001;104:E9005–E9006.

INDEX